Access to Public Health Services and Challenges to Healthcare Management

Access to Public Health Services and Challenges to Healthcare Management

Guest Editors

Isabella Piassi Dias Godói
Carlos Podalirio Borges de Almeida

MDPI

Basel • Beijing • Wuhan • Barcelona • Belgrade • Novi Sad • Cluj • Manchester

Guest Editors
Isabella Piassi Dias Godói
Institute of Pharmaceutical Sciences
Federal University of Rio de Janeiro
Macaé
Brazil

Carlos Podalirio Borges de Almeida
Faculty of Public Health
Federal University of Sul e Sudeste do Pará
Marabá
Brazil

Editorial Office
MDPI AG
Grosspeteranlage 5
4052 Basel, Switzerland

This is a reprint of the Special Issue, published open access by the journal *International Journal of Environmental Research and Public Health* (ISSN 1660-4601), freely accessible at: https://www.mdpi.com/journal/ijerph/special_issues/Z9EBB656TM.

For citation purposes, cite each article independently as indicated on the article page online and as indicated below:

Lastname, A.A.; Lastname, B.B. Article Title. *Journal Name* **Year**, *Volume Number*, Page Range.

ISBN 978-3-7258-6260-3 (Hbk)
ISBN 978-3-7258-6261-0 (PDF)
https://doi.org/10.3390/books978-3-7258-6261-0

Contents

About the Editors

Isabella Piassi Dias Godói

Isabella Piassi Dias Godói is a Professor at the Institute of Pharmaceutical Sciences at the Federal University of Rio de Janeiro (UFRJ), Brazil. Her research projects focus on Public Health, Health Economics, and Health Technology Assessment (HTA), with an emphasis on challenges in public health service management, the promotion of social participation in health, and the pursuit of rationality and efficiency in health decision-making. She leads an HTA Nucleus in Brazil and coordinates multiple research initiatives in collaboration with Brazilian and international universities. Her work integrates scientific evidence with real-world health system needs to strengthen governance and support policy development.

Carlos Podalirio Borges de Almeida

Carlos Podalirio Borges de Almeida is an Assistant Professor in the Department of Health Management at the Federal University of Minas Gerais (UFMG), Brazil. He is a Permanent Faculty Member of the Graduate Program in Family Health at the Federal University of Sul e Sudeste do Pará (UNIFESSPA). He is affiliated with the Health Management Research Group at UFMG and with the Expanded Center for Interdisciplinary Health Research at the Federal University of Santa Catarina (UFSC). His work focuses on public health, particularly health surveillance and health management. His current research interests include tuberculosis illness experiences, infectious disease epidemiology, primary health care, the health workforce, occupational health, and global health.

Preface

According to the World Health Organization (WHO), the health system needs to offer preventive, promotive, curative, and rehabilitative interventions through a combination of public health actions to the population. It is essential to reinforce that the actions of the health system should be responsive and financially fair while treating people respectfully. Additionally, a health system needs staff, funds, information, and overall guidance and direction to function. The WHO highlights that few countries have systems that can monitor service delivery and that data on population access to essential services are limited. In this context, it is indispensable for countries to develop strategies to better assess aspects such as the accessibility and quality of health services offered to the population, to contribute to health monitoring and the planning process in the healthcare management scenario. In this context, this Special Issue sought to gather studies examining perceptions, evaluations, and analytical approaches related to access to public health services. It welcomed qualitative and quantitative contributions, with particular encouragement for work from low- and middle-income countries, whose health systems often revealed complex challenges and innovative responses. This collection was conceived to offer readers a concise and critical view of contemporary debates on access and quality in public health. The volume aimed to serve as both a scholarly resource and a practical guide, contributing to the advancement of more equitable, efficient, and people-centered health systems.

Isabella Piassi Dias Godói and Carlos Podalirio Borges de Almeida
Guest Editors

International Journal of
Environmental Research and Public Health

MDPI

Article

Users' Perspectives on Primary Care and Public Health Services in the State of Rio de Janeiro, Brazil: A Cross-Sectional Study with Implications for Healthcare Quality Assessment

Igor F. L. Ferraz [1], Mariana C. Raimundo [1], Natalia M. A. M. Barros [1], Jhoyce S. Souza [1], Barbará M. V. Lucio [1], Thiago P. Tenreiro [1], Edna A. Reis [2,3], Danielle Maria de Souza Serio dos Santos [1,3], Luisa A. Chaves [1,3], Brian Godman [4,5,6], Stephen M. Campbell [5,7], Johanna C. Meyer [5,8] and Isabella Piassi D. Godói [1,3,*]

1 Institute of Pharmaceutical Sciences, Federal University of Rio de Janeiro, Avenida Aluízio da Silva Gomes 50—Granja dos Cavaleiros, Macaé 27930-560, RJ, Brazil; igorfradique@gmail.com (I.F.L.F.); maricrespo.r2@gmail.com (M.C.R.); natmmbarros@gmail.com (N.M.A.M.B.); jhoyce.tcc.ufrj@gmail.com (J.S.S.); bah_mvl@hotmail.com (B.M.V.L.); thiagopereira900@gmail.com (T.P.T.); dani.farma84@gmail.com (D.M.d.S.S.d.S.); luisa.arueira@gmail.com (L.A.C.)

2 Department of Statistics, Exact Sciences Institute, Federal University of Minas Gerais, Campus Pampulha, Avenida Antônio Carlos 6627, Belo Horizonte 31270-901, MG, Brazil; ednareis@gmail.com

3 Health Technology Assessment Center—Management, Economics, Health Education and Pharmaceutical Services (GEESFAR/NATS/UFRJ) of the Federal University of Rio de Janeiro, Rio de Janeiro 27930-560, RJ, Brazil

4 Strathclyde Institute of Pharmacy and Biomedical Sciences, University of Strathclyde, Glasgow G1 1XQ, UK; brian.godman@strath.ac.uk

5 Department of Public Health Pharmacy and Management, School of Pharmacy, Sefako Makgatho Health Sciences University, Ga-Rankuwa, Pretoria 0208, South Africa; stephen.campbell@manchester.ac.uk (S.M.C.); hannelie.meyer@smu.ac.za (J.C.M.)

6 Antibiotic Policy Group, Institute for Infection and Immunity, City St. George's, University of London, London SW17 0RE, UK

7 School of Health Sciences, University of Manchester, Manchester M13 9PL, UK

8 South African Vaccination and Immunisation Centre, Sefako Makgatho Health Sciences University, Ga-Rankuwa, Pretoria 0208, South Africa

* Correspondence: isabellapiassi@gmail.com

Abstract

This study focuses on the Unified Health System (SUS) in five regions of the state of Rio de Janeiro, Brazil, one of Brazil's most important states, as part of a comprehensive analysis of a research project, which has generated publications in earlier phases. The objective was to assess users' perceptions of SUS in terms of access to and the quality of public health services, including primary care and pharmaceutical services. A cross-sectional study was conducted using a structured questionnaire comprising 66 questions, administered to a purposive sample of 1000 participants between August 2023 and August 2024. Data were analyzed using Pearson's chi-square test with R software version 4.3. Among the participants, 54.5% were female, 62.5% were aged between 26 and 60 years, and 29% reported having private health insurance. Vaccination services were the most frequently used SUS service (25.1% of respondents). Participants who reported more frequent use of SUS services rated access more positively than those who used them less frequently ($p = 0.002$). The regions that evaluated SUS access and quality most favorably were Middle Paraíba and the metropolitan region, while the Coastal Lowlands region received the most negative assessments. Participants with lower socioeconomic status gave more favorable evaluations of access to public health services ($p = 0.001$). These findings highlight concerns about access to, and the quality of, SUS healthcare services and regional disparities in users' perceptions of SUS services in Rio de Janeiro. The results underscore the importance of social participation as a key element in the evaluation and continuous improvement of responsive public healthcare.

Keywords: Brazil; access; quality; health services; users; public health; healthcare quality assessments

1. Introduction

The 1988 Constitution marked a milestone for public health in Brazil, with Article 196 establishing health as a right for all citizens in Brazil and a duty of the State [1]. Following the institutionalization of the Unified Health System (SUS) in 1990, key principles were defined for the healthcare system. Key principles included universality, comprehensiveness, hierarchical organization, and social participation [2]. Alongside this, foundational guidelines were introduced to improve the diverse range of potential health actions [1,2]. Overall, SUS represents a significant social achievement and a substantial transformation in Brazil's health landscape to improve the population's well-being [1–3]. Managing this universal system involves financial, logistical, and human resources across different autonomous political and administrative entities (federal, state, and municipal). In this arrangement, the municipalities are responsible for providing the majority of health services [1,2]. This decentralization strategy necessitates collaboration and cooperation to align health services with local needs [4].

SUS is organized into different levels of care to enhance the rational use of available resources, which range from Primary Health Care (PHC) and Secondary Care to highly complex and specialized services in Tertiary Care facilities [5]. Within this structure, PHC plays a central role in promoting health and preventing diseases, reducing morbidity and mortality, and serving as the main entry point to health care as well as being the gatekeeper to more complex services when necessary [6]. One of the most socially recognized initiatives under SUS is the National Immunization Program (PNI). Since its inception in 1973, PNI has achieved several milestones, including the eradication of smallpox and the containment of epidemics, including COVID-19 [7].

In Brazil, the composition of primary care teams follows the guidelines of the National Primary Care Policy (PNAB). However, municipalities have the autonomy to structure their teams based on local needs, provided they meet the established minimum standards for PHC [8]. The Family Health Strategy (ESF) is the standard model, with teams comprising family physicians, nurses, community health agents (CHAs), and nursing technicians. It is also recommended that the municipalities include an Oral Health Team (ESB), primarily consisting of dentists and technicians, as well as Multidisciplinary Teams (EMulti), which include professionals such as nutritionists, physiotherapists, psychologists, and social workers [9]. Whilst the presence of a pharmacist is not mandatory in EMulti, their role is crucial in pharmaceutical services to improve the dispensing and management of medicines' use, which directly benefits families served by PHC [10].

Whilst SUS is founded on the principle of universal and comprehensive access to services for the entire population, approximately 25% of the population has a private health insurance plan [11]. Whilst many health insurance beneficiaries have their coverage paid by their employers and not through direct payments [12], one of the main motivations for acquiring private coverage is the perceived greater ease in scheduling appointments with specialists [13]. A key reason is the current obstacles encountered in accessing SUS services, aggravated by increasing demand [14]. There can also be concerns with unequal access of funds across the different regions of Brazil to meet unmet needs, which again impacts the availability of comprehensive healthcare services [15–17].

Social participation is a cornerstone in ensuring that the population's needs and demands are responded to, reflecting the foundational principles of the SUS [18]. In Brazil,

Law No. 8142/1990 establishes social participation as one of the pillars of this universal system, highlighting the value of citizen engagement through mechanisms such as Health Councils and Health Conferences in shaping and strengthening the SUS [2,17]. Other countries with public health systems, including Canada [19] and the United Kingdom [20], also incorporate social participation as a key principle. The importance of public opinion in improving health systems informs SUS planning [21], underscoring the relevance of studies that explore users' perspectives to inform future decision-making.

To collect data and foster discussions on the evaluation of various types of public health services in Brazil, the federal government developed programs such as the 2013 National Survey on the Rational Use of Medicines in Brazil (PNAUM), which aimed to evaluate, at a national level, the use and promotion of the rational use of medicines [22]. Alongside this is the 2011 Program for the Improvement of Access and Quality of Primary Care (PMAQ), which assessed the performance of health teams and the quality of services offered in primary care, aiming at the continuous improvement of care provided to the population [23]. These earlier programs contributed to surveys focusing on medication use, e.g., medication use by age group, difficulties encountered, and other findings in the country [22–27], as well as reflections on the provision of public health services [22–27]. These programs employed questionnaires as data collection tools, which subsequently served as references for the development of further research studies addressing these topics [15–17].

After the discontinuation of the aforementioned programs between 2015 and 2019, few publications [28–30] and/or studies on this topic in Brazil have been published. A systematic review was published in 2024 that focused on the challenges of universality in the SUS and evaluated access to and quality of health services in Brazil, including eight studies conducted before 2020 [28]. Additionally, a survey was published in April 2025, based on a digital questionnaire with a 4.7% response rate that included 2458 participants from various regions of the country, evaluating access to and quality of Primary Health Care. These studies showed that users who most frequently utilize the SUS belong to more socially vulnerable groups [29,30].

However, given the limited number of Brazilian publications assessing users' perceptions of SUS services since 2020 [28,29], low response rates in previous studies [29,30], and the restriction of previous studies to specific topics, e.g., only pharmaceutical services or primary care, more up-to-date research is needed to reflect the importance of social participation in identifying population demands and needs. There is also a need to focus on a broader view of users' perceptions of various aspects of public health across primary care, pharmaceutical services, and challenges associated with access to specialized services. In addition, the state of Rio de Janeiro—a strategic region in Brazil due to its tourism, economic, and cultural significance—faces unique challenges related to access to and quality of SUS services [31].

Consequently, a research project titled "*Assessment of Access and Quality of Public Health Services from the Perspective of the Unified Health System*" has been underway since 2023 at the Federal University of Rio de Janeiro [15–17]. Among the regions and the interior of the state of Rio de Janeiro. Previous phases of the project have been published, including analyses from the Coastal Lowlands [16], the metropolitan region [17], and a municipality in the Northern Fluminense region [15].

This study focuses on the five regions within the state of Rio de Janeiro: metropolitan region, Coastal Lowlands, Northern Fluminense, Mountain, and Middle Paraíba. The research aimed to engage with the population by conducting face-to-face interviews in various high-traffic locations across municipalities in both metropolitan regions and the interior of the state of Rio de Janeiro. This paper aims to analyze the perceptions of residents in these five regions regarding their access to, and the quality of, the public health system, including primary care and pharmaceutical services. Furthermore, the study aims to highlight the disparities observed among the five regions of the state of Rio de Janeiro, Brazil, associated with the provision of services in PHC, specialized care, and the pharmaceutical sector. The study also explores the main challenges faced by SUS users and their perceptions of the pharmacist's role in health services. The findings can be used to give guidance to all key stakeholder groups in Brazil regarding potential ways to improve services in the future.

2. Methods

2.1. Study Design and Setting

A cross-sectional study was conducted to evaluate the perceptions of residents from five regions of the state of Rio de Janeiro (Figure 1)—Metropolitan, Coastal Lowlands, Northern Fluminense, Mountain, and Middle Paraíba—regarding different aspects of SUS services. Because the study had no external funding and no financial resources to support the interviews, a convenience sampling was used. This took into account factors such as ease of access and travel within the municipality selected and the possibility for interviews to be conducted by undergraduate students, i.e., in municipalities where they reside and/or have family members who are part of the research project team.

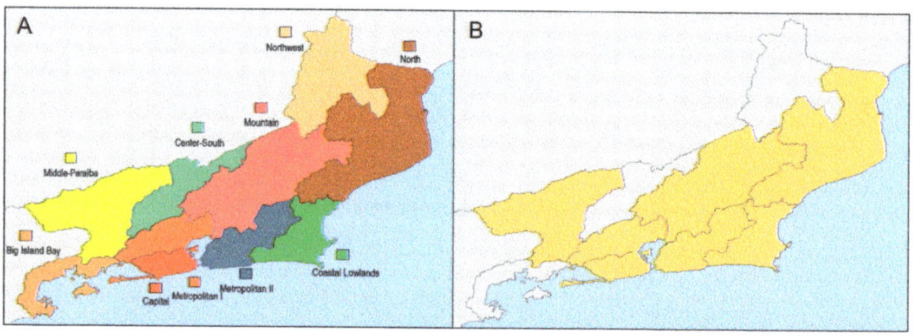

Figure 1. (**A**) Regions of Rio de Janeiro State in Brazil. (**B**) Regions participating in the study. Note: The regions of the state of Rio de Janeiro involved in this study are highlighted in yellow (**B**).

According to IBGE data, the state of Rio de Janeiro has approximately 17 million inhabitants, divided into nine regions and 92 municipalities [32]. For this study, the regions were analyzed according to the political-administrative division into health regions. The metropolitan region (I and II) accounts for 75.4% of the state's population and includes 19 municipalities: Belford Roxo, Duque de Caxias, Itaguaí, Japeri, Magé, Mesquita, Nilópolis, Nova Iguaçu, Queimados, Rio de Janeiro, São João de Meriti, Seropédica, Itaboraí, Maricá, Niterói, Rio Bonito, São Gonçalo, Silva Jardim, and Tanguá [33,34]. Among these, three municipalities were selected as a purposive convenience sample for this study: the state capital (Rio de Janeiro), São Gonçalo, and Duque de Caxias. Together, they represent 68.9% of the region's population.

The Northern Fluminense region comprises 5.7% of the state's population and includes 8 municipalities: Campos dos Goytacazes, Carapebus, Conceição de Macabu, Macaé, Quissamã, São Fidélis, São Francisco de Itabapoana, and São João da Barra [35]. For this study, Campos dos Goytacazes and Macaé were selected as a convenience sample, representing 52.3% of the region's population.

The Coastal Lowlands region accounts for 5.1% of the state's population and includes 9 municipalities: Araruama, Armação dos Búzios, Arraial do Cabo, Cabo Frio, Casimiro de Abreu, Iguaba Grande, Rio das Ostras, São Pedro da Aldeia, and Saquarema [36]. The municipalities of Cabo Frio, Búzios, Rio das Ostras, and São Pedro da Aldeia were chosen as a convenience sample, covering 61.2% of the region's population.

The Middle Paraíba region represents 5.4% of the state's population and includes 12 municipalities: Barra do Piraí, Barra Mansa, Itatiaia, Pinheiral, Piraí, Porto Real, Quatis, Resende, Rio Claro, Rio das Flores, Valença, and Volta Redonda [37]. Questionnaires were collected in all municipalities of this region.

The Mountain region accounts for 6.0% of the state's population and includes 16 municipalities: Bom Jardim, Cachoeiras de Macacu, Cantagalo, Carmo, Cordeiro, Duas Barras, Guapimirim, Macuco, Nova Friburgo, Petrópolis, Santa Maria Madalena, São José do Vale do Rio Preto, São Sebastião do Alto, Sumidouro, Teresópolis, and Trajano de Morais [38]. In this context, Nova Friburgo, Cantagalo, and Cordeiro were included in the study, representing 21.1% of the region's population.

2.2. Data Collection Instrument

The research instrument was developed by the project team based on previous federal government projects: the National Program for Improving Access and Quality of Primary Care (PMAQ) [23,25–27] and the National Survey on Access, Use, and Promotion of the Rational Use of Medicines (PNAUM) [22,24] (Supplementary Material). In the development phase, the focus was on developing simple, objective, and easy-to-understand questions, following the profile of those adopted in the previously cited instruments [23,25–27]. The final questionnaire consisted of 66 questions, and the same instrument was applied across all five regions of the state of Rio de Janeiro included in this study. Aspects such as difficulties in the use of medicines, types of public health services utilized, and perceptions of SUS and other approaches were included.

The 66 questions were organized into the following four sections: (A) socioeconomic profile and use of health services; (B) clinical condition; (C) use of medicines; and (D) perceptions and use of public health services. It is important to emphasize that only participants who reported using SUS services answered Section D (step two: assessing users' perceptions of access to and quality of SUS services), whereas the previous sections (A, B, and C) were completed by all participants (n = 1000).

Section D aimed to explore participants' perceptions of different aspects of SUS services. It included several questions related to access to and quality of public health services, the types of services most frequently used, the need to seek health care in a municipality other than their place of residence, and other related topics. In addition, we included questions addressing the pharmaceutical context, with particular emphasis on medication use, participants' experiences with medicine usage instructions, the acquisition and use of over-the-counter (OTC) medicines, and other relevant aspects. Additional questions sought to assess whether participants fully understood their prescriptions, including instructions for antibiotic use and polypharmacy.

To enhance the robustness of the questionnaire, it was pre-tested with 30 individuals from the municipality of Macaé (Northern Fluminense Region), near the Federal University of Rio de Janeiro (UFRJ-Macaé). During the pre-test, we confirmed that no questions required modification.

2.3. Data Collection and Inclusion Criteria

The sample size was calculated to estimate a proportion with a maximum margin of error of approximately 3% at a 95% confidence level, assuming the scenario of greatest variability (i.e., when the population proportion equals 0.50). This resulted in an estimated sample size of approximately $n = 1000$ participants, using the equation $n = 1/(d^2)$, distributed among the municipalities proportionally to their population sizes [39].

Because the project had no available funding, municipalities and regions of the state of Rio de Janeiro with greater accessibility and feasibility for the interview team were selected as a purposive convenience sample. Inclusion criteria required participants to be 18 years of age or older. For analyses evaluating the quality of public health services, individuals who reported never having used the SUS were excluded.

Data collection was carried out by undergraduate students from the Institute of Pharmaceutical Sciences at the Federal University of Rio de Janeiro/Macaé, who had been previously trained by the study's coordinating professor. Interviews took place in public and freely accessible areas, generally near healthcare facilities, including municipal pharmacies, hospitals, and Basic Health Units (UBSs). These locations were intentionally selected to maximize the recruitment of participants who were users of the SUS or private health insurance, maximizing the inclusion of diverse experiences and perspectives. It should be noted that the interviewers randomly invited individuals from various high-traffic locations within each selected municipality in order to include participants with different socioeconomic profiles. The recruitment strategy aimed to approach individuals who were likely to have recent or ongoing contact with health services, particularly those present in healthcare settings at the time of data collection.

2.4. Data Analysis

Data analysis consisted of a descriptive assessment of participants' responses, including questions on sample characteristics such as gender, age, education level, household income, and clinical profile, which are presented in tables and graphs. In addition, analyses were performed on utilization patterns and perceptions of public health services, with a primary focus on PHC, and included the specialized care and pharmaceutical services. To present the income profile of the interviewees, values in BRL were converted to USD using the exchange rate provided by the Central Bank of Brazil (2025), which was USD 1 = BRL 5.87 [34,40].

Additionally, users' experiences in the pharmaceutical context were evaluated, covering the entire process of acquiring and using medicines, including over-the-counter (OTC) and prescription drugs, challenges related to polypharmacy, and patients' perceptions of the pharmacist's role in health care. Variables were summarized using absolute and relative frequencies, and associations between them were analyzed using Pearson's chi-square test. Results were considered statistically significant when the p-value was <0.05. Analyses were conducted using Microsoft Excel 365 and R software, version 4.3.0.

In addition, we evaluated a potential association between participants' gender, educational level, skin color, and family income and their perceptions of access to and quality of SUS services.

2.5. Ethical Aspects

Participation was voluntary, and research objectives were explained to participants, including a reading of the Informed Consent Form (ICF). Individuals who agreed to participate signed two copies of the ICF, one retained by the participant and the other by the researcher. Once the form was signed, the questionnaire was administered.

The present study was approved by the Ethics and Research Committee of the Federal University of Rio de Janeiro/Macaé Campus (CAAE: 68864623.6.0000.5699).

3. Results

3.1. Participant Characteristics

Based on the analysis of the 1000 questionnaires, it was observed that the sample was predominantly female (66.2%), with an average age range of 25 to 45 years (41.5%), and most participants had completed high school (33.8%).

The majority of participants reported using SUS services (92.1%), as shown in Table 1.

Table 1. Characteristics of study participants (n = 1000).

Variable	n	(%) *
Gender *		
Female	659	66.2%
Male	337	33.8%
Age Profile (years old)		
18–25	166	16.6%
26–45	415	41.5%
46–60	255	25.5%
More than 60	163	16.3%
Race/skin color **		
White	385	39.4%
Black	196	20.0%
Brown	390	40.0%
Other	6	0.6%
Education level ***		
Never attended school	15	1.5%
Incomplete elementary school	141	14.5%
Completed elementary school	72	7.4%
Incomplete high school	56	5.7%
Completed high school	390	40.0%
Incomplete college	145	15%
Completed college or more	156	16.0%
Family Income **** (Number of times the minimum wage *****)		
Up to 1	161	18.4%
1–2	221	26.0%
2–3	216	25.4%
3–5	264	19.3%
5–10	72	8.5%
10–20	14	1.6%
>20	3	0.4%
Use of SUS services—Yes	927	93.6%
Has a private health plan—Yes	314	31.7%

Notes: * Gender: 0.4% of participants did not answer these questions ("don't know/don't want to answer"); ** Race/Skin Color: 2.3% of participants did not answer these questions ("don't know/don't want to answer"); *** Education level: 2.5% of participants did not answer these questions ("don't know/don't want to answer"); **** Family income: 14.9% of participants did not answer these questions ("don't know/don't want to answer"); ***** Minimum wage in 2024: BRL 1412.00 (US $254.41).

Among the services offered by SUS used by the participants, vaccination and medical consultations were the most frequently utilized services (25.1% and 23.6%, respectively), followed by the acquisition of medications (14.5%), as illustrated in Figure 2.

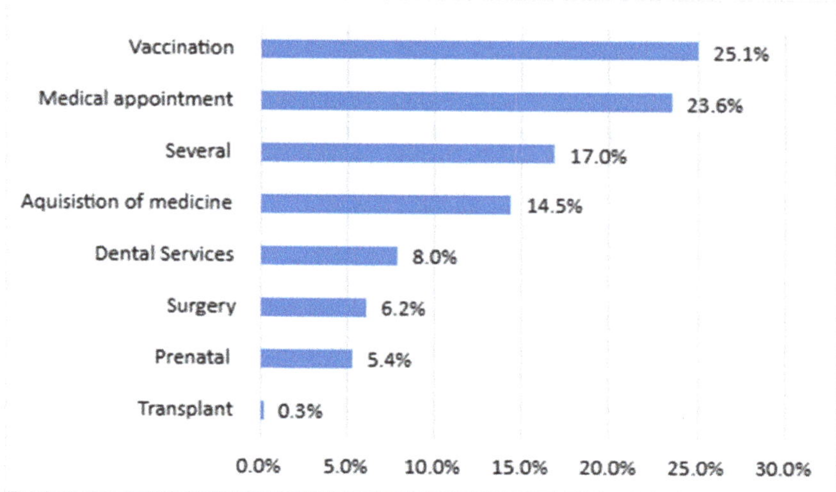

Figure 2. Most commonly used SUS services reported by users from the State of Rio de Janeiro ($n = 1000$). Note: Respondents were allowed to report more than one difficulty.

25.3% of the sample reported having no difficulties in obtaining or using their medications. However, the greatest challenges identified were remembering the time to take medications (22.1%), obtaining the medication (13.3%), and adjusting medication use with their work routine (11.3%), as shown in Figure 3.

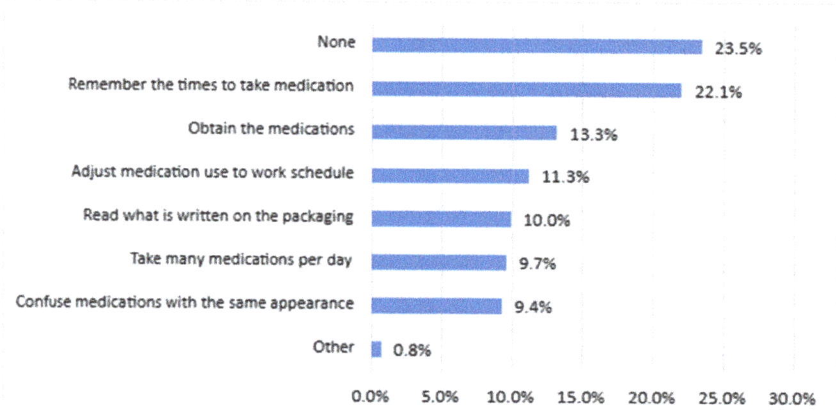

Figure 3. Difficulties reported by respondents associated with the use of medicines ($n = 1000$). Note: respondents could record more than one service.

3.2. Responses from SUS Users

990 (99%) of the sample reported that they currently use or have previously used SUS and thus answered questions relating to the second part of the questionnaire. When asked about medical consultations, 47.4% stated that they rely solely on SUS services, 33.3% use both SUS and private health insurance, and 14.0% reported using only private health insurance for consultations. The remaining 5.3% of respondents did not answer these questions (don't know/don't want to answer).

Most SUS users consider it indispensable and essential, with this view shared by those who always use the system (90.8%) as well as those who use it rarely (82.1%). Among those who always use the system, 40.6% rated access to SUS services as good and 31.9% as neither good nor bad. Occasional and non-users rated access as neither good nor bad (39.0% and 47.8%, respectively). When asked about the quality of services, those who always use the system described it as very good/good, while the most negative evaluations came from those who rarely or never use the system (24.2%), as shown in Table 2.

Table 2. Perceptions of SUS users regarding the relevance, access to, and quality of the public health services (n = 990).

Relevance of SUS n (%) *				
Frequency	**Indispensable**	**Complementary**	**Indifferent**	***p*-Value**
Always	364 (90.8%)	29 (7.2%)	8 (2.0%)	0.056
Frequently	112 (86.2%)	16 (12.3%)	2 (1.5%)	
Sometimes	219 (85.9%)	27 (10.%)	9 (3.5%)	
Rarely	156 (82.1%)	24 (12.6%)	10 (5.3%)	
ALL	851 (87.2%)	96 (9.8%)	29 (3.0%)	

Access to SUS Services n (%) **						
Frequency	**Very Good**	**Good**	**Neither Good nor Bad**	**Bad**	**Very Bad**	***p*-Value**
Always	32 (8.2%)	159 (40.6%)	125 (31.9%)	54 (13.8%)	22 (5.6%)	0.002
Frequently	6 (4.8%)	55 (44.0%)	43 (34.4%)	13 (10.4%)	8 (6.4%)	
Sometimes	10 (4.0%)	68 (27.3%)	97 (39.0%)	55 (22.1%)	19 (7.6%)	
Rarely	10 (7.6%)	48 (36.4%)	38 (28.8%)	24 (18.2%)	12 (9.1%)	
Never	1 (2.2%)	10 (21.7%)	22 (47.8%)	8 (17.4%)	5 (10.9%)	
ALL	59 (6.3%)	340 (36.0%)	325 (34.4%)	154 (16.3%)	66 (7.0%)	

Quality of SUS Services n (%) ***				
Frequency	**Very Good/Good**	**Neither Good nor Bad**	**Bad/Very Bad**	***p*-Value**
Always	196 (48.6%)	135 (33.5%)	72 (17.9%)	0.003
Frequently	66 (50.8%)	49 (37.7%)	15 (11.5%)	
Sometimes	92 (36.7%)	103 (41.0%)	56 (22.3%)	
Rarely/Never	65 (35.7%)	73 (40.1%)	44 (24.2%)	
ALL	419 (43.4%)	360 (37.3%)	187 (19.4%)	

Notes: * 1.4% of participants did not answer these questions ("don't know/don't want to answer"); ** 4.6% of participants did not answer these questions ("don't know/don't want to answer"); *** 2.4% of participants did not answer these questions ("don't know/don't want to answer").

Regarding perceptions of access, the Middle Paraíba and metropolitan regions received the most favorable evaluations, with 57.8% and 56.5% of respondents rating access as very good/good, respectively. In contrast, access was rated poorest (poor/very poor) in the Coastal Lowlands region, with 36.3% of users reporting negative perceptions, as shown in Figure 4. A similar pattern was observed in evaluations of service quality: the Middle Paraíba and metropolitan regions again showed the most positive responses (very good/good) from 57.0% and 53.7% of participants, respectively, while the Coastal Lowlands region had the most negative evaluations, with 30.9% rating quality as poor/very poor.

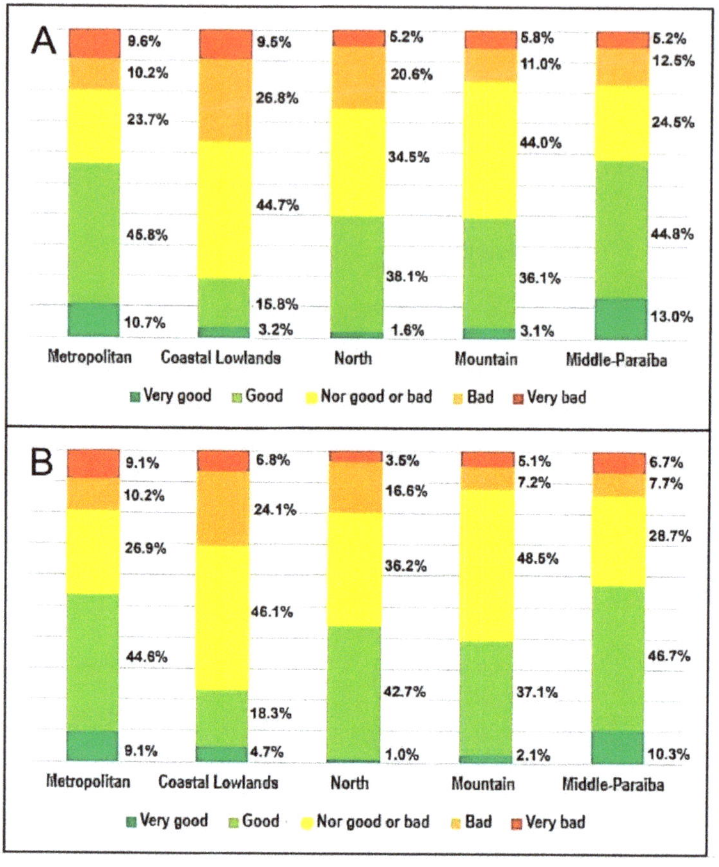

Figure 4. (**A**) Perception of access to SUS services in each region. (**B**) Perception of the quality of health services in each region. ($n = 990$). Notes: 11.7% of participants did not answer this question ("don't know/don't want to answer"); 17.3% of participants did not answer this question ("don't know/don't want to answer").

No statistically significant correlation was observed between perceptions of access to and quality of health services and factors such as gender, family income, or skin color (p-value > 0.05).

More favorable evaluations of access to, and quality of, health services were predominantly reported by participants with lower household incomes, with a significant association found between household income and perceptions of access to SUS services ($p = 0.001$), according to Table 3. Among respondents earning less than the minimum wage, 56.0% rated access as "very good" or "good." Regarding service quality, 53.5% of participants in this income group rated it as "very good" or "good," whereas 45.8% of those earning more than three minimum wages rated it as "neither good nor bad."

Table 3. Views of SUS users regarding the access to and quality of the public health services associated with family income (n = 990).

Access to SUS Services n (%)				
Family Income (Number of Times the Minimum Wage)	**Very Good/Good**	**Nor Good nor Bad**	**Bad/Very Bad**	**p-Value**
Up to 1	88 (56.0%)	35 (22.3%)	34 (21.7%)	0.001
1–2	80 (37.7%)	76 (35.8%)	56 (26.4%)	
2–3	85 (42.1%)	70 (34.6%)	47 (23.3%)	
3–4	53 (34.2%)	62 (40.0%)	40 (25.8%)	
>4	28 (33.3%)	39 (46.4%)	17 (20.3%)	
TOTAL *	334 (41.2%)	282 (34.8%)	194 (24.0%)	
Quality of SUS Services n (%)				
Family Income (Number of Times the Minimum Wage)	**Very Good/Good**	**Nor Good nor Bad**	**Bad/Very Bad**	**p-Value**
Up to 1	85 (53.5%)	49 (30.8%)	25 (15.7%)	0.164
1–2	90 (41.5%)	80 (36.9%)	47 (21.6%)	
2–3	87 (41.0%)	84 (39.6%)	41 (19.3%)	
3–4	62 (39.5%)	63 (40.1%)	32 (20.4%)	
>4	29 (34.9%)	38 (45.8%)	16 (19.3%)	
TOTAL **	353 (42.6%)	35 (37.9%)	161 (19.5%)	

Notes: * 81.8% of participants did not answer these questions ("don't know/don't want to answer"); ** 55.5% of participants did not answer these questions ("don't know/don't want to answer").

Regarding how medications are obtained, 47.6% of participants reported acquiring them exclusively from private pharmacies, 40.5% obtained their medications from both private and public pharmacies, and only 9.7% reported acquiring them exclusively from public pharmacies. When asked about the role of pharmacists, the majority of those who obtained medications through the public system (either exclusively or partially) considered the pharmacist's role essential (82.7%), while 12.3% found it indifferent. Among those who acquired medications solely through private pharmacies, 58.1% viewed the pharmacist as essential, whereas 41.9% considered their role indifferent.

Among those who acquired medications from public pharmacies only (n = 497), 26.8% reported never receiving guidance on how to use them, and 53.7% stated they had never received instructions on how to store their medicines. Furthermore, 40.1% said there was at least one staff member available at the pharmacy to answer questions about medications, while 41.8% said they had never encountered a pharmacist at public health units, as shown in Table 4.

Table 4. Views of SUS users regarding acquiring medications in public pharmacies (n = 497).

Questions	Answers %					
	Always	**Frequently**	**Sometimes**	**Rarely**	**Never**	**Total**
When you pick up medications at public pharmacies of the SUS, do the staff who dispense the medications provide information and/or guidance on how to use them? *	146 (29.8%)	107 (21.9%)	67 (13.7%)	38 (7.8%)	131 (26.8%)	489 (100.0%)
When picking up medications at public pharmacies of the SUS, do you receive guidance on how to store them at home? **	68 (14.0%)	45 (9.2%)	64 (13.2%)	48 (9.9%)	261 (53.7%)	486 (100.0%)

Table 4. *Cont.*

Questions	Answers %					
	Always	Frequently	Sometimes	Rarely	Never	Total
Is the pharmacist or another staff member at public pharmacies of the SUS available when you need to ask questions about medications? ***	170 (40.1%)	87 (20.5%)	82 (19.3%)	25 (5.9%)	60 (14.2%)	424 (100.0%)
Have you ever encountered a pharmacist at the public facility you visit (ESF, UBS, or medication dispensing unit)? ****	61 (15.7%)	76 (19.6%)	57 (14.7%)	32 (8.2%)	162 (41.8%)	388 (100.0%)

Notes: * 1.6% of participants did not answer this question ("don't know/don't want to answer"); ** 2.2% of participants did not answer this question ("don't know/don't want to answer"); *** 14.7% of participants did not answer this question ("don't know/don't want to answer"); **** 21.9% of participants did not answer this question ("don't know/don't want to answer").

4. Discussion

Public health services offered by SUS play a vital role for the Brazilian population, especially through primary care, which serves as the main entry point to the healthcare system. This paper shows that 93.3% of the sample reported using SUS, with those who most frequently used SUS services rating access more positively than those who used SUS less (p-value = 0.002). Participants with lower socioeconomic status also provided more favorable assessments of access to public health services ($p = 0.001$). Moreover, 25.1% of respondents reported using SUS for vaccination and 23.6% for medical consultations, highlighting its role in the health system.

These findings resonate with recent data from across Brazil [30], which highlights the importance of SUS in serving socially vulnerable groups and the most disadvantaged populations. This underscores the need for public policies that promote equity and address socioeconomic and geographic disparities to improve access to and quality of public health services. A high family income was the main characteristic observed in the profile of the population that reported not using SUS services, with 6.4% in this study, focusing on the state of Rio de Janeiro, and 10.7% in a national sample [29,30].

Among frequent users of SUS services, 90.8% view it as indispensable, while 82.1% of those who rarely use it share the same opinion. However, when asked about access, users who reported "always" or "frequently" using SUS expressed more favorable perceptions, with 40.6% and 44.6% rating it as "good," respectively. These findings align with others, which showed that despite recognized issues in health services, users often express satisfaction with the available services [41,42].

When questioned about the quality of SUS services, 50.8% of frequent users rated the system as "very good," while 44% gave a neutral evaluation ("neither good nor bad"). In contrast, among those who rarely use public healthcare services, 24.2% rated it as "poor." These results suggest that those who use the SUS services tend to have a more positive perception compared to those who use it less frequently and may instead rely on private health plans. Similar results were seen in 2019 [41]. This is similar to the findings of the São Paulo State Department of Health, where 60.6% of hospitalized users rated the care they received as good [43]. However, 74% of those surveyed stated they faced some type of barrier when accessing healthcare services. These combined findings underscore the challenges faced by the SUS in meeting the growing demand for quality care.

In 2018, 39% of patients with chronic diseases obtained their medications from public pharmacies, with the majority of people obtaining their medicines from private pharmacies (including popular pharmacy programs) or a combination of public and private sources [44]. This study found that only 9.7% of respondents reported acquiring medications from public facilities. This disparity may be attributable to regional variations, indicating suboptimal access to medicines in public facilities within the state of Rio de Janeiro. Furthermore, given that the popular pharmacy program is administered through private pharmacies [45], respondents may have reported obtaining medications from private pharmacies even if they were procured via this public policy initiative. We will be following this up in future studies.

Among participants who obtained medications from public pharmacies in this study, the majority (82.7%) recognized the role of pharmacists as essential, even though the broader role of pharmacies is often underestimated by the public [10].

When asked about receiving guidance when obtaining medications, 26.85% of respondents stated that they had never received such guidance, and 53% reported never having received information on how to store medications or the necessary precautions. Additionally, 48.1% had never seen a pharmacist providing guidance in a UBS, Family Health Strategy (ESF), or dispensing location. A study conducted during the pandemic showed that although 95% of people perceive the pharmacist as a healthcare professional, 68.6% did not seek guidance from them, and 53.4% had never seen one [46]. This indicates an apparent disconnect between the perceived role of the pharmacist and the full utilization of their services. The lack of pharmacist presence in UBS and ESF contributes to this situation, with only 15% of UBS having a pharmacist. In the units that do have these professionals, there is better medication distribution and greater availability [46]. These findings provide guidance to community pharmacies going forward to help improve medicine use in the country and underscore the importance of continued investment in this critical health sector [47].

While 93.3% of participants reported using SUS, 31.7% reported having private health insurance, above the national average of 25%, according to the National Regulatory Agency for Private Health Insurance and Plans [48]. The higher percentage of participants who have private health insurance, compared to that expected in the country, may be associated with a better socioeconomic status and/or formal employment profile in our sample. Many Brazilians have private health insurance, based on facilities and/or benefits involving their respective companies (e.g., multinationals, state-owned companies, and service sector). Income concentration and employment opportunities are some of the incentives with which individuals seek private health coverage for their families [12]. Notably, the Coastal Lowlands and the North Fluminense regions reported the highest reliance on SUS. This is not only due to socioeconomic factors but also because the access to, and quality of, public healthcare services often influence whether users turn to private services instead [49].

The five regions in the state of Rio de Janeiro revealed varying perceptions of the health system. The Lagos region rated access and quality more negatively compared to the metropolitan region, which showed more favorable evaluations. This was also seen in the Norte Fluminense region, where a larger share of the population uses private health insurance, whereas the metropolitan region relies more heavily on the public system. Furthermore, some regions, including the Coastal Lowlands and Mountains, face shortages of UBS and ESF services. A related study conducted within this same research project in the Coastal Lowlands region [16] demonstrated that the lack of Primary Health Care units, as well as the absence of pharmacists in facilities such as UBS, has negatively impacted the population's perception of access to and quality of health services. In addition to the findings of this study and others conducted by the same research group, it is important to note that although users' perceptions are somewhat positive, public opinion can be significantly influenced by digital media [50]. In this context, negative aspects such as delays in care and medical errors receive greater visibility, while the system's strengths and achievements are often downplayed or overlooked [50]. As a result, SUS has become a target of political and social attacks that threaten its structure and put at risk the continuation of one of the most important programs in the country's history, representing a step backward in light of the progress already made in public health [50]. Consequently, it is essential to understand social demands and, above all, to develop strategies that ensure SUS is responsive to population needs and in receipt of broad social support.

Among our results, we observed that 10.5% of participants had a family income of ≥ five times the minimum wage, 60% self-identified as Black or Brown, and only 16.3% were elderly (>60 years old), according to the Brazilian classification [51]. Data from the latest demographic census of Rio de Janeiro indicate that the combined percentage of the Black and Brown population was higher than other groups across all regions of the state [32,52], with a higher proportion of women and a lower percentage of individuals over 60 [32,52], characteristics also observed in our study. Some published studies, although they did not include statistical analyses correlating respondents' perceptions of SUS services with socioeconomic characteristics (i.e., income and education), generally observed a predominance of participants who self-identified as Black and/or brown, along with a low percentage of individuals with higher education and/or higher income [42,53,54], which is a demographic profile similar to our study.

We acknowledge that this study has some limitations, including the use of purposive convenience sampling. This strategy was adopted due to the impossibility of conducting probability sampling in a large and heterogeneous target population, composed of hundreds of thousands of SUS users. Given the lack of a unified and accessible registry of these users for random selection purposes, the questionnaire was administered to participants who were in or near health services at the time of data collection. Although this approach limits the statistical generalization of the findings to the entire SUS user population, it is frequently employed in applied health research [39,55], particularly when investigating subjective perceptions and experiences, as in the assessment of access to and quality of health services [56,57]. Furthermore, strict inclusion and exclusion criteria were applied, and efforts were made to ensure diversity in the sociodemographic profiles of participants, which we believe contributes to the internal validity of the study. In addition, considering that the study involved undergraduate students from a public university in Brazil and that the project had no available funding, the municipalities and regions of the state of Rio de Janeiro selected for participation were those with greater accessibility and feasibility in terms of transportation, accommodation, and food, allowing interviews to be conducted by a team of volunteer interviewers. Due to logistical challenges, it was not possible to include all municipalities or some localities that could have enhanced regional representation, as in the case of the mountain region, which accounts for approximately 21% of the population. Nonetheless, we prioritized areas with greater socioeconomic relevance, aiming to foster meaningful reflections on the topic within the state context. Furthermore, as a descriptive study, it has certain limitations, such as focusing on describing the findings rather than testing hypotheses or explaining mechanisms, which limits the potential for generalization [58]. However, considering the scarcity of publications on the topics addressed, coupled with the appreciable numbers of participants in this study, we believe our findings will contribute to future discussions on the regional challenges of promoting public health services within a universal system.

Overall, we believe our study offers valuable contributions to the planning and development of public health initiatives, particularly in the context of one of Brazil's most important states as well as the other regions in Brazil facing similar challenges. Research efforts and initiatives such as projects or strategies that foster dialogue and promote the "active listening" of SUS users are essential for informed decision-making by health managers. These insights into user experiences can help guide the implementation and improvement of services to better meet the needs of the population. The results may also be of interest to other countries that face socioeconomic challenges and share the goal of expanding access to quality health services for their populations.

5. Conclusions

The research showed that the population of Rio de Janeiro state perceives the SUS as an essential public service, and access to and the quality of services are evaluated highly, especially by its most frequent users. It also revealed significant regional disparities within the state, particularly regarding services provided by Primary Health Care (PHC) and pharmaceutical services. Promoting research and strategies that foster continuous, constructive dialogue between the population and decision-makers is essential for developing more effective public policies tailored to local needs. To maintain the quality of health service delivery, continuous, constructive dialogue between the population and decision-makers is needed, emphasizing the importance of local engagement in ensuring both access to and the quality of services delivered by municipalities within the Brazilian federal context.

This study covered five of the seven regions of one of Brazil's largest states. Despite being located in the Southeast, a region with more favorable socioeconomic conditions compared to the North and Northeast, user perceptions indicate that many difficulties and challenges persist, such as the provision of specialized care, especially in inland areas such as the Coastal Lowlands region. These findings reflect the real challenges faced by users and have implications for public management so that principles such as universality and comprehensiveness can be effectively achieved in practical settings.

The poor results of access to medicines in Rio de Janeiro state public facilities in comparison to national research necessitate more research to be performed to investigate this further. Finally, the need for the presence of pharmacists in community pharmacies, UBS, and ESF has been highlighted given their capacity to positively influence health indicators and the quality of life of users in alignment with the constitutional principles on which the SUS was founded.

Supplementary Materials: The following supporting information can be downloaded at: https://www.mdpi.com/article/10.3390/ijerph22091424/s1, Survey Instrument.

Author Contributions: Conceptualization, I.P.D.G.; methodology, I.F.L.F., M.C.R., E.A.R., and I.P.D.G.; software, I.F.L.F., M.C.R., E.A.R., and I.P.D.G.; validation, I.F.L.F., M.C.R., N.M.A.M.B., J.S.S., B.M.V.L., T.P.T., D.M.d.S.S.d.S., L.A.C., B.G., S.M.C., J.C.M., I.P.D.G., and I.F.L.F.; formal analysis, I.F.L.F., M.C.R., N.M.A.M.B., J.S.S., B.M.V.L., T.P.T., D.M.d.S.S.d.S., L.A.C., B.G., S.M.C., J.C.M., and I.P.D.G.; investigation, I.F.L.F., E.A.R., and I.P.D.G.; resources, I.F.L.F., M.C.R., N.M.A.M.B., J.S.S., B.M.V.L., T.P.T., D.M.d.S.S.d.S., L.A.C., B.G., S.M.C., J.C.M., and I.P.D.G.; data curation, I.F.L.F., E.A.R., and I.P.D.G.; writing original draft preparation, I.F.L.F., M.C.R., N.M.A.M.B., J.S.S., B.M.V.L., T.P.T., D.M.d.S.S.d.S., L.A.C., B.G., S.M.C., J.C.M., and I.P.D.G. All authors have read and agreed to the published version of the manuscript.

Funding: This research received no external funding.

Data Availability Statement: The original contributions presented in this study are included in the article and supplementary material. Further inquiries can be directed to the corresponding author.

Conflicts of Interest: The authors have no relevant affiliations or financial involvement with any organization or entity with a financial interest in or financial conflict with the subject matter or materials discussed in the manuscript. This includes employment, consultancies, honoraria, stock ownership or options, expert testimony, grants or patents received or pending, or royalties. No writing assistance was utilized in the production of this manuscript.

References

1. Brasil. Lei nº 8.080, de 19 de Setembro de 1990. Dispõe Sobre as Condições Para a Promoção, Proteção e Recuperação da Saúde, a Organização e o Funcionamento dos Serviços Correspondentes e dá Outras Providências. Diário Oficial da União, Brasília, DF, 20 September 1990. Available online: https://www.planalto.gov.br/ccivil_03/leis/l8080.htm (accessed on 9 August 2025).
2. Brasil. Lei nº 8.142, de 28 de Dezembro de 1990. Dispõe Sobre a Participação da Comunidade na Gestão do Sistema Único de Saúde (sus) e Sobre as Transferências Intergovernamentais de Recursos Financeiros na Área da Saúde e dá Outras Providências. Diário Oficial da União, Brasília, DF, 31 December 1990. Available online: https://www.planalto.gov.br/ccivil_03/leis/l8142.htm (accessed on 9 August 2025).
3. Organisation for Economic Co-operation and Development (OECD). *OECD Reviews of Health Systems: Brazil 2021*; OECD Publishing: Paris, France, 2021; Available online: https://www.oecd.org/en/publications/oecd-reviews-of-health-systems-brazil-2021_146d0dea-en.html (accessed on 5 August 2025).
4. Physis. Regionalização em Saúde no Brasil: Uma Análise da Percepção dos Gestores de Comissões Intergestores Regionais. *Physis Rev. Saúde Coletiva* **2022**, *32*, 1–23. [CrossRef]
5. Ministério da Saúde. *Portaria nº 4.279, de 30 de Dezembro de 2010. Estabelece Diretrizes Para a Organização da Rede de Atenção à Saúde no Âmbito do Sistema Único de Saúde (sus)*; Diário Oficial da União, Ministério da Saúde: Brasília, Brazil, 2010.
6. Elidio, G.A.; Sallas, J.; Pacheco, F.C.; de Oliveira, C.; Guilhem, D.B. Atenção primária à saúde: A maior aliada na resposta à epidemia da dengue no Brasil. *Rev. Panam. Salud Publica* **2024**, *48*, e47. [CrossRef] [PubMed]
7. Bousquat, A.; Akerman, M.; Mendes, A.; Louvison, M.; Frazão, P.; Narvai, P.C. Pandemia de covid-19: O SUS mais necessário do que nunca. *Revista USP* **2021**, *1*, 13–26. [CrossRef]
8. Brasil. *Ministério da Saúde. Política Nacional de Atenção Básica*; Ministério da Saúde: Brasília, Brazil, 2017. Available online: https://bvsms.saude.gov.br/bvs/publicacoes/politica_nacional_atencao_basica_2017.pdf (accessed on 17 June 2025).
9. Ministério da Saúde. *Estratégia e-Multi: Equipes Multiprofissionais na Atenção Primária à Saúde*; Ministério da Saúde: Brasília, Brazil, 2022.
10. Peixoto, R.T.; Campos, M.R.; Luiza, V.L.; Mendes, L.V. O farmacêutico na Atenção Primária à Saúde no Brasil: Análise comparativa 2014-2017. *Saúde Debate* **2022**, *46*, 358–375. Available online: https://revista.saudeemdebate.org.br/sed/article/view/6410 (accessed on 17 June 2025). [CrossRef]
11. Ministério da Saúde. Agência Nacional de Saúde Suplementar. ANS Divulga Dados de Beneficiários Referentes a Agosto de 2024. Brasília, Brazil. 2024. Available online: https://www.gov.br/ans/pt-br/assuntos/noticias/numeros-do-setor/ans-divulga-dados-de-beneficiarios-referentes-a-agosto-de-2024 (accessed on 10 October 2024).
12. Souza Júnior, P.R.B.; Szwarcwald, C.L.; Damacena, G.N.; Stopa, S.R.; Vieira, M.L.F.P.; Almeida, W.S.; Oliveira, M.M.; Sardinha, L.M.V.; Macário, E.M. Cobertura de plano de saúde no Brasil: Análise dos dados da Pesquisa Nacional de Saúde 2013 e 2019. *Ciência Saúde Coletiva* **2021**, *26*, 2529–2541. [CrossRef]
13. Instituto de Estudos para Políticas de Saúde. Estado do Rio Tem a pior Cobertura de Atenção Básica do sus no país; Piauí, a melhor: Veja o ranking. [S.l.: S.n.]. 2025. Available online: https://ieps.org.br/estado-do-rio-tem-a-pior-cobertura-de-atencao-basica-do-sus-no-pais-piaui-a-melhor-veja-o-ranking/ (accessed on 15 January 2025).
14. Economist Impact. The Road to Health Inclusivity: From Policy to Practice. 2023. Available online: https://impact.economist.com/projects/health-inclusivity-index/documents/the_road_to_health_inclusivity_health_inclusivity_index_2023_economist_impact_final.pdf (accessed on 9 August 2025).
15. Dornas, B.S.S.; Reis, E.A.; Campos, A.A.O.; Godói, I.P.D. Percepções sobre os serviços de saúde pública em macaé-rj: Um estudo transversal. *Rev. Saúde Pública Paraná* **2024**, *7*, 1–20. [CrossRef]
16. Souza, J.S.; Reis, E.A.; Godman, B.; Campbell, S.M.; Meyer, J.C.; Sena, L.W.P.; Godói, I.P.D. Users' perceptions of access to and quality of unified health system services in brazil: A cross-sectional study and implications to healthcare management challenges. *Int. J. Environ. Res. Public Health* **2024**, *21*, 721. [CrossRef]
17. Raimundo, M.C.; Reis, E.A.; Ferraz, I.F.L.; Borges de Almeida, C.P.; Godman, B.; Campbell, S.M.; Meyer, J.C.; Godói, I.P.D. Users' perceptions of access to and quality of public health services in brazil: A cross-sectional study in metropolitan rio de janeiro, including pharmaceutical services. *Int. J. Environ. Res. Public Health* **2025**, *22*, 967. [CrossRef]
18. Picorelli, L.F. o papel da participação comunitária no sus. *Rev. Direito Med.* **2019**, *1*, 1–20. Available online: https://www.mpgo.mp.br/portal/arquivos/2022/06/01/13_19_11_463_O_papel_da_participa_o_comunit_ria_no_SUS.pdf (accessed on 17 January 2025).
19. Caring for Canadians: Canada's Future Health Workforce—The Canadian Health Workforce Education, Training and Distribution Study. 2025. Available online: https://www.canada.ca/en/health-canada/services/health-care-system/health-human-resources/workforce-education-training-distribution-study.html (accessed on 6 August 2025).
20. HS England. Working in Partnership with People and Communities: Statutory Guidance. London: NHS England, Updated 2023. Available online: https://www.england.nhs.uk/long-read/working-in-partnership-with-people-and-communities-statutory-guidance/ (accessed on 6 August 2025).

21. Vital Strategies, Umane, Universidade Federal de Pelotas (UFPel), Resolve to Save Lives. More Data Better Health: Acesso e Percepção da População Brasileira Sobre a Atenção Primária à Saúde, Módulo 1. São Paulo, Brazil. 2025. Available online: https://www.vitalstrategies.org (accessed on 6 August 2025).
22. Gadelha, C.A.; Costa, K.S.; Nascimento, J.M., Jr.; Soeiro, O.M.; Mengue, S.S.; Motta, M.L.; Carvalho, A.C. PNAUM: Integrated approach to pharmaceutical services, science, technology and innovation. *Rev. Saude Publica* **2016**, *50* (Suppl. 2), 3s. [CrossRef]
23. Fardousi, N.; Nunes da Silva, E.; Kovacs, R.; Borghi, J.; Barreto, J.O.; Kristensen, S.R.; Sampaio, J.; Shimizu, H.E.; Gomes, L.B.; Russo, L.X.; et al. Performance bonuses and the quality of primary health care delivered by family health teams in brazil: A difference-in-differences analysis. *PLoS Med.* **2022**, *19*, e1004033. [CrossRef]
24. Mengue, S.S.; Bertoldi, A.D.; Boing, A.C.; Tavares, N.U.L.; Pizzol, T.D.S.D.; Oliveira, M.A.; Arrais, P.S.D.; Ramos, L.R.; Farias, M.R.; Luiza, V.L.; et al. National survey on access, use and promotion of rational use of medicines (PNAUM): Household survey component methods. *Rev. Saude Publica* **2016**, *50* (Suppl. 2), 4s. [CrossRef]
25. Mello, L.A.F.; Tonini, T.; Sousa da Silva, A.; Dutt-Ross, S.; de Souza Velasque, L. Evaluation of primary health care units in the Rio de Janeiro city according to results of pmaq 2012. *J. Ambul. Care Manag.* **2017**, *40*, S71–S82. [CrossRef] [PubMed]
26. Protasio, A.P.L.; Gomes, L.B.; Machado, L.D.S.; Valença, A.M.G. User satisfaction with primary health care by region in Brazil: 1st cycle of external evaluation from PMAQ-AB. Satisfação do usuário da Atenção Básica em Saúde por regiões do Brasil: 1° ciclo de avaliação externa do PMAQ-AB. *Ciência Saúde Coletiva* **2017**, *22*, 1829–1844. [CrossRef] [PubMed]
27. Protasio, A.P.; Gomes, L.B.; Machado, L.D.; Valença, A.M. Factors associated with user satisfaction regarding treatment offered in Brazilian primary health care. *Cad. Saúde Publica* **2017**, *33*, e00184715. [CrossRef]
28. Medeiros, T.M.; Valerio, F.R.; Silva, M.F.B.; Santos, P.L.; Tenório, B.A.; Branco, S.M.C.; Pereira, M.F.; Sá, A.S.; Costa, N.K.A.; Soares, L.C.L.; et al. Desafios da universalidade no sus: Avaliação do acesso e qualidade dos serviços de saúde no brasil. *Cad. Pedag.* **2024**, *21*, e5102. [CrossRef]
29. UMANE. Estudo Inédito Revela Percepção Sobre Acesso e Qualidade da Atenção primária à Saúde. Available online: https://biblioteca.observatoriosaudepublica.com.br/blog/saude-publica-no-brasil-atencao-primaria/ (accessed on 9 August 2025).
30. Vital Strategies, UMANE, Universidade Federal de Pelotas, Instituto Devive, Resolve to Save Lives. Mais Dados Mais saúde–Atenção Primária à Saúde. Brasil. 2025. ISBN 978-65-85591-09-6. Available online: https://pesquisa.atlasintel.org (accessed on 8 August 2025).
31. Campos, D.S. Saúde e políticas sociais no rio de janeiro brasil: História, caminhos e tendências. *Cad. Saúde Pública* **2019**, *35*, e00065119. [CrossRef]
32. Instituto Brasileiro de Geografia e Estatística (IBGE). Censo Demográfico Brasileiro de 2022. Rio de Janeiro, Brazil. 2022. Available online: https://censo2022.ibge.gov.br/panorama/ (accessed on 15 August 2024).
33. Governo do Estado do Rio de Janeiro. *Diagnóstico de saúde da região metropolitana I*; Secretaria de Saúde: Rio de Janeiro, Brazil, 2020.
34. Governo do Estado do Rio de Janeiro. *Diagnóstico de saúde da região metropolitana II*; Secretaria de Saúde: Rio de Janeiro, Brazil, 2020.
35. Governo do Estado do Rio de Janeiro. *Diagnóstico de saúde da região norte*; Secretaria de Saúde: Rio de Janeiro, Brazil, 2020.
36. Governo do Estado do Rio de Janeiro. *Diagnóstico de saúde da região baixada litorânea*; Secretaria de Saúde: Rio de Janeiro, Brazil, 2020.
37. Governo do Estado do Rio de Janeiro. *Diagnóstico de saúde da região médio paraíba*; Secretaria de Saúde: Rio de Janeiro, Brazil, 2020.
38. Governo do Estado do Rio de Janeiro. *Diagnóstico de saúde da região serrana*; Secretaria de Saúde: Rio de Janeiro, Brazil, 2020.
39. Althubaiti, A. Sample size determination: A practical guide for health researchers. *J. Gen. Fam. Med.* **2022**, *24*, 72–78. [CrossRef]
40. Brasil. *Histórico de Cotação*; Banco Central do Brasil: Brasília, Brazil, 2025. Available online: https://www.bcb.gov.br/estabilidadefinanceira/historicocotacoes (accessed on 15 April 2025).
41. Instituto Brasileiro de Geografia e Estatística (IBGE). Pesquisa Nacional de Saúde 2019: Informações Sobre Domicílios, Acesso e Utilização dos Serviços de Saúde. IBGE: Rio de Janeiro, Brazil, 2020. Available online: https://biblioteca.ibge.gov.br/visualizacao/livros/liv101748.pdf (accessed on 10 May 2025).
42. Cantalino, J.L.R.; Scherer, M.D.D.A.; Soratto, J.; Schäfer, A.A.; Anjos, D.S.O.D. Satisfação dos usuários em relação aos serviços de Atenção Primária à Saúde no Brasil. *Rev. Saúde Pública* **2021**, *55*, 22. Available online: https://revistas.usp.br/rsp/article/view/186498 (accessed on 17 June 2025). [CrossRef]
43. São Paulo (Estado). Secretaria de Estado da Saúde. Pesquisa de Satisfação dos Usuários do sus/sp. São Paulo, Brazil. 2023. Available online: https://fedap.com.br/2023/09/12/governo-de-sp-lanca-pesquisa-de-satisfacao-dos-usuarios-do-sus-paulista/ (accessed on 10 May 2025).
44. Matta, S.R.; Bertoldi, A.D.; Emmerick, I.C.M.; Fontanella, A.T.; Costa, K.S.; Luiza, V.L. Fontes de obtenção de medicamentos por pacientes diagnosticados com doenças crônicas, usuários do Sistema Único de Saúde. *Cad. Saúde Pública* **2018**, *34*, e00073817. [CrossRef]

45. Oliveira, M.A.; Luiza, V.L.; Tavares, N.U.L.; Mengue, S.S.; Arrais, P.S.D.; Farias, M.R.; Pizzol, T.D.S.D.; Ramos, L.R.; Bertoldi, A.D. Access to medicines for chronic diseases in Brazil: A multidimensional approach. *Rev. Saude Publica* **2016**, *50* (Suppl. 2), 6s. [CrossRef]
46. Lacerda, M.G.C.; Sampaio, J.P.S.; Dourado, C.S.M.E. Percepção Da População Sobre O Papel Do Farmacêutico No Contexto Da Pandemia Do Novo Coronavírus. *Res. Soc. Dev.* **2021**, *10*, e54310918304. [CrossRef]
47. Marinho, L.N.; Campbell, S.M.; Amaral, I.B.S.T.; Reis, R.S.; Godman, B.; Meyer, J.C.; Godói, I.P.D. Public health financing in Brazil (2019–2022): An analysis of the national health fund and implications for health management. *Front. Public Health* **2025**, *13*, 1568351. [CrossRef]
48. Agência Nacional de Saúde Suplementar (ANS). Dados Econômico-Financeiros do Setor de Planos de Saúde: 1° Trimestre de 2025. Brasília, Brazil. 2025. Available online: https://www.gov.br/ans (accessed on 10 May 2025).
49. Mahmood, S.; Sequeira, R.; Siddiqui, M.M.U.; Herkenhoff, M.B.A.; Ferreira, P.P.; Fernandes, A.C.; Sousa, P. Decentralization of the health system-experiences from Pakistan, Portugal and Brazil. *Health Res. Policy Syst.* **2024**, *22*, 61. [CrossRef] [PubMed]
50. Santos, R.T.; Franco, T.A.V.; Pitthan, R.G.V.; Cabral, L.M.S.; Cotrim, D.F.; Gomes, B.C. Saúde pública e comunicação: Impasses do SUS à luz da formação democrática da opinião pública. *Ciência Saúde Coletiva* **2022**, *27*, 1547–1556. [CrossRef] [PubMed]
51. Brasil. Lei n° 10.741, de 1° de Outubro de 2003. Dispõe Sobre o Estatuto da Pessoa Idosa e dá Outras Providências. Diário Oficial da União, Brasília, Brazil, 1 October 2003. Available online: https://www.planalto.gov.br/ccivil_03/leis/2003/l10.741.htm (accessed on 31 August 2025).
52. Secretaria de Saúde do Estado do Rio de Janeiro. População Residente Estudo de Estimativas Populacionais por Município, Idade e Sexo 2000–2024-Pactuada pela SES-RJ. Rio de Janeiro, Brazil. 2024. Available online: https://sistemas.saude.rj.gov.br/tabnetbd/dhx.exe?populacao/pop_populacao_ripsa2024.def (accessed on 10 May 2025).
53. Instituto Brasileiro de Geografia e Estatística (IBGE). *Pesquisa Nacional de Saúde 2019: Atenção Primária à Saúde e Informações Antropométricas*; IBGE: Rio de Janeiro, Brazil, 2020; Available online: https://www.pns.icict.fiocruz.br/wp-content/uploads/2021/02/liv101758.pdf (accessed on 31 August 2025).
54. Novais, M.; Martins, C.B. Perfil dos Beneficiários de Planos e SUS e o Acesso a Serviços de Saúde–PNAD 2003 e 2008. Instituto de Estudos de Saúde Suplementar-IESS. 2010. Available online: https://www.iess.org.br/sites/default/files/2021-04/TD35.pdf (accessed on 31 August 2025).
55. Ahmed, S.K. Research Methodology Simplified: How to Choose the Right Sampling Technique and Determine the Appropriate Sample Size for Research. *Oral Oncol. Rep.* **2024**, *12*, 100662. [CrossRef]
56. Hulley, S.B.; Cummings, S.R.; Browner, W.S.; Grady, D.G.; Newman, T.B. *Delineando a Pesquisa clínica: Uma Abordagem Epidemiológica*, 4th ed.; Artmed: Porto Alegre, Brazil, 2013.
57. Gil, A.C. *Métodos e Técnicas de Pesquisa Social*, 7th ed.; Atlas: São Paulo, Brazil, 2019.
58. Aggarwal, R.; Ranganathan, P. Study designs: Part 2-Descriptive studies. *Perspect. Clin. Res.* **2019**, *10*, 34–36. [CrossRef]

International Journal of
Environmental Research and Public Health

MDPI

Article

Applying Design Thinking for Co-Designed Health Solutions: A Case Study on Chronic Kidney Disease in Regional Australia

Anita Stefoska-Needham [1,2,*], Jessica Nealon [1], Karen Charlton [1], Karen Fildes [1] and Kelly Lambert [1]

1 School of Medical, Indigenous and Health Sciences, University of Wollongong, Wollongong 2522, Australia; jnealon@uow.edu.au (J.N.); karenc@uow.edu.au (K.C.); kfildes@uow.edu.au (K.F.); klambert@uow.edu.au (K.L.)
2 School of Health Sciences, University of New South Wales, Sydney 2052, Australia
* Correspondence: a.stefoska-needham@unsw.edu.au

Abstract

(1) Background: This paper outlines key issues to consider when implementing Design Thinking methodology in health-based qualitative research to achieve a meaningful outcome. The purpose is to share our learnings with others. (2) Methods: Using the case study of an Australian region with high rates of chronic kidney disease, we describe a design-led methodological approach (co-design) that ensures end users remain central to research for the lifespan of the project; from conception of the research question and protocol design, through to solution generation and change implementation. (3) Results: Representation of the four Design Voices—people with lived experience, expertise, intent, and design knowledge—was imperative to minimise bias towards researchers as the main drivers of the project. A commitment to the five core elements of design thinking (empathising, defining, ideating, prototyping, and testing) was maintained throughout the research. Empathising through direct interaction with users was crucial to creating a meaningful understanding of their problems and challenges. Ideation ensured user-centred solution generation, with solutions aligned with addressing the 'real' problem and creating an improved future state. (4) Conclusions: Incorporation of Design Thinking principles in health research is a valuable adjunct to traditional qualitative methodologies, with the potential to facilitate meaningful outcomes for people in our community experiencing a wicked health problem.

Keywords: design-led thinking; codesign; consumer; chronic kidney disease; qualitative research

1. Introduction

Chronic kidney disease (CKD) poses a significant public health burden in Australia [1]. In the Illawarra and Shoalhaven region of New South Wales, the prevalence of CKD is around 9% [2]. In 2018, researchers in the Health Impacts Research Centre (HIRC) at the University of Wollongong, New South Wales, embarked on a multidisciplinary research programme to investigate reasons for the high rates of CKD, and to design potential interventions to prevent or slow the progression of the disease in the region. Community engagement was recognised as an important starting point in this endeavour, the specific aim of which was to better understand the diverse experiences of people living with CKD, their family members, carers, and health care providers. To achieve this aim, researchers within HIRC were committed to implementing an *authentic* co-design process that was underpinned by the principle of 'design thinking', a lesser-known approach among academic health researchers generally, but more broadly recognised in business, technology, and service design sectors. Design Thinking, also known as design-led thinking, emerged prominently in these fields as a structured yet flexible approach for addressing complex challenges [3]. Its emphasis on empathy, ideation, and iterative problem-solving has been widely adopted to improve user experiences and drive organisational change. More recently, health and social care research has begun to adopt design-led principles, recognising their potential to address multifaceted or "wicked" problems that resist simple solutions. Unlike traditional top-down research approaches, design-led thinking is explicitly participatory and user-centred, positioning lived experience as a critical form of evidence alongside clinical or academic expertise [4,5]. This framing helps to bridge the gap between health service users and providers by generating solutions that are not only theoretically desirable but also practically feasible and economically viable [6]. In the context of chronic conditions such as CKD, where care pathways are fragmented and experiences vary widely, design-led thinking can uncover hidden barriers and co-create person-centred innovations that align with the realities of diverse stakeholders.

Therefore, using the complex problem of high CKD rates in the Illawarra and Shoalhaven regions of Australia as an example, this viewpoint paper outlines some key issues to consider when implementing design thinking methodology in health-based qualitative research. We intend to share our learnings with the broader academic health services research community so that others may also successfully use codesign. The concept of design thinking is defined, and its potential value in research that explores a complex health problem in the community is showcased. Suggestions for successfully incorporating design thinking into traditional qualitative research methodologies are also made. Finally, we suggest that Design Thinking is elevated from being considered as a technology/innovation-specific tool for solution generation to a valuable adjunct to traditional qualitative research methodologies, with the potential to facilitate meaningful outcomes for people in our community experiencing a multifarious health problem.

2. Materials and Methods

2.1. Overview of Design Thinking

Design Thinking encompasses an iterative and human-centred approach to solving complex problems [3] by promoting empathy for those experiencing the problem, and thereby encouraging the creation of human-centred, also known as user-centred, solutions [4,5]. Traditionally, the Design Thinking approach has been successfully implemented within technology and business sectors to enhance products and improve services, and relies strongly on collaborative multidisciplinary teams working together with the end users to achieve desired outcomes, or to design a valuable solution [6]. These "users" are generally people in the community who may engage in a product or service, such as customers. In employing Design Thinking, establishing the nexus between what is desirable from a human perspective with what is technologically feasible and economically viable, is pivotal because the most valuable idea or solution to a problem is the one that meets all three criteria [7] (Figure 1). This methodological approach, often described as 'design-led', reflects the underpinning Design Thinking principles.

Typically, this process requires repeated cycles of brainstorming with all key stakeholders, including end-users, to generate ideas for a potential solution, followed by testing to identify potential barriers, which then may feed back into further ideation. Eventually, through this iterative process, the most valuable solution or idea is generated [8,9]. Tom Brown of Stanford University, one of the seminal proponents of Design Thinking, proposes that solution generation through Design Thinking is achieved across five stages: (i) empathising, (ii) defining, (iii) ideating, (iv) prototyping, and (v) testing [4] (Figure 2).

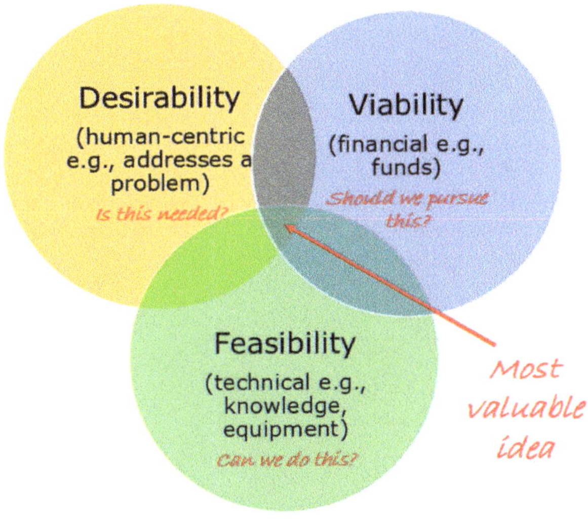

Figure 1. The three design lenses: desirability, viability, and feasibility to guide the selection of the most valuable idea or solution (adapted from [7]). The most valuable idea or solution to a problem is the one that meets all three criteria.

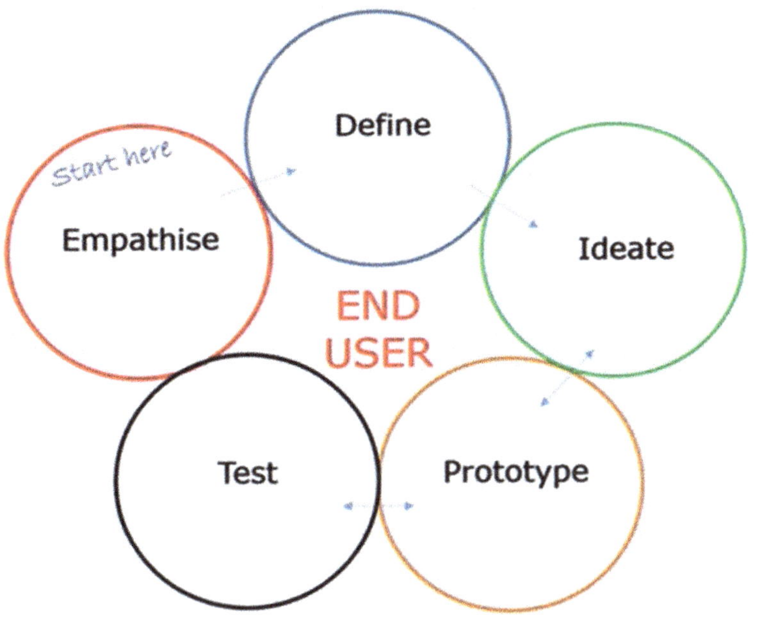

Figure 2. The five phases of Design Thinking, adapted from Stanford University's Design Thinking Model: a strategy for authentic and innovative user-centric solution generation [4].

Empathising relates to direct interaction with users, as an instinctive, emotional, affective, shared, and mirrored experience [5] crucial to making sense of things and creating meaning [10]. It helps to understand a need or a problem from the perspective of the end-user. The "define" phase allows reflection on the articulated need or problem in the "empathise" phase, as a means to devise a plan for a solution. The "ideation" phase includes creative brainstorming and innovative solution generation, and may include research on how to translate the solution into reality. During the "prototype" phase, an authentic and tangible solution is brought to life, often through numerous, rapidly generated user-centred prototypes. In the "test" phase, review and feedback of the prototype are received to ensure it meets the end-users' needs, and includes iterations and refinements to the prototype, resulting in its final implementation or launch. According to Brown [4], to ensure that design-led activities are authentic requires the representation of four Design Voices throughout the process: the voice of intent (senior stakeholders), the voice of experience (the users), the voice of expertise (domain experts), and the voice of design (external facilitator guiding the process authentically) (Figure 3). Representation of all four Design Voices throughout the project minimises bias towards one voice over another.

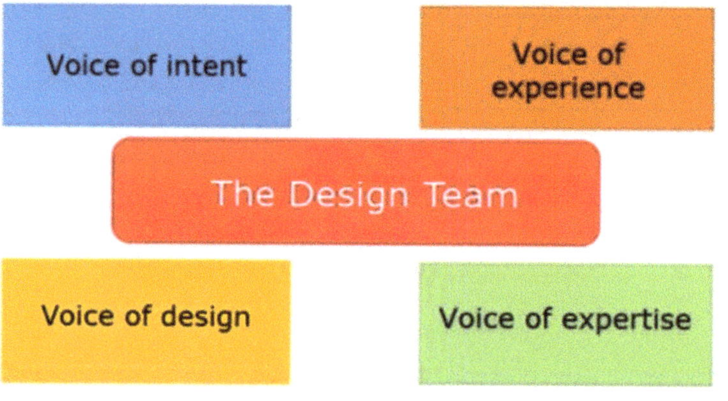

Figure 3. The Design Voices (adapted from and used with permission from ThinkPlace Global, [11]) represent four key groupings of stakeholders which are important for the design and execution of an effective co-design project.

From a pragmatic perspective, a number of tools are commonly used to collect data in design-led projects, including workshops, interviews, surveys, storyboarding, personas, and journey maps, depending on the needs and preferences of the users involved. For example, personas are fictional characters that are created based on research data, and are useful to embed empathy and to create an improved experience for the target group [12,13]. They are widely used in product design to create reliable and realistic representations of a key audience or target group for reference [14], but are also emerging in traditional qualitative research [15]. A journey map is a visual representation of a persona's experiences and interactions over time, and helps to develop an understanding of how these experiences and interactions may be improved [16].

For many years, Design Thinking has also been used for social innovation, across different community segments to solve complicated and complex problems (also referred to as wicked problems) [17]. Globally, governments and private businesses alike have recognised the value of engaging with the community to design services and products that involve people who use or are affected by that service or product [18]. In health care systems, Design Thinking has also been used to restructure patient-oriented clinical services, aiming to improve patient journeys and clinical outcomes [19–21]. Typically, the process of implementing Design Thinking methodologies is referred to as "co-design" in the health research literature [8]. Stakeholders involved in redesigning health system-related processes may include patients and their families and carers, clinicians, nursing staff, executives, and operational managers [22]. By coming together to co-design a solution, multi-stakeholder perspectives are represented, with no one voice being more dominant or important than the other. Chronic kidney disease (CKD) is a complex, even wicked, public health problem in Australia [1] and is well-suited to a design-led approach in finding a solution to the broad health and economic challenges it presents to communities. CKD refers to all conditions of the kidney, lasting at least three months, where there is evidence of kidney damage and/or reduced kidney function, regardless of the specific diagnosis of disease or condition causing the disease [23]. CKD is associated with an increased risk of morbidity and mortality [24], as well as significant economic costs, as high as $9.9 billion Australian dollars per year. Of concern is the overrepresentation of CKD amongst the Aboriginal and Torres Strait Islander community [1]. CKD is a multifaceted condition that not only affects multiple metabolic pathways [23], but it has impacts on the mental health of patients [25] and is usually associated with considerable co-morbidity and ageing [26]. This complexity makes CKD difficult to manage, both from the perspective of the patient, the patient's family/carers, as well as health care providers.

Person-centred health care is recommended for the management of CKD due to the multifactorial nature of the condition; however, there is evidence to suggest that this standard is not being achieved consistently across Australia [21]. Person-centred health care is defined as "health care that involves the patient, their carer and family; and is respectful of and responsive to the preferences, needs and values of patients and consumers" [27]. Shortfalls in the delivery of CKD person-centred health care in Australia have emerged through reported gaps in treatment targets and failures to meet other recommended health indicators of optimal clinical care, such as treatment of anaemia [28]. Missed or late diagnosis of CKD and late referral of at-risk patients to nephrologists have also been documented [29]. Patient activation, described as an individual's knowledge, skills, and confidence for managing their health and health care [30], is an essential component of the successful delivery of person-centred health care. In people with CKD, low levels of patient activation have been reported, especially in patients with co-morbidities, older patients, and those with *worse* self-reported health [31,32]. Low patient activation is associated with poor participation and engagement in an individual's own health care, which challenges the core pillars of the person-centred health care philosophy.

Integrated care is also important for the management of CKD. This approach has been shown to have favourable impacts on people's self-management and their short-term clinical outcomes, as well as on CKD progression over time [33–35]. Key benefits of integrated care include improved communication between health professionals, clarity among primary care practitioners around guidelines, referral to specialist care, and more time available for individualised education [36]. Neale et al. [37] identified provider-related barriers to integrated care, such as confusion with clinical guidelines, inadequate financial reimbursement for screening, and lack of supportive primary care technology. Hence, the redesign of CKD services must consider integrative care as a core activity or philosophy.

2.2. Community Engagement Is Essential in the Design of Person-Centred Health Care for People Living with CKD

To better achieve person-centred health care and thereby increase patient activation in CKD, it is important to meaningfully engage the community affected by CKD, including patients, carers, family, and health care practitioners (and numerous other stakeholders). This holistic approach has greater potential to offer a better understanding of existing challenges and help to identify opportunities for improvement. From a health perspective, co-design (underpinned by Design Thinking) is a way of "improving health care services for patients by bringing together all stakeholders and consumers in partnership, to develop health services that best meet the needs of consumers and carers in the most effective way possible" [38]. The commitment to and support of co-design in health is also reflected at the state health department level with the formation of the Agency for Clinical Innovation (ACI) (NSW, Australia), commissioned to engage patients and consumers to design, promote and implement a person-centred approach to health care in NSW using co-design methodologies [38]. Recently, kidney care services in Victoria and New South Wales have been co-designed with people with CKD, their families/carers, and health practitioners [21], with potential for nationwide roll-out, though this is yet to be confirmed.

3. Results

In the Health Impacts Research Centre (University of Wollongong, Wollongong, NSW, Australia) CKD project [39], community engagement was identified as a key strategic research priority. Thus, a specific community engagement hub was created that included researchers skilled in qualitative research, key stakeholders working in CKD from the Local Health District, members of the community, and other stakeholders, according to Design Thinking principles. The results are published elsewhere [39]. The community engagement hub worked alongside a hub of researchers conducting epidemiological research, as well as a hub of researchers performing systematic reviews of the literature, as part of a multi-disciplinary approach to understanding why CKD rates are high relative to other regions of Australia.

The execution of the design-led HIRC CKD project followed a number of key steps reflecting the important principles of Design Thinking (see Figure 4). Stakeholders were assembled that reflected the four Design Voices, and an intent meeting was held to set expectations to guide the project for the duration of its lifecycle. The intent meeting included the facilitation of activities designed to (i) elicit insights from end users in an empathetic way that draws upon lived experiences to better define the current state and existing challenges, and (ii) offer users opportunities to ideate and propose (prototype) solutions to their perceived problem and challenges.

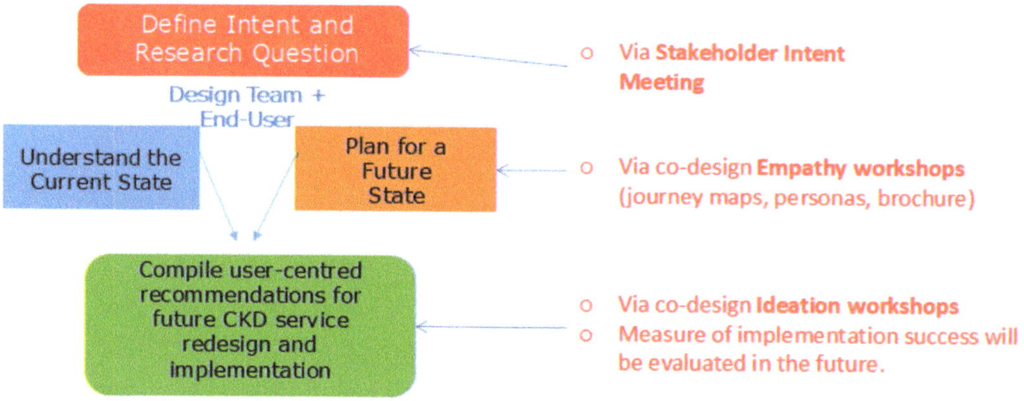

Figure 4. Overview of the CKD co-design project underpinned by Design Thinking methodologies, from defining the project intent to developing recommendations for the redesign of new CKD services in the Illawarra–Shoalhaven region.

The key steps are broadly described here:

Step 1: Recruitment of Stakeholders to Represent the Four Design Voices

For the recruitment of the four representative Design Voices in the HIRC CKD project, purposive sampling was employed. Purposive sampling is the intentional selection of participants based on their ability to provide detailed and extensive information about the phenomenon under investigation [40]. The voice of intent was represented by senior stakeholders, including HIRC directors (n = 2) and executive members (n = 5), as well as HIRC CKD project managers (n = 4). The voice of experience was represented by the patients (with a formal CKD diagnosis across the spectrum of disease stages), and their family/carers living in the Illawarra-Shoalhaven region. The participants were recruited from the Local Health District Renal Units and general medical practices, where study posters and flyers were showcased in consulting and waiting rooms to promote the project. The voice of expertise was represented by nurses, doctors, allied health professionals, alongside researchers (members of HIRC at the University of Wollongong with an interest in health research). Eligible secondary and tertiary health care practitioners were required to be actively practising as secondary or tertiary health care practitioners based in the Illawarra-Shoalhaven region. They were directly contacted by one of the HIRC CKD project researchers to seek their voluntary participation. Finally, the voice of design was represented by an external facilitator guiding the co-design process authentically. The ongoing representation of the four Design Voices throughout the project was crucial to remaining authentic to the co-design process and minimising bias. Figure 5 represents the four Design Voices overseeing the HIRC CKD project.

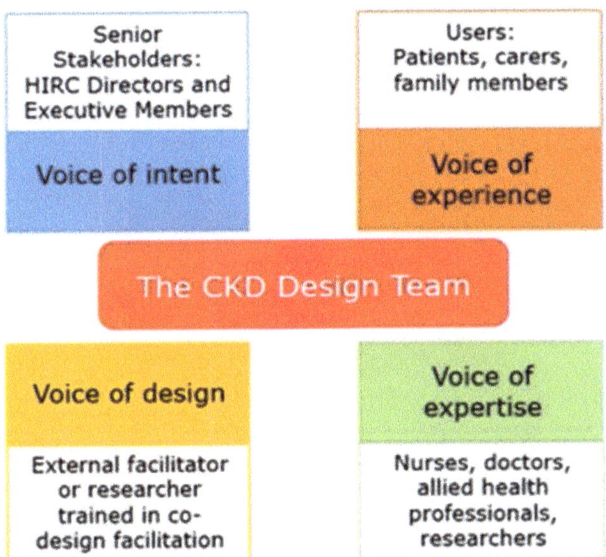

Figure 5. The Design Team, comprising key stakeholders representing the four Design Voices underpinning the HIRC CKD Project. The *voice of intent* was represented by HIRC directors, executive members, and project managers. The *voice of experience* was represented by the patients and their family/carers. The *voice of expertise* was represented by researchers and medical and allied health professionals. The *voice of design* was represented by an expert co-design facilitator.

Step 2: Defining the Project's Intent, Problem Statement, and Setting Expectations

Following the collation of the four Design Voices, the voice of intent representatives led a meeting to define the project's intent, involving stakeholders representing all Design Voices. The intent of the project was defined as follows: "*to understand the current state for people living with CKD, their family and carers, in the Illawarra-Shoalhaven region, and use these insights to recommend changes to achieve a future state with improved patient/user journeys and more empathetic renal services that meet the complex needs of its varied users.*" To add rigour to the methodological approach, the appropriateness of the project's intent was tested through the three lenses of Design Thinking: desirability (is the project needed by end users?/is it valuable?), is it viable (do we have the financial means to conduct the project activities?), is it feasible (do we have the experience and expertise to conduct the work?). For the purposes of this project, end users included people with CKD and their families/carers, as well as health care professionals working within Illawarra-Shoalhaven renal services. Stakeholders at the intent meeting deemed that all three Design Thinking criteria were satisfied, and hence, the project received consensus agreement for launch.

The main value and output of the intent meeting was the design of a research question together with all relevant stakeholders, rather than researchers proposing the question exclusively. Traditional academic approaches to research design typically start with a predetermined research question that is seldom tested or validated with stakeholders, and is most certainly proposed in isolation from the collective Design Voices. The research question often emerges from identified gaps in the previously published literature or prior research activities. This approach is therefore unlikely to be an authentic reflection of co-design or design-led principles, as it is biased towards one stakeholder, that being the researcher [41]. This is therefore a major, though less acknowledged or recognised, limitation of current qualitative research purporting to be "co-designed".

The intent meeting also offered an early-stage opportunity to identify other stakeholders to include within the four Design Voices, to ensure the project maintained its authenticity to co-design and methodological rigour throughout the duration of the research period. Following the initial intent meeting, the research question and protocol underpinning the HIRC CKD project were formally drafted and validated with representatives of all the Design Voices, and approval from the University of Wollongong Human Research Ethics Committee was received (HE2018/348).

Step 3: Empathising with the End Users to Collect Valuable Insights (Data) and Define the Problem, and Ideate Potential Solutions

Through a series of workshops facilitated by the *voice of design* (external facilitator and trained HIRC researchers), insights from people with CKD, family members, carers, health researchers, and health care providers (representing both the *voice of experience* and *voice of expertise*) were conducted over a two-year period in 2018 and 2019. In addition, telephone interviews were conducted with some stakeholders who were unable to attend the workshops. The first workshops were called *Empathy Workshops* to reflect the purpose of building empathy with the users to better understand their experiences, and their perspectives on the current state and problem. The second round of workshops was called *Ideation Workshops*, which represented opportunities for users to ideate or brainstorm solutions.

3.1. Empathy Workshops

For each small group discussion at the workshops, a 'scribe' was allocated to capture key points on Post-it notes (Figure 6). Each small group consisted of people with similar experiences, such as people on dialysis, people with a kidney transplant, or health professionals. Segmentation of groups enabled potential power imbalances to be minimised. The scribe was usually a HIRC researcher acting in their role as the voice of design, under the broader guidance of the external facilitator. These Post-it notes were then attached to a wall chart representing elements of a user journey through kidney care services in the Illawarra-Shoalhaven region. The user journey wall chart comprised four themes or subheadings: (i) narrative or background story; (ii) user satisfaction points; (iii) pain points or challenges; and (iv) ideas for change (see Figure 6). The users within each small group sorted the Post-it notes into the four categories. Photographs of each of the small groups' wall charts were taken for further data analysis by researchers who conducted thematic analysis to identify, analyse, and report themes within the data [42]. Thematic analysis summarises and systemises the content of the qualitative data and is one of the most widely used approaches in health research [43]. As thematic analysis involves active researcher interpretation, reflexivity was used to enhance rigour and transparency [44]. This included regular self-reflection and team discussions to consider how researchers' backgrounds and perspectives might shape data interpretation. Findings of this analysis, published in full elsewhere [39], indicate there are challenges with timely access to kidney care services and a need to dismantle health professional silos that lack good interdisciplinary communication.

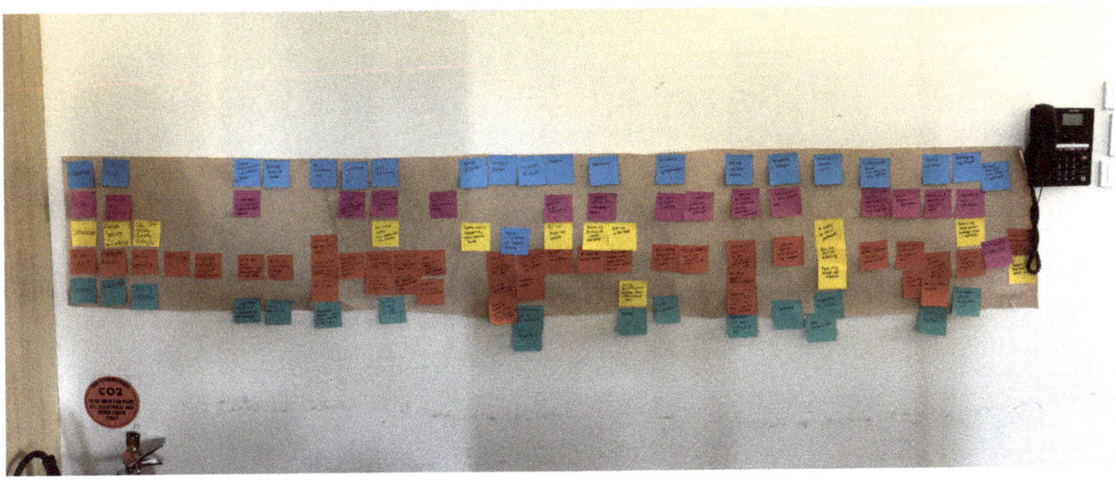

Figure 6. Image of Post-it notes generated by scribes with consumers during the co-design process. These notes represent the user perspectives and experiences, arranged on a wall chart to form user journeys. The notes are grouped according to four themes: narrative (or background story), user satisfaction points, challenges, and ideas for change.

3.2. Personas

All users attending the workshops created their own personas using a fictitious name but based on their personal experiences and background, emotions, desires, barriers, and supports. In addition, users shared their own personas with other users within their small groups at the workshops. Users were also encouraged to specifically share their personal interactions with local health services. Their key insights were recorded on Post-it notes again by the external facilitator or researcher. The users then placed these Post-it notes back on the journey map wall chart, and a photograph was taken to enable all journey maps to undergo further analysis by researchers following the workshops. Researchers were also tasked with grouping similar individual personas to produce "aggregated personas" to reflect the different users engaging with Illawarra-Shoalhaven CKD services. Personas of individuals with CKD, their families and caregivers, healthcare providers (including medical doctors, general practitioners, nephrologists, nurses, and allied health professionals), and others were developed, each representing different perspectives. An example of a persona is shown in Figure 7.

Name: Jeffrey **Age:** 75 years 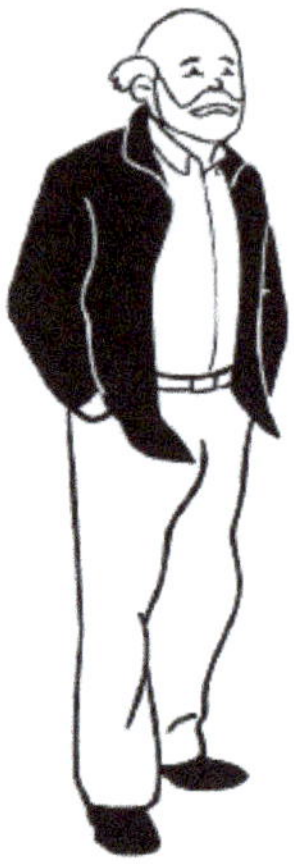 **Occupation:** Retiree **Quote:** *"I refuse to be tied up to a machine and all the burden that comes with it."*	**Background:** I am a retired miner. I was diagnosed with Type 2 diabetes when I was in my 50s. My wife would help manage my diabetes by cooking the right foods for me and accompanying me for walks because she knows that I don't like to exercise. At age 65, I had a heart attack, then my GP put me on a health care plan to see a diabetic educator, dietitian, exercise physiologist, optometrist, and podiatrist. I had a different appointment almost every day. My GP ran many tests and told me that I also had stage 3 chronic kidney disease. I was referred to a nephrologist, and I expected that I would be put on some kind of intervention, but instead, I was told I would have end-stage kidney disease within a few months. I was given rudimentary advice on my diet and left wondering how I could have let my kidneys get that bad. At every appointment, my wife and I would ask the doctors for advice on how to manage my kidney disease and my type 2 diabetes. I am now 75 years old. I still have stage 3 chronic kidney disease and have since been diagnosed with hypertension and prostate cancer. I still don't know if I am doing enough to avoid end-stage kidney disease.

I am feeling
- concerned that I'm taking too many medications that could be impacting my kidneys,
- confused on how to manage all my different diseases, and
- scared of going to the specialist and being told that I suddenly have in-stage kidney disease

My goals are
- to effectively manage all of my diseases,
- to have a holistic approach to my health care, and
- to ensure that all the medications I am taking are not making my health worse

Barriers to reaching my goals are
- limited resources available and the resources that are available sometimes contradict each other, and
- a limited number of appointments subsidising the GP care plan and different brand names for medications.

My supports are
- my wife for helping me through this journey, and
- my GP for being patient when explaining the invent information to me and my wife.

Figure 7. Example of a persona of an older CKD patient using a fictitious name. The persona is based on the patient's personal experiences and background, emotions, desires, perceived barriers, and supports.

3.3. Ideation Workshops

A few months after the *Empathy Workshops*, all users were invited back to a new round of workshops to ideate and brainstorm solutions or changes required to improve services and experiences for people living with CKD in the Illawarra-Shoalhaven region. Following similar methodologies as described for the *Empathy* workshops, a number of improvements to services were identified, enabling researchers to more accurately describe a potential future state for all users.

After the *Ideation* workshop, a pamphlet was produced to summarise the outcomes discussed (Supplementary Materials, File S1). To validate the contents of the pamphlet as an accurate reflection of users' thoughts and feelings, face-to-face meetings were held with a sub-group of users who had attended the *Ideation* workshops, in their home or at the University of Wollongong. Any feedback or gaps were taken into account, and the pamphlet was updated. This cross-checking activity with end users reflected the project's ongoing commitment to authentic co-design that aims to continually place the end user at the centre throughout the research process.

3.4. Interviews

Attendance at the workshops by primary and tertiary health care professionals was low due to work commitments. To overcome this gap, semi-structured interviews were conducted with a purposive sample of nephrologists, general practitioners, renal and general practice nurses, dietitians, and social workers, at a time that was convenient to them [36]. Design Thinking methodology encourages the employment of different tools in order to capture all stakeholders' experiences and insights, and to be guided by their individual needs, so that pragmatic barriers such as non-attendance due to work commitments do not limit the representation of key stakeholders. Insights from the workshops proved valuable when constructing the question guides for use in the interviews, representing another advantage of the design-led approach that promotes cycles of iteration and refinement. The verbatim interview transcripts were analysed using a relativist ontological position and a directed content analysis approach by three independent researchers, who reached consensus on key themes. These themes confirmed that the delivery of person-centred care for people with CKD was important among all health care professionals; however, a deficit in shared understanding of the disease within and between disciplines was identified, and a major barrier to an integrated approach to delivery of health care to individuals living with early-stage kidney disease [36].

4. Discussion

In summary, data from discussions at empathy and ideation workshops and interviews afforded HIRC CKD researchers, alongside end-users, the opportunity to more meaningfully describe what a desirable future state for people living with CKD in the Illawarra-Shoalhaven region may look like. This future state would be inclusive of empathetic and personalised experiences through an integrated kidney care service, notably involving more seamless communication and patient management by primary, secondary, and tertiary health care providers. Specifically, the pamphlet summarising the ideation sessions, alongside findings emerging from all the different activities in workshops and interviews, will be used as collateral in future discussions with health service decision makers to encourage the redesign and re-imagination of kidney care services in the Illawarra-Shoalhaven region. This final step ensures that attention, respect, and empathy towards end users' perspectives and recommendations for service improvements are fully afforded.

Positioning the design-led chronic kidney disease case-study within a traditional theoretical research framework

From an academic perspective, the HIRC CKD project falls under the high-level framework of "Implementation Research" (IR), a field of health research that has been shown to contribute to more effective public health, clinical policies, and programme designs [45] (Figure 8). IR is a scientific enquiry into questions concerning implementation or "the act of fulfilling or carrying out an intention" and is especially concerned with the users of the research, not merely the production of knowledge [45]. There is a wide range of implementation-specific research methods, including qualitative methods (grounded theory, ethnography, phenomenology, case studies and narrative approaches, key informant interviews, and focus groups), quantitative methods (cross-sectional surveys), and mixed methods (a combination of qualitative and quantitative methods) [45]. Specifically, the HIRC CKD project is underpinned by key principles of Participatory Action Research

(PAR), a specific type of IR. PAR refers to a number of different research methods that emphasise participation and action (such as implementation), using methods that involve iterative processes of reflection and action, "carried out with and by the local people, rather than on them" [46]. In PAR, the control of the process rests with the participants, which includes people with CKD, their families/carers, health care practitioners, domain experts, and academics/researchers in the case of the proposed research project.

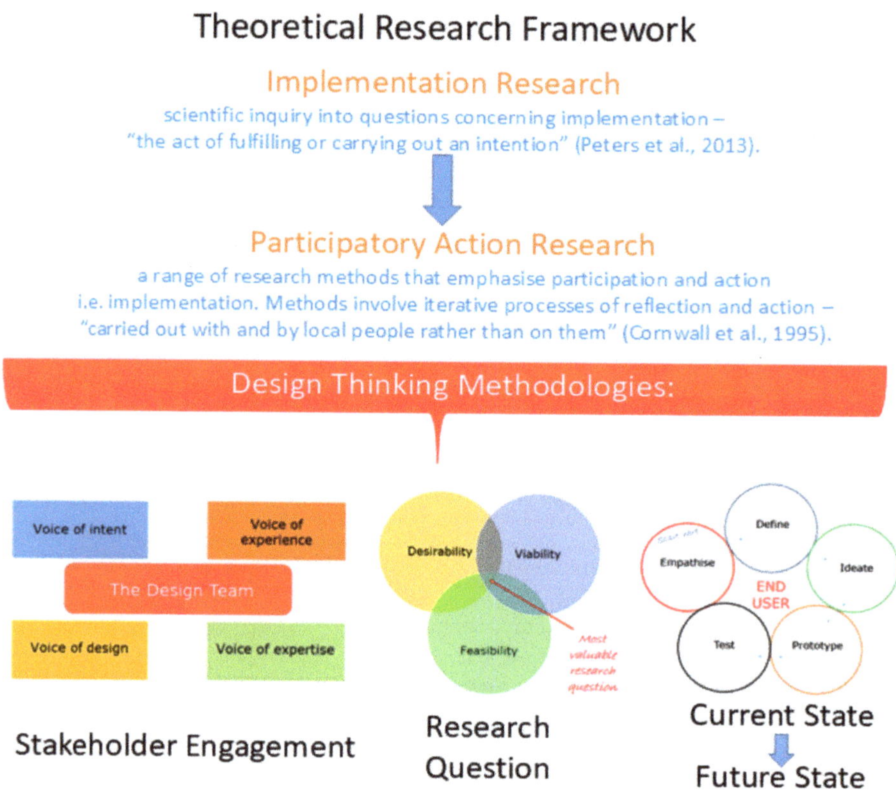
Theoretical Research Framework
Implementation Research
scientific inquiry into questions concerning implementation –
"the act of fulfilling or carrying out an intention" (Peters et al., 2013).
Participatory Action Research
a range of research methods that emphasise participation and action
i.e. implementation. Methods involve iterative processes of reflection and action –
"carried out with and by local people rather than on them" (Cornwall et al., 1995).
Design Thinking Methodologies:
Voice of intent
Voice of experience
The Design Team
Voice of design
Voice of expertise
Stakeholder Engagement
Desirability
Viability
Feasibility
Most valuable research question
Research Question
Define
Empathise
Ideate
END USER
Test
Prototype
Current State
Future State

Figure 8. Conceptual schematic of the CKD Co-Design Project. This figure illustrates how the project was underpinned by Design Thinking methodologies and situated within the broader context of Implementation and Participatory Action Research, described by Peters et al. [45] and Cornwall et al. [46]. The schematic represents the integration of practical actions (e.g., problem definition, ideation, prototyping, iteration) with theoretical frameworks, highlighting how these approaches merge to guide the co-design process.

Improvements to traditional qualitative research, which purports to be "co-designed", can be made through a commitment to applying the core principles of authentic Design Thinking. This means aiming to, firstly, conduct an intent meeting with end users and people who represent all four Design Voices at the start of a project to help clarify what the problem is and to define what the current state is, whilst pondering what the future state might look like. This helps to identify the gaps and gives some ideas about what changes might be necessary. It also helps to better define the problem statement and identify additional key stakeholders across the four Design Voices to ensure the best approach. It also means co-designing the research question rather than having researchers propose the question from the outset based on perceived gaps from previous literature or work.

Finally, it means to always maintain representation of all four Design Voices throughout the duration of the project to minimise bias. Challenges with these recommendations may be the greater initial time investment, for example, even before the research question is proposed. From an ethics perspective, there may be concerns that stakeholders are approached to help define the project intent and research question prior to the research being approved by an ethics committee. Delineation between engagement prior to "official" research commencing may be required. Finally, because cycles of iteration are a core part of the design thinking process, research protocol changes may be more frequent, and this could have implications for ethics committees that require reporting and approval of any amendments. The precise nature of the expected "looping" and potential iterations should therefore be stated within original ethics applications to mitigate this. Increasingly, advocacy for authentic co-design is growing to empower both researchers and participants, service providers and service users, policy makers and community members [47].

Limitations

While the design-led approach offers valuable opportunities to co-create meaningful health solutions, several limitations should be acknowledged. First, authentic co-design requires extensive stakeholder engagement across the four Design Voices. This can be resource- and time-intensive, often demanding substantial coordination before a formal research protocol is approved. Such requirements may not be feasible in all health research contexts, particularly where funding, staffing, or timelines are constrained. Second, the iterative and cyclical nature of Design Thinking can pose challenges for ethics approval processes, since frequent refinements to protocols and outputs may necessitate multiple amendments. This tension between the flexibility of Design Thinking and the rigidity of institutional governance frameworks can limit methodological agility. Third, participation bias may arise. Stakeholders who are more motivated, available, or vocal may be overrepresented, while harder-to-reach groups (e.g., people with advanced disease, carers with limited availability, or marginalised communities) may have less influence in shaping outcomes. This could inadvertently undermine the equity aims of co-design. Finally, translating co-designed ideas into sustainable health service change remains a challenge. Even when solutions are desirable and feasible, systemic constraints, such as workforce shortages, siloed care structures, and limited resources, may hinder their implementation at scale. Future research should therefore explore mechanisms to embed co-designed outputs into policy and service redesign in a sustainable manner.

5. Conclusions

This paper describes how a commitment to key principles of Design Thinking can more authentically achieve co-designed research outcomes, aiming to explore a complex health problem in the community. Using the case study of high CKD rates in the Illawarra and Shoalhaven regions of Australia, we showcased a design-led methodological approach that ensures end-users remain at the centre of all research throughout the project's lifespan, from the conception of the research question and protocol to solution generation and change implementation. Representation of the four Design Voices with appropriate stakeholders throughout the research project is imperative to minimise bias towards researchers as the main research orchestrators. This paper showed that empathising through direct interaction with users is crucial to making sense and creating meaning of users' problems and their challenges. Ideation ensures user-centred solution generation, which is likely to be closer to addressing the real problem and creating an improved future state. The future planned prototyping/testing phases for this project will offer further validation of the user-centred ideas and solutions. Through this case study, we encourage the incorporation of Design

Thinking principles for solution generation in health research as a valuable adjunct to traditional qualitative research methodologies, with the potential to facilitate meaningful outcomes for people in our community experiencing a wicked health problem anywhere in the world.

Supplementary Materials: The following supporting information can be downloaded at: https://www.mdpi.com/article/10.3390/ijerph22101475/s1. File S1: Workshop findings Report for participants.

Author Contributions: Conceptualization, A.S.-N., K.F., J.N., and K.L.; formal analysis, K.F., J.N., A.S.-N., and K.L.; data curation, K.F., A.S.-N., and J.N.; writing—original draft preparation, A.S.-N.; writing—review and editing, A.S.-N., J.N., K.C., K.F., and K.L.; funding acquisition, K.C. All authors have read and agreed to the published version of the manuscript.

Funding: This research was funded by the Health Impacts Research Cluster at the University of Wollongong.

Institutional Review Board Statement: Approved by the University of Wollongong Human Research Ethics Committee (Approval number HE2018/348, on 11 September 2018).

Informed Consent Statement: Informed consent was obtained from all subjects involved in the study.

Data Availability Statement: Data available on reasonable request.

Conflicts of Interest: The authors declare no conflicts of interest.

References

1. Australian Bureau of Statistics. Health Conditions Prevalence, 2020–2021. Available online: https://www.abs.gov.au/statistics/health/health-conditions-and-risks/health-conditions-prevalence/ (accessed on 29 April 2025).
2. Hassan, H.I.C.; Lambert, K.; Moules, S.; Mcalister, B.J.; Murali, K. Mapping CKD Prevalence Burden in a Reportedly High Australian Health District Region: TH-PO1009. *J. Am. Soc. Nephrol.* **2023**, *34*, 373–374. [CrossRef]
3. Rouse, W.B.; Cody, W.R.; Boff, K.R. The human factors of system design: Understanding and enhancing the role of human factors engineering. *Int. J. Hum. Factors Manuf.* **1991**, *1*, 87–104. [CrossRef]
4. Brown, T. Design thinking. *Harv. Bus. Rev.* **2008**, *86*, 84.
5. Carmel-Gilfilen, C.; Portillo, M. Designing With Empathy: Humanizing Narratives for Inspired Healthcare Experiences. *HERD Health Environ. Res. Des. J.* **2015**, *9*, 130–146. [CrossRef]
6. Chasanidou, D.; Gasparini, A.A.; Lee, E. Design Thinking Methods and Tools for Innovation. In *Design, User Experience, and Usability: Design Discourse*; Lecture Notes in Computer Science; Marcus, A., Ed.; Springer: Cham, Switzerland, 2015; Volume 9186. [CrossRef]
7. Brown, T. Design Thinking Defined. Available online: https://designthinking.ideo.com/ (accessed on 29 April 2025).
8. Roberts, J.P.; Fisher, T.R.; Trowbridge, M.J.; Bent, C. A design thinking framework for healthcare management and innovation. *Healthcare* **2016**, *4*, 11–14. [CrossRef] [PubMed]
9. Searl, M.M.; Borgi, L.; Chemali, Z. It is time to talk about people: A human-centered healthcare system. *Health Res. Policy Syst.* **2010**, *8*, 35. [CrossRef]
10. Devecchi, A.; Guerrini, L. Empathy and Design. A new perspective. *Des. J.* **2017**, *20*, S4357–S4364. [CrossRef]
11. ThinkPlace Global. Available online: https://www.thinkplace.com.au/ (accessed on 29 April 2025).
12. Floyd, I.R.; Cameron Jones, M.; Twidale, M.B. Resolving Incommensurable Debates: A Preliminary Identification of Persona Kinds, Attributes, and Characteristics. *Artifact* **2008**, *2*, 12–26. [CrossRef]
13. Holden, R.J.; Kulanthaivel, A.; Purkayastha, S.; Goggins, K.M.; Kripalani, S. Know thy eHealth user: Development of biopsychosocial personas from a study of older adults with heart failure. *Int. J. Med. Inform.* **2017**, *108*, 158–167. [CrossRef]
14. Pruitt, J.; Adlin, T. *The Persona Lifecycle: Keeping People in Mind Throughout Product Design*; Elsevier: Amsterdam, The Netherlands, 2010.
15. Stefoska-Needham, A.; Fildes, K.; Atkinson, J.; Nealon, J.; Charton, K.; Gutker, M.; Lambert, K.; Anna, L.; Smyth, M.; Walton, K. SUN-247 Experiencing chronic kidney disease: Perspectives of individuals living with chronic kidney disease, their family members, carers and health professionals. *Kidney Int. Rep.* **2019**, *4*, S262. [CrossRef]
16. Stickdorn, M.; Hormess, M.E.; Lawrence, A.; Schneider, J. *This Is Service Design Doing: Applying Service Design Thinking in the Real World*; O'Reilly Media, Inc.: Sevastopol, CA, USA, 2018.
17. Buchanan, R. Wicked problems in design thinking. *Des. Issues* **1992**, *8*, 5–21. [CrossRef]

18. Binder, T.; Brandt, E.; Gregory, J. Design participation(-s)—A creative commons for ongoing change. *CoDesign* **2008**, *4*, 79–83. [CrossRef]
19. Altman, M.; Huang, T.T.; Breland, J.Y. Design thinking in health care. *Prev. Chronic Dis.* **2018**, *15*, E117. [CrossRef] [PubMed]
20. Donetto, S.; Tsianakas, V.; Robert, G. *Using Experience-Based Co-Design (EBCD) to Improve the Quality of Healthcare: Mapping Where We Are Now and Establishing Future Directions*; King's College London: London, UK, 2014; pp. 5–7. Available online: https://www.semanticscholar.org/paper/Using-Experience-based-Co-design-(EBCD)-to-improve-Donetto-Tsianakas/259c2ebc8e3e39c42c4a1ac50df8ccd2f1e04994 (accessed on 29 April 2025).
21. Lo, C.; Zimbudzi, E.; Teede, H.; Cass, A.; Fulcher, G.; Gallagher, M.; Kerr, P.G.; Jan, S.; Johnson, G.; Mathew, T. Models of care for co-morbid diabetes and chronic kidney disease. *Nephrology* **2018**, *23*, 711–717. [CrossRef]
22. Robert, G.; Cornwell, J.; Locock, L.; Purushotham, A.; Sturmey, G.; Gager, M. Patients and staff as codesigners of healthcare services. *BMJ* **2015**, *350*, g7714. [CrossRef]
23. Levey, A.S.; de Jong, P.E.; Coresh, J.; El Nahas, M.; Astor, B.C.; Matsushita, K.; Gansevoort, R.T.; Kasiske, B.L.; Eckardt, K.U. The definition, classification, and prognosis of chronic kidney disease: A KDIGO Controversies Conference report. *Kidney Int.* **2011**, *80*, 17–28. [CrossRef]
24. Tonelli, M.; Wiebe, N.; Guthrie, B.; James, M.T.; Quan, H.; Fortin, M.; Klarenbach, S.W.; Sargious, P.; Straus, S.; Lewanczuk, R.; et al. Comorbidity as a driver of adverse outcomes in people with chronic kidney disease. *Kidney Int.* **2015**, *88*, 859–866. [CrossRef]
25. Palmer, S.; Vecchio, M.; Craig, J.C.; Tonelli, M.; Johnson, D.W.; Nicolucci, A.; Pellegrini, F.; Saglimbene, V.; Logroscino, G.; Fishbane, S. Prevalence of depression in chronic kidney disease: Systematic review and meta-analysis of observational studies. *Kidney Int.* **2013**, *84*, 179–191. [CrossRef] [PubMed]
26. Sullivan, M.K.; Rankin, A.J.; Jani, B.D.; Mair, F.S.; Mark, P.B. Associations between multimorbidity and adverse clinical outcomes in patients with chronic kidney disease: A systematic review and meta-analysis. *BMJ Open* **2020**, *10*, e038401. [CrossRef] [PubMed]
27. Australian Commission on Safety and Quality in Health Care. Patient Centred Care: Improving Quality and Safety Through Partnerships with Patients and Consumers. Available online: https://www.safetyandquality.gov.au/publications-and-resources/resource-library/patient-centred-care-improving-quality-and-safety-through-partnerships-patients-and-consumers (accessed on 29 April 2025).
28. Hill, C.J.; Cardwell, C.R.; Patterson, C.C.; Maxwell, A.P.; Magee, G.M.; Young, R.J.; Matthews, B.; O'Donoghue, D.J.; Fogarty, D.G. Chronic kidney disease and diabetes in the national health service: A cross-sectional survey of the U.K. national diabetes audit. *Diabet. Med.* **2014**, *31*, 448–454. [CrossRef]
29. Lenz, O.; Mekala, D.P.; Patel, D.V.; Fornoni, A.; Metz, D.; Roth, D. Barriers to successful care for chronic kidney disease. *BMC Nephrol.* **2005**, *6*, 11. [CrossRef]
30. Hibbard, J.H.; Mahoney, E.R.; Stockard, J.; Tusler, M. Development and testing of a short form of the patient activation measure. *Health Serv. Res.* **2005**, *40*, 1918–1930. [CrossRef]
31. Lo, C.; Teede, H.; Ilic, D.; Russell, G.; Murphy, K.; Usherwood, T.; Ranasinha, S.; Zoungas, S. Identifying health service barriers in the management of co-morbid diabetes and chronic kidney disease in primary care: A mixed-methods exploration. *Fam. Pract.* **2016**, *33*, 492–497. [CrossRef]
32. Zimbudzi, E.; Lo, C.; Ranasinha, S.; Gallagher, M.; Fulcher, G.; Kerr, P.G.; Russell, G.; Teede, H.; Usherwood, T.; Walker, R.; et al. Predictors of Health-Related Quality of Life in Patients with Co-Morbid Diabetes and Chronic Kidney Disease. *PLoS ONE* **2016**, *11*, e0168491. [CrossRef] [PubMed]
33. Nicoll, R.; Robertson, L.; Gemmell, E.; Sharma, P.; Black, C.; Marks, A. Models of care for chronic kidney disease: A systematic review. *Nephrology* **2018**, *23*, 389–396. [CrossRef] [PubMed]
34. Thanachayanont, T.; Chanpitakkul, M.; Hengtrakulvenit, J.; Watcharakanon, P.; Wisansak, W.; Tancharoensukjit, T.; Kaewsringam, P.; Leesmidt, V.; Pongpirul, K.; Lekagul, S.; et al. Effectiveness of integrated care on delaying chronic kidney disease progression in rural communities of Thailand (ESCORT-2) trials. *Nephrology* **2021**, *26*, 333–340. [CrossRef] [PubMed]
35. Yang, F.J.; Hou, Y.H.; Chang, R.E. The Impact of a Social Networking Service-Enhanced Smart Care Model on Stage 5 Chronic Kidney Disease: Quasi-Experimental Study. *J. Med. Internet Res.* **2020**, *22*, e15565. [CrossRef]
36. Fildes, K.; Stefoska-Needham, A.; Atkinson, J.; Lambert, K.; Lee, A.; Pugh, D.; Smyth, M.; Turner, R.; Wallace, S.; Nealon, J. Optimising health care for people living with chronic kidney disease: Health-professional perspectives. *J. Ren. Care* **2022**, *48*, 168–176. [CrossRef]
37. Neale, E.P.; Middleton, J.; Lambert, K. Barriers and enablers to detection and management of chronic kidney disease in primary healthcare: A systematic review. *BMC Nephrol.* **2020**, *21*, 83. [CrossRef]
38. NSW Government Agency for Clinical Innovation. Patient Experience and Consumer Engagement: A Framework for Action. Available online: https://aci.health.nsw.gov.au/__data/assets/pdf_file/0013/502240/Guide-Build-Codesign-Capability.pdf (accessed on 29 April 2025).

39. Fildes, K.; Nealon, J.; Charlton, K.; Lambert, K.; Lee, A.; Pugh, D.; Smyth, M.; Stefoska-Needham, A. Collaborative codesign: Unveiling concerns and crafting solutions for healthcare with health professionals, carers and consumers with chronic kidney disease. *Kidney Dial.* **2025**, *5*, 22. [CrossRef]
40. van Rijnsoever, F.J. (I Can't Get No) Saturation: A simulation and guidelines for sample sizes in qualitative research. *PLoS ONE* **2017**, *12*, e0181689. [CrossRef]
41. Rudman, H.; Bailey-Ross, C.; Kendal, J.; Mursic, Z.; Lloyd, A.; Ross, B.; Kendal, R.L. Multidisciplinary exhibit design in a Science Centre: A participatory action research approach. *Educ. Action Res.* **2018**, *26*, 567–588. [CrossRef]
42. Braun, V.; Clarke, V. Using thematic analysis in psychology. *Qual. Res. Psychol.* **2006**, *3*, 77–101. [CrossRef]
43. Castleberry, A.; Nolen, A. Thematic analysis of qualitative research data: Is it as easy as it sounds? *Curr. Pharm. Teach. Learn.* **2018**, *10*, 807–815. [CrossRef] [PubMed]
44. Braun, V.; Clarke, V. Conceptual and design thinking for thematic analysis. *Qual. Psychol.* **2022**, *9*, 3–26. [CrossRef]
45. Peters, D.H.; Adam, T.; Alonge, O.; Agyepong, I.A.; Tran, N. Implementation research: What it is and how to do it. *BMJ* **2013**, *347*, f6753. [CrossRef] [PubMed]
46. Cornwall, A.; Jewkes, R. What is participatory research? *Soc. Sci. Med.* **1995**, *41*, 1667–1676. [CrossRef]
47. Donetto, S.; Pierri, P.; Tsianakas, V.; Robert, G. Experience-based co-design and healthcare improvement: Realizing participatory design in the public sector. *Des. J.* **2015**, *18*, 227–248. [CrossRef]

International Journal of
Environmental Research and Public Health

MDPI

Article

Impact of Combined Hypertension and Diabetes on the Prevalence of Disability in Brazilian Older People—Evidence from Population Studies in 2013 and 2019

Rafaela Gonçalves Ribeiro-Lucas [1], Barbara Niegia Garcia de Goulart [2,*] and Patricia Klarmann Ziegelmann [1,2]

1 Postgraduate Program in Cardiology and Cardiovascular Sciences, Universidade Federal do Rio Grande do Sul (UFRGS), Porto Alegre 90610-264, Brazil; rafaelaglribeiro@gmail.com (R.G.R.-L.); patricia.ziegelmann@ufrgs.br (P.K.Z.)

2 Postgraduate Program in Epidemiology, Universidade Federal do Rio Grande do Sul (UFRGS), Porto Alegre 90035-003, Brazil

* Correspondence: bngoulart@gmail.com

Abstract

Disability in basic and instrumental activities of daily living (BADL and IADL) reflects functional decline in older adults and can be associated with chronic conditions like type 2 diabetes (T2DM) and hypertension (SAH). This cross-sectional study utilized data from the 2013 and 2019 Brazilian National Health Surveys to investigate the associations between T2DM, SAH, and disability levels. Exposures were self-reported diagnoses and outcomes were classified as independent, moderate, or severe. Multivariable Poisson regression models, with robust variance estimates, estimated adjusted prevalence ratios (PRa), accounting for sociodemographic variables and the survey design. In 2013, the absence of diabetes and hypertension was associated with a lower prevalence (PRa = 0.70; 95% CI: 0.58–0.85) of moderate disability in BADL when compared with the presence of only one of the conditions. On the other hand, the coexistence of T2DM and SAH was associated with a higher prevalence (PRa = 1.39; 95% CI: 1.01–1.91). A similar result was found in 2019 with the addition that coexistence was also associated with a higher prevalence of severe disability in BADLs (PRa = 1.82; 95% CI: 1.59–2.07). For IADL, the absence of T2DM and SAH was associated with a lower prevalence of severe disability in 2013 and 2019 and a lower prevalence of moderate disability only in 2019. However, coexistence showed a higher prevalence in both degrees of disability and both years of the survey. These findings highlight the impact of T2DM and SAH on disability in older people. Therefore, it is crucial to develop targeted strategies for vulnerable subgroups to enhance functional independence in aging populations.

Keywords: aged; chronic disease; disability studies

1. Introduction

Chronic noncommunicable diseases (NCDs), such as type 2 diabetes mellitus (T2DM) and systemic arterial hypertension (SAH), represent a major challenge to global public health. According to the Global Burden of Disease (GBD) study, these conditions are among the leading causes of morbidity and mortality worldwide. SAH is the foremost risk factor for cardiovascular diseases, contributing substantially to global mortality and disability-adjusted life years (DALYs) [1]. T2DM also ranks among the primary conditions associated with high rates of mortality and disability [2]. Both T2DM and SAH are key risk factors for cardiovascular diseases, which remain the leading cause of death in Brazil [3]. This global scenario places a significant burden on healthcare systems, increasing the demand for outpatient care, pharmacological treatment, and hospitalization [4].

According to the Brazilian National Health Survey (2019 PNS), the prevalence of SAH increased with age, reaching 56.6% among people aged 65 to 74 and 62.1% among those aged 75 or over [5]. Likewise, the prevalence of T2DM was 21.9% for people aged 65 to 74. For those aged 75 or over, the percentage was 21.1% [5]. In Brazil, the impact of aging on functionality is significant, as approximately 9.5% (or 3.3 million) of people aged 60 or over reported functional limitations in performing activities of daily living [6]. The mechanisms underlying the relationship between SAH, T2DM, and disability involve several pathophysiological factors that increase cardiovascular events and mortality [7]. In the case of diabetes, disability can be attributed to chronic inflammation and its micro- and macrovascular complications, such as neuropathy, peripheral vascular disease, retinopathy, and stroke, which directly compromise the mobility and functionality of individuals [8].

In a systematic review with meta-analysis, which aimed to estimate the magnitude of the association between diabetes/prediabetes and disability in adults, it was found that diabetes was associated with a high prevalence of both basic activities of daily living (BADL) disability (OR = 1.82; 95% CI 1.63–2.04) and instrumental activities of daily living (IADL) disability (OR = 1.65; 95% CI 1.55–1.74) [9]. On the other hand, a representative population study of the elderly Chinese population with SAH shows that the prevalence of disability for BADL or IADL was observed to increase proportionally with the increase in the number of comorbidities (OR = 1.76; 95% CI 1.321–2.367 for one comorbidity and OR = 3.66; 95% CI 2.819–4.763 for two comorbidities) [10].

Reis-Júnior and collaborators (2024), using data from the Brazilian National Health Surveys (2013 PNS), found that the prevalence of BADL disability is higher among the elderly (>=60 years) with SAH when compared to those without (PR = 1.60; 95% CI 1.43–1.79), as well as there being a greater prevalence of IADL disability (PR = 1.41; 95% CI 1.28–1.54) [11]. However, to date, we have not found studies evaluating the specific concomitant combination of hypertension and diabetes associated with functional disability, leaving it unclear how this combination affects the functional capacity. Thus, this study aimed to evaluate whether the combination of diabetes and hypertension is a factor associated with BADL and IADL disabilities in the population of non-institutionalized older Brazilians, using data from two representative surveys of the Brazilian population (2013 and 2019 PNS).

2. Materials and Methods

This study is based on data from the Brazilian National Health Survey (PNS) collected in 2013 and 2019. The PNS is an epidemiological surveillance initiative designed to monitor the health of the Brazilian population. This is a cross-sectional household survey study with complex sampling, conducted by the Oswaldo Cruz Foundation (Fiocruz, Rio de Janeiro, Brazil), the Brazilian Institute of Geography and Statistics (IBGE, Rio de Janeiro, Brazil), and the Ministry of Health (MS, Brasília, Brazil). The complex probabilistic cluster sampling plan with three stages ensures the national and regional representativeness of the survey [12].

Both editions of the PNS survey maintained a similar sampling design. To ensure comparability, the sample weights from 2013 were recalculated using updated population projections by sex and age, released by the IBGE in 2018. Small changes were made, including adjustments to household sample sizes and an expansion of the minimum age range for individual interviews [5]. The PNS questionnaire was divided into three parts in both editions: the first collects information about the household; the second gathers data on all household residents; and the third addresses individual questions from a randomly selected resident. Changes have been made to some questions and/or response categories. The data collection in both surveys was carried out using mobile devices. Additionally, the PNS questionnaire underwent cognitive test evaluations and a pilot study. Also, they were duly reviewed and approved by the National Research Ethics Committee (CONEP/CNS), as per opinions No. 328.159 issued on 8 July 2013 and No. 3.529.376 on 23 August 2019 [13]. All participants signed informed consent forms in two copies. More details about the PNS methodology are described in specific articles [12–15].

For this study, we included data from elderly individuals aged 60 or over who responded to the third part of the questionnaire in both editions of the PNS. Participants who did not answer the question about a self-reported medical diagnosis of T2DM and SAH were excluded from the analysis. All data used were anonymized and publicly available. Therefore, according to the National Health Council Resolution 466/12, this study does not require Ethics Committee approval. This manuscript will be reported based on the STROBE Statement for cross-sectional studies [16].

The exposure of interest is the self-reported medical diagnosis of T2DM and SAH. The variable created has three categories: only T2DM or SAH, both, or neither. This study focused on two main outcomes: Basic Activities of Daily Living (BADL) and Instrumental Activities of Daily Living (IADL) disabilities. For the BADL assessment, individuals were queried on their ability to perform tasks such as eating, bathing, using the toilet, dressing, walking between rooms, lying down, and sitting alone. Responses ranged from "No difficulty" to "Unable", categorized into binary variables (0 for no difficulty, 1 for any degree of difficulty). A BADL score was derived by summing these variables, and then the subjects were categorized as independent (6 points), moderate (3–5 points), or severe (0–2 points). To align with the original scale, a "transfer" variable was created by combining "lying down" and "sitting" responses.

For the IADL assessment, individuals were asked about managing tasks such as shopping, managing finances, taking medication, attending medical appointments, and using transportation alone. An IADL score was similarly created with cut-offs of independent (5 points), moderate (3–4 points), or severe (0–2 points). Notably, these scales were adapted from the Katz scale [17], modified in the PNS to assess difficulty rather than dependence.

Further modifications included the adaptation of the IADL question regarding medication management between the 2013 and 2019 PNS surveys, addressing swallowing, scheduling, and remembering medication. NA values were considered "no difficulty", following consultations with aging specialists and the Ministry of Health's technical area on Elderly Health.

The response categories of the Katz and Lawton scales [17] were aligned with the Washington Group Short Set on Functioning (WG-SS), designed to standardize functional limitation assessments globally. This framework, beginning with "Do you have difficulty in...", offers four response options: no difficulty, some difficulty, a lot of difficulty, and cannot do at all. This standardization supports international and longitudinal comparisons, vital for monitoring health disparities [18].

The classification of functional disability levels (independent, moderate dependency, and severe dependency) was based on the Medication and Quality of Life in Frail Older Persons (MedQoL) Research Group's methodology, which established cut-off points through a systematic review and expert panel consensus [19]

Based on the specialized literature on the subject [20–22], the following variables were chosen for the adjusted analyses: sex, age group (60–69, 70–79, 80–89, and 90+), region of the country, marital status, education level, and ethnicity. Appendix A presents the operational definitions of those variables at the baseline, as well as the new categorizations

(Table A1), along with the adherence of this study to the STROBE criteria (Table A2) and with the raw data (Tables A3–A6).

Data were described using absolute and relative frequencies. Prevalence was estimated using binomial and multinomial models. The contribution of TDM2 and SAH to disability was analyzed separately for BADL and IADL. The association between the exposure factor and each disability was assessed using the adjusted Poisson regression model with a robust estimation of the variance. The prevalence and prevalence ratios were weighted according to the complex sample plan of the PNS. Data importation, variable manipulation, data frame creation, statistical analyses, and data visualization were performed using R software, version R-4.4.2, and RStudio version 2024.12.0+467, utilizing the Comprehensive R Archive Network (CRAN) repository packages: readr, ggplot2, PNSIBGE, dplyr, tidyr, crosstable, survey, foreign, lmtest, sandwich, multcomp, and geobr.

3. Results

3.1. Sample Description

For the PNS 2013 analysis, individuals aged 18 years or older were included, totaling 60,202 respondents who answered the third individual questionnaire. After filtering the data to include only elderly individuals aged 60 years or older, 11,177 participants were identified and were considered to estimate the prevalence. Excluding individuals without answers to T2DM or SAH, 10,537 were considered for the association analysis. In the 2019 PNS edition, those numbers were 94,114; 22,728; and 21,968 (Figure 1).

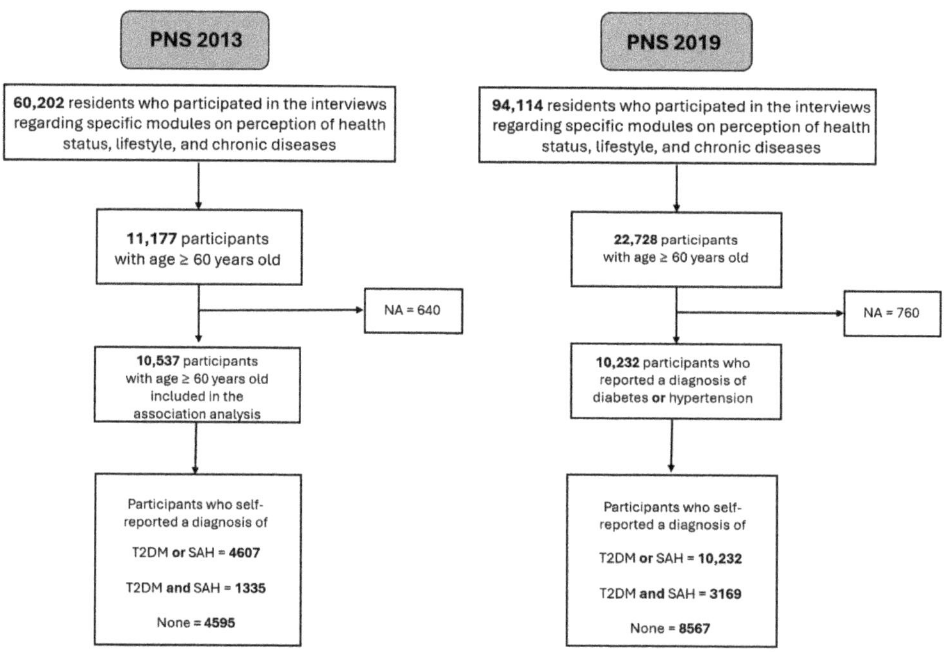

Figure 1. Flowchart of study participants, Brazilian National Health Survey, 2013 and 2019.

3.2. Brazilian National Health Survey (2013 PNS) Sample Description

The sample was composed mostly of females (pw = 56.4%) who were black (pw = 44.8%), without a partner (pw = 46.5%), with elementary school as a minimum level of education (pw = 70.7%), a resident of an urban region (pw = 85.2%), and with a mean age of 69 years (SD 7.88). Among the participants, 4607 were diagnosed with hypertension or diabetes (pw 44.3%), 1335 with both conditions (pw = 13.6%), and 4595 (pw = 42.1%) without any of these diseases. Regarding BALD functionality, 9424 were independent (they had no difficulty performing activities), 1197 had moderate disability, and 556 had severe disability. In contrast, in the IADL, 7893 were independent (they had no difficulty performing activities), 1540 had moderate disability, and 1744 had severe disability (Table 1).

Table 1. Prevalence of moderate and severe dependence in basic activities of daily living (BADLs) and instrumental activities of daily living (IADLs) according to sociodemographic characteristics in Brazilian older adults who participated in the Brazilian National Health Survey (2013 PNS).

	2013 PNS						
	BALD				IADL		
Variable	**Total Population**	**Independent**	**Moderate**	**Severe**	**Independent**	**Moderate**	**Severe**
	n = 11,177	**n = 9424**	**n = 1197**	**n = 556**	**n = 7893**	**n = 1540**	**n = 1744**
Chronic Disease							
Diabetes or Hypertension	4607 (44.3)	3794 (43.6)	567 (48.1)	246 (47.7)	3091 (42.9)	677 (46.8)	839 (48.5)
Both	1335 (13.6)	1021 (12.2)	208 (20.6)	106 (21.6)	786 (15.7)	242 (15.7)	307 (18.8)
None	4595 (42.1)	4055 (44.2)	366 (31.3)	174 (30.6)	3543 (18.8)	536 (37.4)	516 (32.7)
NA	640	554	56	30	473	85	82
Age							
60–69	6238 (56.6)	5590 (60.2)	512 (44.0)	136 (22.5)	5148 (66.2)	618 (39.5)	472 (25.6)
70–79	3441 (29.8)	2859 (29.3)	391 (32.2)	191 (34.3)	2220 (27.0)	631 (40.4)	590 (34.2)
80–89	1293 (11.6)	877 (9.2)	243 (19.6)	173 (32.9)	494 (6.3)	261 (17.9)	538 (30.8)
90+	205 (2.0)	98 (1.3)	51 (4.2)	56 (10.3)	31 (0.5)	30 (2.2)	144 (9.4)
Sex							
Female	6622 (56.4)	5508 (55.7)	754 (57.9)	360 (63.6)	4421 (53.8)	993 (59.0)	1208 (66.3)
Male	4555 (43.6)	3916 (44.3)	443 (42.1)	196 (36.4)	3472 (46.2)	574 (41.0)	536 (33.7)
Race							
White	5314 (53.8)	4477 (53.9)	569 (53.3)	268 (52.0)	3816 (54.5)	696 (53.4)	802 (50.5)
Black	5701 (44.8)	4807 (44.5)	615 (46.2)	279 (47.1)	3957 (43.8)	822 (45.5)	822 (48.7)
Others	160 (1.4)	139 (1.6)	12 (0.5)	9 (1.0)	119 (1.7)	21 (1.1)	20 (0.7)
NA	0	0	0	0	1	1	0
Marital Status							
With partner	4808 (53.5)	4207 (55.4)	444 (48.9)	753 (32.7)	3725 (58.0)	553 (45.6)	350 (39.0)
Without partner	6369 (46.5)	5217 (44.6)	157 (51.1)	399 (67.3)	4168 (42.0)	987 (54.4)	1214 (61.0)
Education level							
Until elementary school	7738 (70.7)	6337 (68.4)	953 (82.2)	448 (84.2)	4997 (64.6)	1,26 (84.4)	1481 (87.3)
High school or more	3439 (29.3)	3087 (31.6)	244 (17.8)	108 (84.2)	2896 (35.4)	280 (15.6)	263 (12.7)
Region							
Urban	8999 (085.2)	7575 (85.5)	953 (81.2)	471 (87.3)	6401 (86.2)	1211 (82.8)	1387 (82.5)
Rural	2178 (14.8)	1849 (14.5)	244 (18.8)	85 (12.7)	1492 (13.8)	329 (17.2)	357 (82.5)

NA = not applicable; Source: Brazilian National Health Survey, 2013.

3.3. Brazilian National Health Survey (PNS 2019) Sample Description

The 2019 sample shows similar characteristics: the majority was female (pw = 56.7%), black (pw = 47.7%), without a partner (pw = 49.3%), with elementary school as the level of education (pw = 63.3%), residents of an urban region (pw = 85.5%), and with a mean age of 70 years (SD 7.85) (Table 2). Among the participants, 10,232 were diagnosed with hypertension or diabetes (47.5%), 3169 with both conditions (15.2%), and 8567 (37.3%) without any of these diseases. About BALD functionality, 18,141 were independent (they had no difficulty performing activities), 3040 had moderate disability, and 1547 had severe disability. On the other hand, for the IADL, 2967 were independent (they had no difficulty performing activities), 14,354 had moderate disability, and 5407 had severe disability.

Table 2. Prevalence of moderate and severe dependence in basic activities of daily living (BADL) and instrumental activities of daily living (IADL) according to sociodemographic characteristics in Brazilian older adults who participated in the Brazilian National Health Survey (2019 PNS).

Variable	2019 PNS						
	BALD				IADL		
	Total Population	Independent	Moderate	Severe	Independent	Moderate	Severe
	n = 22,728	n = 18,141	n = 3040	n = 1547	n = 2967	n = 14,354	n = 5407
Chronic Disease							
Diabetes or Hypertension	10,232 (47.5)	8053 (47.0)	1470 (51.4)	709 (45.0)	326 (13.0)	7193 (52.1)	2713 (51.5)
Both	3169 (15.2)	2176 (13.3)	628 (20.8)	365 (26.2)	37 (1.2)	1988 (15.3)	1144 (21.8)
None	8567 (37.3)	7283 (39.7)	853 (27.7)	431 (28.8)	2324 (85.8)	4827 (32.6)	1416 (26.7)
NA	760	629	89	42	280	346	134
Age							
60–69	12,555 (56.3)	10,756 (60.7)	1345 (44.9)	454 (28.7)	2154 (74.0)	8788 (62.6)	1613 (29.7)
70–79	7157 (30.1)	5584 (29.3)	1091 (35.2)	482 (29.5)	692 (21.8)	4469 (30.0)	1996(34.8)
80–89	2580 (11.5)	1652 (9.2)	508 (16.8)	420 (27.2)	115 (3.9)	1036 (7.1)	1429 (27.6)
90+	436 (2.1)	149 (0.8)	96 (3.1)	191 (14.6)	6 (0.3)	61 (0.3)	369 (7.9)
Sex							
Female	12,535 (56.7)	9654 (54.6)	1918 (64.5)	963 (64.6)	9654 (54.6)	1918 (64.5)	963 (64.6)
Male	10,193 (43.3)	8487 (45.4)	1122 (35.5)	584 (35.4)	8487 (45.4)	1122 (35.5)	584 (35.4)
Race							
White	9901 (50.5)	7948 (50.9)	1287 (48.0)	666 (50.7)	1155 (48.5)	6544 (52.0)	2202 (47.5)
Black	12,456 (47.7)	9890 (47.1)	1709 (50.9)	857 (47.6)	1755 (49.2)	7562 (46.1)	3139 (51.1)
Others	369 (1.8)	301 (1.9)	44 (1.2)	24 (1.7)	56 (2.2)	247 (1.9)	66 (1.3)
NA	2	0	0	0	1	1	0
Marital Status							
With partner	9946 (50.7)	8221 (52.6)	1233 (45.8)	492 (37.5)	1433 (55.4)	6726 (54.3)	1787 (38.2)
Without partner	12,782 (49.3)	9920 (47.4)	1807 (54.2)	1055 (62.5)	1534 (44.6)	7628 (45.7)	3620 (61.8)
Education level							
Until elementary school	14,987 (63.3)	11,445 (59.6)	2307 (76.5)	1235 (79.1)	1929 (58.6)	8612 (57.6)	4446 (81.4)
High school or more	7741 (36.7)	6696 (40.4)	733 (23.5)	312 (20.9)	1038 (41.4)	5742 (42.4)	961 (18.6)
Region							
Urban	17,313 (85.5)	13,750 (85.4)	2361 (86.2)	1202 (84.7)	2066 (81.6)	11,228 (87.3)	4019 (82.5)
Rural	5415 (14.5)	4391 (14.6)	679 (13.8)	345 (15.3)	901 (18.4)	3126 (12.7)	1388 (17.5)

NA = not applicable; Source: Brazilian National Health Survey, 2019.

3.4. Disability Prevalences

Figure 2 illustrates the spatial distribution by the state of the prevalence of BADL and IADL among older adults in Brazil for both 2013 and 2019. While disability in BADLs ranged from 15% to 25% (Figure 2, map A), disability in IADL presented a higher range, between 20% and 40% (Figure 2, map C).

Geographically, it is observed that the states with the highest disability prevalence of BADL also tend to have a high prevalence of IADL. As illustrated in maps A and B, disability in BADL ranged from 12% to 24%. In 2013, the state with the lowest prevalence was Rondônia, at 8.72%, and the state with the highest prevalence was Alagoas, at 24.01%.

In 2019, the state with the lowest prevalence of BALD disability was Amapá (13.38%) and the highest was Piauí (25.25%). In 2013, regarding the prevalence of disability in IADL, the lowest prevalence was observed in the southern region at 24.92%, followed by the southeast region at 25.64%, the midwest at 28.98%, the north at 31.46%, and the northeast at 34.93%. Likewise, in BALD, the state with the lowest prevalence was Rondônia, at 19.18%, and the state with the highest prevalence was Paraíba, at 42.04%. In 2019, the region with the lowest prevalence of IADL disability was the north, at 83.83%, followed by the midwest (87.26%), northeast (87.59%), southeast (88.33%), and south (89.40%). In 2019, the state with the lowest prevalence of IADL disability was Pará (80.32%) and the highest was Rio Grande do Sul (90.38%).

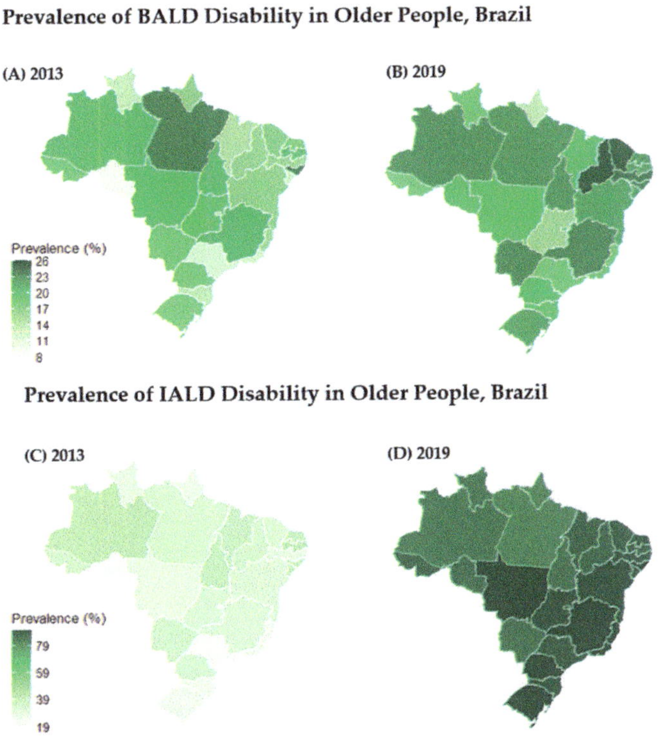

Figure 2. Map of the prevalence of BADL and IALD disability in older people in Brazil, according to data from the Brazilian National Health Survey, 2013 and 2019. Source: Brazilian National Health Survey, 2013 and 2019 | Graphics: Drawn by the authors.

3.5. Association Between T2DM/SAH and BADL/IADL

In 2013, the absence of diabetes and hypertension was associated with a lower prevalence (PRa = 0.70; 95% CI: 0.58–0.85) of moderate disability in BADL when compared with the presence of only one of the conditions (Table 3). On the other hand, the coexistence of T2DM and SAH was associated with a higher prevalence (PRa = 1.39; 95% CI: 1.01–1.91). A similar result was found in 2019 with the addition that coexistence was also associated with a higher prevalence of severe disability in BADL (PRa = 1.82; 95% CI: 1.59–2.07) (Table 3). For IADL, the absence of T2DM and SAH was associated with a lower prevalence of severe disability in 2013 (PRa = 0.79; 95% CI: 0.69–0.90) and 2019 (PRa = 0.77; 95% CI: 0.73–0.81) and a lower prevalence of moderate disability only in 2019 (PRa = 0.76; 95% CI: 0.75–0.77) (Table 4).

Table 3. Association between diabetes and hypertension with moderate and severe BALD disability adjusted for education, sex, marital status, region, and age in Brazilian older adults, Brazilian National Health Survey 2013 and 2019.

BALD	**2013 PNS**				**2019 PNS**			
Variables	**Moderate**		**Severe**		**Moderate**		**Severe**	
	PrAdj (CI 95%)	***p* Value**	**PrAdj (CI95%)**	***p* Value**	**PrAdj (CI 95%)**	***p* Value**	**PrAdj (CI95%)**	***p* Value**
Chronic Disease								
Only one	1		1		1		1	
Both	1.39 (1.01–1.91)	0.04	1.45 (0.85–2.47)	0.16	1.20 (1.07–1.36)	<0.001	1.82 (1.59–2.07)	<0.001
None	0.70 (0.58–0.85)	<0.001	0.79 (0.51–1.11)	0.15	0.75 (0.66–0.84)	<0.001	0.92 (0.82–1.04)	0.20

Table 3. *Cont.*

BALD	2013 PNS				2019 PNS			
Variables	Moderate PrAdj (CI 95%)	*p* Value	Severe PrAdj (CI95%)	*p* Value	Moderate PrAdj (CI 95%)	*p* Value	Severe PrAdj (CI95%)	*p* Value
Elementary vs. High school or more	1.64 (1.29–2.11)	<0.001	1.63 (1.15–4.02)	0.005	1.72 (1.56–1.91)	<0.001	1.52 (1.32–1.74)	<0.001
Female vs. Male	0.97 (0.80–1.18)	0.82	1.01 (0.65–1.56)	0.95	1.29 (1.19–1.40)	<0.001	1.08(0.95–1.24)	0.21
Not married vs. married	1.05 (0.85–1.30)	0.60	1.73(1.06–2.83)	0.02	1.00 (0.91–1.09)	0.94	1.27 (1.11–1.45)	<0.001
Urban vs. rural	0.77 (0.62–0.95)	0.01	1.11 (0.70–1.76)	0.63	1.15 (1.14–1.45)	0.01	0.96 (0.86–1.07)	0.54
Age (in years)								
60–69	1		1		1		1	
70–79	1.27 (1.03–1.57)	0.02	2.53 (1.59–4.02)	<0.001	1.28 (0.89–0.90)	<0.001	1.69 (1.46–1.96)	<0.001
80–89	1.99 (1.58–2.52)	<0.001	5.63 (3.36–9.43)	<0.001	1.58 (1.39–1.79)	<0.001	3.84 (3.26–4.53)	<0.001
90+	2.47 (1.78–3.43)	<0.001	10.41 (6.68–16.21)	<0.001	1.56 (1.22–1.99)	<0.001	11.1 (9.64–12.8)	<0.001

PrAdj: Adjusted Prevalence Ratio; 95% CI: 95% Confidence Interval; Source: Brazilian National Health Survey, 2013 and 2019.

Table 4. Adjusted analysis of the association between chronic diseases and moderate and severe dependence in Brazilian older adults in IADL, National Health Survey 2013 and 2019.

IADL	PNS 2013				PNS 2019			
Variables	Moderate PrAdj (95%CI)	*p* Value	Severe PrAdj (95%CI)	*p* Value	Moderate PrAdj (95%CI)	*p* Value	Severe PrAdj (95%CI)	*p* Value
Chronic Disease								
Only one	1	1	1	1	1	1	1	1
Both	1.03 (0.83–1.28)	0.73	1.23 (1.05–1.44)	0.008	0.92 (0.91–0.93)	<0.001	1.29 (1.23–1.34)	<0.001
None	0.89 (0.75–1.05)	0.18	0.79 (0.69–0.90)	0.006	0.76 (0.75–0.77)	<0.001	0.77 (0.73–0.81)	<0.001
Female vs. Male	0.97 (0.82–1.14)	0.71	1.32 (1.14–1.53)	<0.001	0.96 (0.95–0.97)	<0.001	1.34 (1.27–1.42)	<0.001
Urban vs. Rural	0.96 (0.79–1.16)	0.69	0.89 (0.79–1.00)	0.055	1.08 (1.07–1.10)	<0.001	0.87(0.84–0.90)	<0.001
Elementary vs. High school or more	2.00 (1.64–2.44)	<0.001	2.04 (1.77–2.37)	<0.001	0.85 (0.85–0.86)	<0.001	1.82 (1.71–1.94)	<0.001
Not married vs. married	1.32 (1.10–1.60)	0.003	1.22(1.06–1.41)	0.005	0.93 (0.92–0.94)	<0.001	1.19 (1.14–1.26)	<0.001
Black race	0.92 (0.79–1.08)	0.22	1.14 (1.00–1.29)	0.04	0.95 (0.94–0.96)	<0.001	1.06 (1.03–1.10)	<0.001
Other races	0.79 (0.54–0.1.15)	0.35	0.65 (0.45–0.92)	0.01	0.98 (0.94–1.01)	0.24	0.73 (0.58–0.98)	0.04
Age (in years)								
60–69	1		1		1		1	
70–79	1.71 (1.42–2.07)	<0.001	2.28 (1.91–2.72)	<0.001	0.90 (0.88–0.90)	<0.001	1.88 (1.76–2.00)	<0.001
80–89	1.88 (1.52–2.32)	<0.001	5.07 (4.33–5.94)	<0.001	0.57 (0.55–0.59)	<0.001	3.69 (3.47–3.92)	<0.001
90+	1.34 (0.75–2.39)	0.30	8.52 (7.36–9.87)	<0.001	0.12 (0.10–0.15)	<0.001	5.65 (5.32–6.00)	<0.001

PrAdj: Adjusted Prevalence Ratio; 95% CI: 95% Confidence Interval; Source: Brazilian National Health Survey, 2013 and 2019.

4. Discussion

Our findings demonstrate that the absence of diabetes and hypertension plays a protective role in preserving functional independence among older adults in Brazil. Compared to individuals with only one chronic disease (diabetes or hypertension), those without either condition consistently showed a lower prevalence of functional disability, especially in IADL. On the other hand, individuals with both diabetes and hypertension combined experienced higher prevalence rates of BADL disability, moderate in 2013 and severe in 2019, highlighting the burden of multimorbidity in this population. Furthermore, the spatial distribution of disability prevalence reveals a consistent pattern of geographic disparity, particularly in the north and northeast regions of Brazil. These regions not only exhibited the highest prevalence of BADL disability in both years, but also showed a marked increase in IADL disability, with several states approaching the upper limit of the prevalence scale.

Associations between T2DM and hypertension are expected since they share several similar pathophysiological mechanisms, including the inadequate activation of the renin–angiotensin–aldosterone system, oxidative stress caused by the excessive production of reactive oxygen species, inflammatory processes, impaired insulin-mediated vasodilation, the increased activation of the sympathetic nervous system, dysfunction of innate and adaptive immune responses, and abnormalities in renal sodium handling [20].

Our results, along with previous findings in Brazilian populations [11,21–27] and in other populations worldwide [28–32], reflect the understanding that aging is a progressive process that leads to a decline in the physiological function in all organic systems and, together with the presence of chronic diseases such as diabetes and hypertension, can significantly impair essential daily activities of older adults [33], including limitations in walking, standing, sitting, or lifting objects due to diabetic neuropathy, infections, amputations, or cardiovascular diseases [34].

Although our study is not suitable for investigating causality, our results are in line with a recent Mendelian Randomization study that demonstrated that frailty doubles the chances of developing T2DM, supporting the hypothesis of a bidirectional causal relationship between T2DM and frailty [35].

The biggest strength of this study is its representative population base, as the data were extracted from the Brazilian National Health Survey of 2013 and 2019. The PNS is a comprehensive national survey driven by the IBGE in partnership with the Ministry of Health, using probabilistic complex sampling to ensure the representation of the Brazilian population. Using two versions of the same survey allowed for a temporal analysis of health conditions, identifying trends and changes in prevalence over the period evaluated. Thus, the findings reflect the country's epidemiological scenario with high external validity. Another strength of this study is the standardization of data collection methods, ensuring comparability between the periods analyzed. The PNS uses structured questionnaires administered by trained interviewers, reducing measurement bias and ensuring the quality of the information. The inclusion of sociodemographic, behavioral, and health service access data allows for the appropriate adjustment of the analysis statistics, reducing potential confounding factors and strengthening inferences about the determinants of hypertension, diabetes, and disabilities.

The limitations of our study include the presentation of small sample sizes in some categories, especially among older people (90+), which may introduce survival bias, as well as a small sample size in the "other races" category. Added to this, other limitations include the formulation of the exposition, as only the self-report variable diagnosis was used to consider a case. There is evidence in the literature that the prevalence of diabetes can change dramatically when using other criteria points, such as considering the values of hemoglobin laboratory tests to be glycated and using the exclusion variable for the diagnosis of gestational diabetes [36].

In the context of our study, survivorship bias may have led to an underestimation of both the prevalence and the functional impact of diabetes and hypertension. This occurs because the study population consists only of individuals who survived into older age and were available to participate in the survey. As a result, those who experienced more severe forms of the disease, especially individuals with early-onset diabetes or major complications such as amputations, myocardial infarction, or stroke, may have died prematurely and are, therefore, not represented in the sample. Consequently, the associations observed may reflect a subset of individuals with less severe or better-controlled disease, leading to attenuated estimates of risk and an under-representation of the true burden of disability attributable to these conditions.

Additionally, this bias may help explain the decreasing prevalence ratios with advancing age observed in our data. The oldest age groups may appear "healthier," not necessarily because they are unaffected, but because only the healthiest among them have survived, while those more severely impacted by chronic diseases were systematically excluded by mortality. In Picon and collaborators' study, they have shown that there are disparities in the prevalence of hypertension in different outlines, such as national and telephone surveys [37]; therefore, as our study is a national household survey, this may be related to an underestimation of the prevalence evaluated.

The results of this study contribute to a growing body of evidence highlighting the functional repercussions of chronic conditions such as diabetes and hypertension among older adults in Brazil. These findings reinforce the need for integrated public health strategies that move beyond disease control to encompass functional health and autonomy as key outcomes in aging populations. In this context, policies aimed at early detection, comprehensive care, and multidisciplinary management of chronic diseases become essential to slow the progression of disability. Additionally, the disproportionate burden of functional decline among socioeconomically and racially marginalized groups underscores the urgency of addressing health disparities. Developing targeted, equity-oriented interventions that prioritize accessibility and continuity of care may mitigate long-term consequences and improve the quality of life of vulnerable older adults. By recognizing functionality as a central component of healthy aging, public health actions can better align with the complex and multidimensional needs of this population [38].

5. Conclusions

This population-based study with adults living in Brazil of 60 years and older demonstrated that the combination of chronic conditions, such as diabetes and hypertension, significantly impacts the functional capacity of older individuals, with varying magnitudes depending on the different levels of functional commitment (BALD and IADL). Unlike previous research on Brazilians, which does not explore the specific combination of diabetes and hypertension comorbidities from a population perspective. This study highlights the relevance of this specific combination, demonstrating that its influence on disability in older populations occurs in a differentiated way, reinforcing the need to consider it in clinical and epidemiological research.

The comparison between BALD and IADL suggests that the loss of functionality occurs progressively, starting with difficulties in more complex activities and progressing to limitations in basic activities as frailty increases. This pattern reinforces the need for early interventions aimed at preserving independence in IADL to delay or prevent the progression of disability to BADL, which can result in greater dependence and an overload on health and social care systems.

The findings of this study have practical implications that extend beyond epidemiological observation. From a clinical standpoint, they support the growing recognition that older adults should be stratified not only by the presence of chronic diseases, but also by the severity of their functional limitations. This approach is especially relevant in geriatric medicine and rehabilitation, where multimorbidity and functional decline frequently coexist and demand individualized, multidimensional interventions. In public health surveillance, our results reinforce the need to monitor the functional impacts of diabetes and hypertension over time, informing resource allocation and the design of targeted programs for high-risk older adults. Furthermore, these findings align with a shift in disability paradigms from a purely medical model focused on disease to a more integrated perspective that incorporates the social model and the human rights model. This broader framework emphasizes autonomy, inclusion, and equity in health care for older adults and supports the development of policies that address functional limitations not only as medical outcomes, but also as social determinants of participation and well-being. Future research should explore how clinical care pathways and public health strategies can be restructured to reflect this multidimensional understanding of disability and aging, contributing to more just and effective care systems.

Author Contributions: Conceptualization, R.G.R.-L. and P.K.Z.; Methodology, B.N.G.d.G. and P.K.Z.; Formal analysis, R.G.R.-L. and P.K.Z.; Data visualization, R.G.R.-L.; Writing—original draft preparation, R.G.R.-L.; Writing—review and editing, R.G.R.-L., B.N.G.d.G. and P.K.Z. All authors have read and agreed to the published version of the manuscript.

Funding: The authors received funding from the Coordination for the Improvement of Higher Education Personnel (CAPES), a foundation linked to the Ministry of Education of Brazil. Rafaela Ribeiro-Lucas had a Master's degree fellowship from CAPES, number: 001.

Institutional Review Board Statement: The 2013 PNS and 2019 studies were duly reviewed and approved by the National Research Ethics Committee (CONEP/CNS), as per opinions No. 328.159 issued on 8 July 2013 and No. 3.529.376 on 23 August 2019.

Informed Consent Statement: Informed consent was obtained from all subjects involved in this study.

Data Availability Statement: The PNS is a national household-based survey where data are made available openly and free of charge to any individual. The data are available in a publicly accessible repository. Since our study was conducted with these secondary data, the repository of the two databases can be found at the link [https://www.ibge.gov.br/estatisticas/sociais/saude/9160-pesquisa-nacional-de-saude.html?=&t=downloads] (accessed on 27 May 2025).

Conflicts of Interest: The authors declare that the research was conducted in the absence of any commercial or financial relationships that could be construed as a potential conflict of interest.

Abbreviations

The following abbreviations are used in this manuscript:

95%CI	95% Confidence Interval
BADL	Basic Activities of Daily Living
DALY	Disability-Adjusted Life Years
GBD	Global Burden of Disease
IADL	Instrumental Activities of Daily Living
IBGE	Instituto Brasileiro de Geografia e Estatística
NCDs	Chronic noncommunicable diseases
NHS	National Health Survey
PNS	Pesquisa Nacional de Saúde
PRa	Prevalence-Ratio-Adjusted (ou conforme sua definição específica)
Pw	Probability weight
SAH	Systemic Arterial Hypertension
T2DM	Type 2 Diabetes Mellitus

Appendix A

Table A1. Definition of the operational study adjustment variables in the baseline and the new categorizations.

Variable	Definitions in the Original Study	New Categorizations
Age	In years	In years
Sex	Male	Masculine
	Female	Feminine
Education	Uneducated Incomplete elementary school	Incomplete elementary education
	Complete elementary Incomplete medium Complete medium Incomplete higher education Completed higher education	Completed elementary education

Table A1. *Cont.*

Variable	Definitions in the Original Study	New Categorizations
Race	White Yellow Brown Black Indigenous	White Black Others
Region	Rural Urban	Rural Urban
Marital status	Married Divorced Separate Single Widower	Married Not married
Type 2 Diabetes Mellitus	Self-reported medical diagnosis	0—does not have diabetes 1—has diabetes
Systemic Arterial Hypertension	Self-reported medical diagnosis	0—no hypertension 1—has hypertension
	No difficulty There is little difficulty It has great difficulty Cannot	0—cannot, has much difficulty, and has little difficulty 1—No difficulty
IADL	No difficulty There is little difficulty It has great difficulty Cannot	0—Cannot, has much difficulty, and has little difficulty 1—No difficulty

Table A2. Adherence of this study to the STROBE criteria.

Item No.	STROBE Recommendation	Location in the Manuscript (Page, Paragraph)
1(a)	Indicate the study's design with a commonly used term in the title or the abstract	Title (p. 1, 1)
1(b)	Provide in the abstract an informative and balanced summary of what was carried out and what was found	Abstract (p. 1,1)
2	Explain the scientific background and rationale for the investigation being reported	Introduction (p. 1, 1–4)
3	State-specific objectives, including any prespecified hypotheses	Final of the introduction (p. 2, 4)
4	Present key elements of the study design early in the paper	Materials and Methods (p. 2, 1–2)
5	Describe the setting, locations, and relevant dates, including periods of recruitment, exposure, follow-up, and data collection	Materials and Methods (p. 3, 3)
6(a)	Give the eligibility criteria, and the sources and methods of selection of participants	Materials and Methods (p. 3, 4)
7	Clearly define all outcomes, exposures, predictors, potential confounders, and effect modifiers. Give diagnostic criteria, if applicable	Materials and Methods (p. 3, 4–6)
8	For each variable of interest, give sources of data and details of methods of assessment (measurement). Describe the comparability of assessment methods if there is more than one group	Materials and Methods (p. 3, 5–6)
9	Describe any efforts to address potential sources of bias	Does not apply
10	Explain how the study size was arrived at	Materials and Methods (p. 2, 2)
11	Explain how quantitative variables were handled in the analyses. If applicable, describe which groupings were chosen and why	Materials and Methods (p. 3, 5–6)

Table A2. *Cont.*

Item No.	STROBE Recommendation	Location in the Manuscript (Page, Paragraph)
12(a)	Describe all statistical methods, including those used to control for confounding	Materials and Methods (p. 3, 7)
12(b)	Describe any methods used to examine subgroups and interactions	Does not apply
12(c)	Explain how missing data were addressed	Materials and Methods (p. 3, 5)
12(d)	If applicable, describe analytical methods taking account of sampling strategy	Materials and Methods (p. 2, 7)
12(e)	Describe any sensitivity analyses	Does not apply
13(a)	Report numbers of individuals at each stage of study (e.g., potentially eligible, examined for eligibility, included, analyzed)	Results (p. 4, 1)
13(b)	Give reasons for non-participation at each stage	Results (p. 4, 1)
13(c)	Consider use of a flow diagram	Results (p. 4, 1)
14(a)	Give characteristics of study participants (e.g., demographic, clinical, and social) and information on exposures and potential confounders	Results (p. 6 and 8)
14(b)	Indicate number of participants with missing data for each variable of interest	Results (p. 6 and 8)
15	Report numbers of outcome events or summary measures	Results (p. 6 and 8)
16(a)	Give unadjusted estimates and, if applicable, confounder-adjusted estimates and their precision (e.g., 95% confidence interval). Make clear which confounders were adjusted for and why they were included	Results (3 and Table 4)
16(b)	Report category boundaries when continuous variables were categorized	Methods (p. 3, 4)
16(c)	If relevant, consider translating estimates of relative risk into absolute risk for a meaningful time period	Does not apply
17	Report other analyses completed, e.g., subgroup analyses and sensitivity analyses	Does not apply
18	Summarise key results with reference to study objectives	Discussion (p. 13)
19	Discuss limitations of the study, taking into account sources of potential bias or imprecision	Discussion (p. 13, 4–5)
20	Give a cautious overall interpretation of results considering objectives, limitations, multiplicity of analyses, results from similar studies, and other relevant evidence	Discussion and conclusions (p. 13, 5–6; p. 14, 4)
21	Discuss the generalizability (external validity) of the study results	Conclusions (p. 14, 1)
22	Give the source of funding and the role of the funders for the present study	p. 15, 2

Table A3. Descriptive table of raw Basic Activities of Daily Living (BADL) data in 2013 PNS.

Categories	K001 To Eat	K004 To Bath	K007 Bathroom Use	K010 To Dress Up	K013 To Walk	K016 + K019 Transfer
No difficulty	10,667 (95.44)	10,469 (93.67%)	10,536 (94.27%)	10,239 (91.61%)	10,290 (92.06%)	20,573 (92.03)
There is little difficulty	316 (2.83)	354 (3.17)	352 (3.15)	551 (4.93)	522 (4.67)	1161 (5.19)
It has great difficulty	125 (1.12%)	180 (1.61%)	139 (1.24%)	215 (1.92%)	222 (1.99%)	360 (1.61%)
Cannot	69 (0.62%)	174 (1.56%)	150 (1.34%)	172 (1.54%)	143 (1.28%)	260 (1.16%)

Table A4. Description of raw data on Instrumental Activities of Daily Living (IADL) in 2013 PNS.

Categories	K022 Shopping	K025 Finances	K028 Medicines	K031 Doctor	K034 Transport
No difficulty	9302 (83.22%)	9891 (88.49%)	8211 (73.46%)	8646 (77.36%)	8732 (78.12%)
There is little difficulty	678 (6.07%)	478 (4.28%)	391 (3.50%)	1151 (10.30%)	921 (8.24%)
It has great difficulty	457 (4.09%)	263 (2.35%)	205 (1.83%)	630 (5.64%)	639 (5.72%)
Cannot	740 (6.62%)	545 (4.88%)	245 (2.19%)	750 (6.71%)	885 (7.92%)
Does not use medication	-	-	2125 (19.01%)	-	-

Table A5. Description of raw Basic Activities of Daily Living (BADL) data in 2019 PNS.

Categories	K001 To Eat	K004 To Bath	K007 Bathroom Use	K010 To Dress Up	K013 To Walk	K016 + K019 Transfer
No difficulty	21,613 (95.09%)	21,061 (92.67%)	20,681 (90.99%)	20,052 (88.23%)	20,289 (89.27%)	39,898 (87.77%)
There is little difficulty	697 (3.07%)	936 (4.12%)	1086 (4.78%)	1749 (7.70%)	1405 (6.18%)	3576 (7.87%)
It has great difficulty	250 (1.10%)	374 (1.65%)	372 (1.64%)	590 (2.60%)	517 (2.27%)	1.015 (2.23%)
Cannot	168 (0.74%)	357 (1.57%)	589 (2.59%)	337 (1.48%)	517 (2.27%)	967 (2.13%)

Table A6. Description of raw data on Instrumental Activities of Daily Living (IADL) in 2019 PNS.

Categories	K022 Shopping	K025 Finances	K028 Remedy	K031 Doctor	K034 Transport
No difficulty	18,473 (81.28%)	19,722 (86.77%)	602 (2.65%)	16,956 (74.60%)	16,916 (74.43%)
There is little difficulty	1768 (7.78%)	1293 (5.69%)	482 (2.12%)	2578 (11.34%)	2383 (10.48%)
It has great difficulty	963 (4.24%)	607 (2.67%)	1295 (5.70%)	1226 (5.39%)	1367 (6.01%)
Cannot	1524 (6.71%)	1106 (4.87%)	16896 (74.34%)	1968 (8.66%)	2062 (9.07%)
Does not use medication	-	-	3453 (15.19%)	-	-

References

1. GBD Compare. Available online: http://vizhub.healthdata.org/gbd-compare (accessed on 21 April 2025).
2. GBD 2021 Diseases and Injuries Collaborators. Global incidence, prevalence, years lived with disability (YLDs), disability-adjusted life-years (DALYs), and healthy life expectancy (HALE) for 371 diseases and injuries in 204 countries and territories and 811 subnational locations, 1990–2021: A systematic analysis for the Global Burden of Disease Study 2021. *Lancet* **2024**, *403*, 2133–2161.
3. Oliveira, G.M.M.D.; Brant, L.C.C.; Polanczyk, C.A.; Malta, D.C.; Biolo, A.; Nascimento, B.R.; Souza, M.D.F.M.D.; Lorenzo, A.R.D.; Fagundes Júnior, A.A.D.P.; Schaan, B.D.; et al. Cardiovascular Statistics—Brazil 2023. *Arq. Bras. Cardiol.* **2024**, *121*, e20240079. [CrossRef]
4. Muzy, J.; Campos, M.R.; Emmerick, I.; Silva, R.S.D.; Schramm, J.M.D.A. Prevalência de diabetes mellitus e suas complicações e caracterização das lacunas na atenção à saúde a partir da triangulação de pesquisas. *Cad. Saúde Pública* **2021**, *37*, e00076120. [CrossRef] [PubMed]
5. Instituto Brasileiro de Geografia e Estatística (IBGE). *Pesquisa Nacional de Saúde, 2019: Ciclos de Vida*; IBGE: Rio de Janeiro, Brazil, 2021.

6. Instituto Brasileiro de Geografia e Estatística (IBGE). *Pesquisa Nacional de Saúde: 2019: Percepção do Estado de Saúde, Estilos de Vida, Doenças Crônicas e Saúde Bucal: Brasil e Grandes Regiões*; IBGE: Rio de Janeiro, Brazil, 2021.
7. Chen, G.; McAlister, F.A.; Walker, R.L.; Hemmelgarn, B.R.; Campbell, N.R.C. Cardiovascular Outcomes in Framingham Participants with Diabetes: The Importance of Blood Pressure. *Hypertension* **2011**, *57*, 891–897. [CrossRef]
8. Tsai, Y.H.; Chuang, L.L.; Lee, Y.J.; Chiu, C.J. How Does Diabetes Accelerate Normal Aging? An Examination of ADL, IADL, and Mobility Disability in Middle-aged and Older Adults with and Without Diabetes. *Diabetes Res. Clin. Pract.* **2021**, *182*, 109114. [CrossRef] [PubMed]
9. Wong, E.; Backholer, K.; Gearon, E.; Harding, J.; Freak-Poli, R.; Stevenson, C.; Peeters, A. Diabetes and risk of physical disability in adults: A systematic review and meta-analysis. *Lancet Diabetes Endocrinol.* **2013**, *1*, 106–114. [CrossRef] [PubMed]
10. Qian, J.; Ren, X. Association between comorbid conditions and BADL/IADL disability in hypertension patients over age 45: Based on the China health and retirement longitudinal study (CHARLS). *Medicine* **2016**, *95*, e4536. [CrossRef]
11. Reis Júnior, W.M.; Ferreira, L.N.; Molina-Bastos, C.G.; Bispo Júnior, J.P.; Reis, H.F.T.; Goulart, B.N.G. Prevalence of functional dependence and chronic diseases in the community-dwelling Brazilian older adults: An analysis by dependence severity and multimorbidity pattern. *BMC Public Health* **2024**, *24*, 140. [CrossRef]
12. Damacena, G.N.; Szwarcwald, C.L.; Malta, D.C.; Souza Júnior, P.R.B.d.; Vieira, M.L.F.P.; Pereira, C.A.; Neto, O.L.d.M.; Júnior, J.B.d.S. O processo de desenvolvimento da Pesquisa Nacional de Saúde no Brasil, 2013. *Epidemiol. Serv. Saúde* **2015**, *24*, 197–206. [CrossRef]
13. Souza Júnior, P.R.B.D.; Szwarcwald, C.L.; Almeida, W.D.S.D.; Damacena, G.N.; Pedroso, M.D.M.; Sousa, C.A.M.D.; Morais, I.D.S.; Saldanha, R.D.F.; Lima, J.; Stopa, S.R. Comparison of sampling designs from the two editions of the Brazilian National Health Survey, 2013 and 2019. *Cad. Saúde Pública* **2022**, *38*, e00164321. [CrossRef]
14. Szwarcwald, C.L.; Malta, D.C.; Pereira, C.A.; Vieira, M.L.F.P.; Conde, W.L.; Souza Júnior, P.R.B.D.; Damacena, G.N.; Azevedo, L.O.; Azevedo e Silva, G.; Theme, M.; et al. Pesquisa Nacional de Saúde no Brasil: Concepção e metodologia de aplicação. *Ciênc. Saúde Coletiva* **2014**, *19*, 333–342. [CrossRef] [PubMed]
15. Stopa, S.R.; Szwarcwald, C.L.; Oliveira, M.M.D.; Gouvea, E.D.C.D.P.; Vieira, M.L.F.P.; Freitas, M.P.S.D. National Health Survey 2019: History, methods and perspectives. *Epidemiol. Serv. Saúde* **2020**, *29*, e2020315. [CrossRef] [PubMed]
16. Skrivankova, V.W.; Richmond, R.C.; Woolf, B.A.R.; Yarmolinsky, J.; Davies, N.M.; Swanson, S.A.; VanderWeele, T.J.; Higgins, J.P.; Timpson, N.J.; Dimou, N.; et al. Strengthening the Reporting of Observational Studies in Epidemiology Using Mendelian Randomization: The STROBE-MR Statement. *JAMA* **2021**, *326*, 1614–1621. [CrossRef] [PubMed]
17. Katz, S. Assessing self-maintenance: Activities of daily living, mobility, and instrumental activities of daily living. *J. Am. Geriatr. Soc.* **1983**, *31*, 721–727. [CrossRef]
18. Altman, B.M. *International Measurement of Disability*; Springer: Cham, Switzerland, 2016.
19. Brefka, S.; Dallmeier, D.; Mühlbauer, V.; von Arnim, C.A.F.; Bollig, C.; Onder, G.; Petrovic, M.; Schönfeldt-Lecuona, C.; Seibert, M.; Torbahn, G.; et al. A Proposal for the Retrospective Identification and Categorization of Older People with Functional Impairments in Scientific Studies-Recommendations of the Medication and Quality of Life in Frail Older Persons (MedQoL) Research Group. *J. Am. Med. Dir. Assoc.* **2019**, *20*, 138–146. [CrossRef]
20. Sowers, J.R. Diabetes mellitus and vascular disease. *Hypertension* **2013**, *61*, 943–947. [CrossRef]
21. Alves, L.C.; Leite, I.d.C.; Machado, C.J. Factors associated with functional disability of elderly in Brazil: A multilevel analysis. *Rev. Saúde Pública* **2010**, *44*, 468–478. [CrossRef]
22. Nunes, J.D.; Saes, M.D.O.; Nunes, B.P.; Siqueira, F.C.V.; Soares, D.C.; Fassa, M.E.G.; Thumé, E.; Facchini, L.A. Functional disability indicators and associated factors in the elderly: A population-based study in Bagé, Rio Grande do Sul, Brazil. *Epidemiol. Serv. Saude* **2017**, *26*, 295–304. [CrossRef]
23. Gavasso, W.C.; Beltrame, V. Functional capacity and reported morbidities: A comparative analysis in the elderly. *Rev. Bras. Geriatr. Gerontol.* **2017**, *20*, 398–408. [CrossRef]
24. Bernardes, G.M.; Mambrini, J.V.d.M.; Lima-Costa, M.F.; Peixoto, S.V. Perfil de multimorbidade associado à incapacidade entre idosos residentes na Região Metropolitana de Belo Horizonte, Brasil. *Ciênc. Saúde Coletiva* **2019**, *24*, 1853–1864. [CrossRef]
25. Aguiar, B.M.; Silva, P.O.; Vieira, M.A.; Costa, F.M.d.; Carneiro, J.A. Evaluation of functional disability and associated factors in the elderly. *Rev. Bras. Geriatr. Gerontol.* **2019**, *22*, e180163. [CrossRef]
26. Schmidt, T.P.; Wagner, K.J.P.; Schneider, I.J.C.; Danielewicz, A.L. Padrões de multimorbidade e incapacidade funcional em idosos brasileiros: Estudo transversal com dados da Pesquisa Nacional de Saúde. *Cad. Saúde Pública* **2020**, *36*, e00241619. [CrossRef] [PubMed]
27. Barbosa, B.R.; Almeida, J.M.d.; Barbosa, M.R.; Rossi-Barbosa, L.A.R. Avaliação da capacidade funcional dos idosos e fatores associados à incapacidade. *Ciênc. Saúde Coletiva* **2014**, *19*, 3317–3325. [CrossRef] [PubMed]
28. Lestari, S.K.; Ng, N.; Kowal, P.; Santosa, A. Diversity in the Factors Associated with ADL-Related Disability among Older People in Six Middle-Income Countries: A Cross-Country Comparison. *Int. J. Environ. Res. Public Health* **2019**, *16*, 1341. [CrossRef] [PubMed]

29. Dunlop, D.D.; Manheim, L.M.; Sohn, M.W.; Liu, X.; Chang, R.W. Incidence of functional limitation in older adults: The impact of gender, race, and chronic conditions. *Arch. Phys. Med. Rehabil.* **2002**, *83*, 964–971. [CrossRef]
30. Zhu, J.; Xu, L.; Sun, L.; Li, J.; Qin, W.; Ding, G.; Wang, Q.; Zhang, J.; Xie, S.; Yu, Z. Chronic Disease, Disability, Psychological Distress and Suicide Ideation among Rural Elderly: Results from a Population Survey in Shandong. *Int. J. Environ. Res. Public Health* **2018**, *15*, 1604. [CrossRef]
31. Oyewole, O.O.; Ale, A.O.; Ogunlana, M.O.; Gurayah, T. Burden of disability in type 2 diabetes mellitus and the moderating effects of physical activity. *World J. Clin. Cases* **2023**, *11*, 3128–3139. [CrossRef]
32. Nolde, J.; Beaney, T.; Carnagarin, R.; Stergiou, G.S.; Poulter, N.R.; Schutte, A.E.; Schlaich, M.P. Regional variation of age-related blood pressure trajectories and their association with blood pressure control rates, disability-adjusted life years and death. *Eur. Heart J.* **2024**, *45* (Suppl. S1), ehae666.2541. [CrossRef]
33. Buford, T.W. Hypertension and aging. *Ageing Res. Rev.* **2016**, *26*, 96–111. [CrossRef]
34. Chiu, C.J.; Wray, L.A. Physical disability trajectories in older Americans with and without diabetes: The role of age, gender, race or ethnicity, and education. *Gerontologist* **2011**, *51*, 51–63. [CrossRef]
35. Gao, Y.; Gao, Y.; Li, Y.; Zhang, Q.; Wang, Y. Causal associations of frailty and type 2 diabetes mellitus: A bidirectional Mendelian randomization study. *Medicine* **2025**, *104*, e41630. [CrossRef] [PubMed]
36. Malta, D.C.; Duncan, B.B.; Schmidt, M.I.; Machado, Í.E.; Silva, A.G.D.; Bernal, R.T.I.; Pereira, C.A.; Damacena, G.N.; Stopa, S.R.; Rosenfeld, L.G.; et al. Prevalência de diabetes *mellitus* determinada pela hemoglobina glicada na população adulta brasileira, Pesquisa Nacional de Saúde. Rev bras epidemiol. *Rev. Bras. Epidemiol.* **2019**, *22* (Suppl. S2), E190006.
37. Picon, R.V.; Fuchs, F.D.; Moreira, L.B.; Fuchs, S.C. Prevalence of hypertension among elderly persons in urban Brazil: A systematic review with meta-analysis. *Am. J. Hypertens.* **2013**, *26*, 541–548. [CrossRef] [PubMed]
38. Berghs, M.; Atkin, K.; Graham, H.; Hatton, C.; Thomas, C. Implications for public health research of models and theories of disability: A scoping study and evidence synthesis. *Public Health Res.* **2016**, *4*, 1–166. Available online: http://www.ncbi.nlm.nih.gov/books/NBK378941/ (accessed on 6 July 2025). [CrossRef]

International Journal of
Environmental Research and Public Health

MDPI

Article

Predictors of Health-Workforce Job Satisfaction in Primary Care Settings: Insights from a Cross-Sectional Multi-Country Study in Eight African Countries

Samuel Muhula [1], Yvonne Opanga [2], Saida Kassim [1,*], Lazarus Odeny [1], Richard Zule Mbewe [1], Beverlyne Akoth [1], Mable Jerop [1], Lizah Nyawira [1], Ibrahima Gueye [1], Richard Kiplimo [1], Thom Salamba [3], Jackline Kiarie [1] and George Kimathi [1]

[1] Amref Health Africa, Headquarters, Nairobi P.O. Box 27691-00506, Kenya; samuel.muhula@amref.org (S.M.); lazarus.odeny@amref.org (L.O.); richard.mbewe@amref.org (R.Z.M.); beverlyne.akoth@amref.org (B.A.); mable.jerop@amref.org (M.J.); lizahnm@gmail.com (L.N.); ibrahima.gueye@amref.org (I.G.); richard.kiplimo@amref.org (R.K.); jackline.kiarie@amref.org (J.K.); george.kimathi@amref.org (G.K.)

[2] Amref Health Africa, Kenya Country Office, Nairobi P.O. Box 30125-00100, Kenya; yvonne.opanga@amref.org

[3] Amref Health Africa, Malawi Country Office, Lilongwe P.O. Box 30768, Malawi; salamba.salamba@amref.org

* Correspondence: saida.kassim@amref.org

Abstract

Job satisfaction in sub-Saharan Africa is crucial as it directly impacts employee productivity, retention, and overall economic growth, fostering a motivated workforce that drives regional development. In sub–Saharan Africa, poor remuneration, limited professional development opportunities, and inadequate working conditions impact satisfaction. This study examined job-satisfaction predictors among health workers in primary healthcare settings across eight countries: Ethiopia, Kenya, Malawi, Senegal, South Sudan, Tanzania, Uganda, and Zambia. A cross-sectional study surveyed 1711 health workers, assessing five dimensions: employer–2employee relationships, remuneration and recognition, professional development, physical work environment, and supportive supervision. The study was conducted from October 2023 to March 2024. The job-satisfaction assessment tool was adopted from a validated tool originally developed for use in low-income healthcare settings. The tool was reviewed by staff from all the country offices to ensure contextual relevance and organization alignment. The responses were measured on a five-point Likert scale: 0: Not applicable, 1: Very dissatisfied, 2: Dissatisfied, 3: Neutral, 4: Satisfied, and 5: Very satisfied. The analysis employed descriptive and multivariable regression methods. Job satisfaction varied significantly by country. Satisfaction with the employer–employee relationship was highest in Zambia (80%) and lowest in Tanzania (16%). Remuneration satisfaction was highest in Senegal (63%) and Zambia (49%), while it was very low in Malawi (9.8%) and Ethiopia (2.3%). Overall, 44% of respondents were satisfied with their professional development, with Uganda leading (62%) and Ethiopia having the lowest satisfaction level (29%). Satisfaction with the physical environment was at 27%, with Uganda at 40% and Kenya at 12%. Satisfaction with supervisory support stood at 62%, with Zambia at 73% and Ethiopia at 30%. Key predictors of job satisfaction included a strong employer–employee relationships (OR = 2.20, $p < 0.001$), fair remuneration (OR = 1.59, $p = 0.002$), conducive work environments (OR = 1.71, $p < 0.001$), and supervisory support (OR = 3.58, $p < 0.001$. Improving the job satisfaction, retention, and performance of health workers in sub-Saharan Africa requires targeted interventions in employer–employee relationships, fair compensation, supportive supervision, and working conditions. Strategies must be tailored to each country's unique challenges, as one-size-fits-all solutions may not be effective. Policymakers should prioritize these factors to build a motivated, resilient workforce, with ongoing research and monitoring essential to ensure sustained progress and improved healthcare delivery.

Keywords: job satisfaction; health workforce; primary healthcare; sub-Saharan Africa

1. Introduction

Job satisfaction reflects an employee's overall attitude towards their job, including their feelings about various aspects of the job or an emotional response defining the degree to which people like their jobs, which may range from extreme satisfaction to extreme dissatisfaction [1]. It significantly influences job performance, commitment, absenteeism, retention, and turnover rates, with dissatisfied health workers often seeking employment out of their speciality [2–4].

Health workers are the cornerstone of effective health systems, playing a pivotal role in achieving Universal Health Coverage (UHC) and delivering quality primary healthcare (PHC) [5]. In low- and middle-income countries (LMICs), job satisfaction among health workers has been identified as a key determinant of their performance, retention, and overall productivity [6]. This is because a satisfied workforce is more likely to provide better patient care, foster trust and ensure the continuity of care within communities. The significance of job satisfaction has garnered increasing attention, particularly in sub-Saharan Africa, where healthcare systems face numerous challenges, including workforce shortages and high turnover rates. Improving health-workforce job satisfaction in resource-limited settings is essential for addressing systemic health challenges and ensuring the sustainability of health services.

Globally, job satisfaction among healthcare workers is influenced by a complex interplay of factors such as working conditions, the organizational environment, job stress, role conflict and ambiguity, role perception and content, and organizational and professional commitment [7]. Studies have consistently shown that factors such as fair remuneration, supportive supervision, adequate resources, and opportunities for career advancement are strongly associated with higher levels of job satisfaction [8]. Recent Gallup statistics on job satisfaction indicated that a substantial proportion of the world's 1 billion full-time workers are disengaged and experiencing declining overall well-being. Specifically, 41% of employees are stressed, with one in five experiencing loneliness, half watching for or actively seeking a new job, and one in four experiencing burnout either "very often" or "always" [9]. Europeans are unhappier with their workplaces than workers in any other region, with only 14% of European employees engaged at work, a figure that is seven percentage points lower than the global average (21%) and nineteen (19) points lower than the U.S. and Canada (33%) [9].

The African context presents unique challenges to health-worker job satisfaction. Frequent infectious-disease outbreaks place significant strain on already overburdened healthcare systems, impacting workers' well-being [10,11]. Less equipped facilities, limited access to essential medicines and supplies, and inadequate infrastructure such as electricity and water, further hinder job satisfaction [12]. In addition, many African countries face severe workforce shortages, leading to heavy workloads and burnout. A study by Muthuri and colleagues conducted in the East Africa Community (EAC) indicates that there are individual, organizational/structural, and societal determinants of healthcare workers' motivation. The systematic review highlighted barriers reported by the health workforce which included a lack of or inadequate monetary support, favoritism, a critical shortage of skilled healthcare professionals leading to a heavy workload, and unrealistic expectations from management and government. Another study reported that 82.3% of respondents in Tanzania were satisfied with their jobs, compared to 71.0% in Malawi, and 52.1% in South Africa. In all three countries, health workers were most satisfied with their job's variety and the opportunity to fully utilize their abilities [13].

While low salaries, a lack of benefits, lack of recognition, and unsafe working environments drive high attrition rates [14,15], these challenges present various opportunities that can be harnessed. There is notable willingness among health workers to further develop skills and knowledge and a proactive search for solutions to enhance stock-outs of drugs and other medical devices. There are also motivational factors to improve the quality of care [14]. Non-financial incentives and human-resources management tools play an important role in motivating health professionals. Acknowledging and addressing professional goals, such as career development, recognition and improving their skillset, can uphold and strengthen the professional ethos of health workers [16]. However, little comparative evidence across sub-Saharan Africa countries that simultaneously examines multiple satisfaction domains exists—a gap that this study addresses.

Between October 2023 and March 2024, a multi-country cross-sectional study was conducted across eight African countries including Ethiopia, Kenya, Malawi, Senegal, South Sudan, Tanzania, Uganda, and Zambia. The eight countries are a representation of the different African regions within sub-Saharan Africa including west, east, and southern Africa. These countries were selected based on their diversity in contexts including sociopolitical and economic. Despite these variations, the eight countries share common challenges among the health workforce including resource constraints, shortages in the health workforce, and inequitable access to healthcare services, driven largely by the differences in the urban and rural populations [17,18].

Ethiopia, categorized as a low-income country, is characterized by a predominantly rural population that relies heavily on agriculture. While the country has demonstrated improvement in key health indicators, literacy levels remain low mostly among women [19]. The national health system is organized around a three-tier structure, with the Health Extension Program driving primary-care service delivery through over 40,000 health extension workers deployed in communities [18,20].

Kenya is categorized as a lower-middle-income country characterized by a rapidly urbanizing population and a relatively diversified economy. There are regional and socioeconomic disparities in relation to healthcare and education access as well as income levels [17]. The health system is devolved across 47 county governments where service delivery responsibilities are delegated. The healthcare network includes community health promoters at the community level, dispensaries, health centers, and referral hospitals both at national and subnational levels. The current healthcare reforms include the establishment of primary-care networks to drive primary healthcare and address chronic challenges faced by the system including periodic health-worker strikes and resource constraints [18,21].

Malawi ranks among the poorest countries globally, with more than 70% of its rural population living below the poverty line [19]. The rural population experiences high levels of undernutrition and food insecurity. The health system is structured around district-level service delivery which heavily relies on donor funding. While community health workers drive primary-care services which are widely utilized, the system struggles with health-workforce shortages, drug stockouts, and inadequate infrastructure [18,22].

Senegal is a lower-middle-income country with a growing economy anchored in agriculture, fisheries, and mining. Despite improvements in health and education, urban rural divides in healthcare access persist [17]. The health system follows a pyramidal structure, comprising health posts, centers, and hospitals. Senegal has implemented an advanced universal health-coverage scheme (Couverture Maladie Universelle) and community health strategies to enhance service delivery [18,23].

South Sudan is recognized as the world's youngest nation. Its health system has been weakened by chronic conflict, political instability, and severe humanitarian challenges. Conflicts have driven the majority of the population to extreme poverty with minimal access to basic services [24]. The health system is underdeveloped, heavily reliant on international aid, and faces chronic shortages of trained personnel and functional health facilities. However, health-services delivery is predominantly provided by non-governmental and faith-based organizations [18,25].

Tanzania has sustained moderate economic growth in recent years but continues to grapple with widespread poverty and a high dependency ratio [17]. The health system is decentralized and structured to provide primary healthcare services through dispensaries and health centers. Community health workers play a pivotal role in delivering preventive and promotive services. Persistent challenges include health-workforce shortages, underfunding, and weak referral systems [18,26].

Uganda has a young and rapidly growing population, with over 75% under the age of 30. While economic performance has improved, poverty and inequality remain significant, particularly in rural regions [19]. The health system is organized into national, regional, district, and community levels. Village Health Teams (VHTs) serve as the first point of contact for health services in many communities. Despite gains in immunization and maternal health, disparities in service quality and access remain [18,27].

Zambia is a lower-middle-income country with substantial mineral wealth, though poverty levels remain high, especially in rural areas [17]. The health system is structured into primary, secondary, and tertiary levels, with an expanding cadre of community health assistants who support service delivery at the grassroots level. While the country has made strides in strengthening health infrastructure and services, it continues to face funding gaps, workforce shortages, and inequities in rural health access [18,28].

The study aimed to inform key strategic directions, including strengthening a fit-for-purpose health workforce for improved skills and productivity. The findings of the study served as a baseline assessment to inform targeted health-workforce interventions, recognizing that each country in sub-Saharan Africa faces unique challenges that require tailored solutions. This study contributes to a growing body of the literature evaluating health-workforce motivation and satisfaction in low- and middle-income countries (LMICs), particularly in sub-Saharan Africa, where human resources for health (HRH) shortages remain a major bottleneck to achieving universal health coverage (UHC) and Sustainable Development Goal 3 [29]. Previous publications in this domain have largely focused on small-scale or country-specific studies, often using qualitative designs or limited sample sizes [30]. Our multi-country, quantitative approach provides a broader comparative perspective, enabling policy-relevant benchmarking across eight countries with differing health-system capacities and reform trajectories.

Governments of the study countries, including Ethiopia, Kenya, Malawi, Senegal, South Sudan, Tanzania, Uganda, and Zambia have recognized health-worker motivation and retention as strategic pillars within their national health-sector strategic plans and HRH policies. For example, Kenya's Human Resources for Health Strategic Plan [31] emphasizes improving working conditions and incentives for primary healthcare workers; similarly, Uganda's Health Workforce Strategy (2020–2030) includes components for enhancing supportive supervision and career progression [32]. These strategies align with the WHO's Global Strategy on Human Resources for Health: Workforce 2030, which underscores job satisfaction as a critical determinant of workforce sustainability and equitable health-service delivery [33].

The relevance of the study is further reinforced by the crucial need to strengthen primary healthcare (PHC) systems in sub-Saharan Africa. As countries shift toward UHC- and PHC-oriented models, frontline health workers must be adequately supported to ensure the continuity of care, improved health outcomes, and community trust [34]. By identifying clear predictors of satisfaction—such as fair remuneration, strong supervisory relationships, and a supportive work environment—this research provides actionable evidence for health-system leaders and donors. These findings can inform targeted investments, particularly through bilateral and multilateral support frameworks like the Global Financing Facility (GFF), PEPFAR, and the Global Fund, all of which increasingly emphasize health-system strengthening.

In addition, by contrasting results with patterns observed in high-income countries, where satisfaction tends to be driven by professional autonomy, career flexibility, and workload balance [35], this study highlights contextual distinctions that are vital for policy design. A one-size-fits-all approach is unlikely to work; therefore, country-level interventions should be tailored to existing health-system bottlenecks, budgetary constraints, and labor-market dynamics. The study's potential impact lies in its capacity to guide reforms that not only reduce health-worker attrition but which also enhance productivity, quality of care, and, ultimately, health equity across the region.

By identifying key factors such as employer–employee relationships, fair remuneration, supportive supervision, and conducive working environments, the study provides evidence-based insights that can guide policy and decision-making. These findings are crucial for policymakers to prioritize specific areas of improvement to foster a motivated, resilient health workforce, which is essential for achieving sustained progress in healthcare delivery. The study also lays the groundwork for future interventions aimed at addressing workforce challenges and ensuring that healthcare systems in the region are equipped to meet the growing demands of the population. Amref Health Africa assessed the levels and predictors of job satisfaction among health workers in primary healthcare settings across these eight countries.

2. Materials and Methods

2.1. Study Design

The baseline evaluation employed a cross-sectional study design that surveyed 1711 healthcare workers from 8 countries where Amref implements health-workforce interventions. The countries were chosen to represent a diverse cross-section of sub-Saharan Africa, encompassing eastern, western, and southern African contexts, rather than being selected purely for convenience based on project coverage. By including countries from different regions, the study aims to capture a broader range of health-workforce challenges and job-satisfaction indicators, offering a more comprehensive understanding of the varying dynamics across the region. This approach allows for the identification of region-specific factors while also enabling cross-country comparisons to inform tailored interventions that can be adapted to each country's unique context. Thus, the inclusion of these countries was a strategic decision to ensure that the findings are relevant and actionable across diverse sub-Saharan African settings. The quantitative methods to assess job satisfaction across five dimensions that were utilized are as follows: employee–employer relationships, remuneration and recognition, professional development, the physical environment and facilities, and supportive supervision.

2.2. Study Sites

This study presents the findings from eight African countries—Ethiopia, Kenya, Malawi, Senegal, South Sudan, Tanzania, Uganda, and Zambia. The countries are in the west, east and south of Africa; Figure 1 shows the geographical locations of these countries.

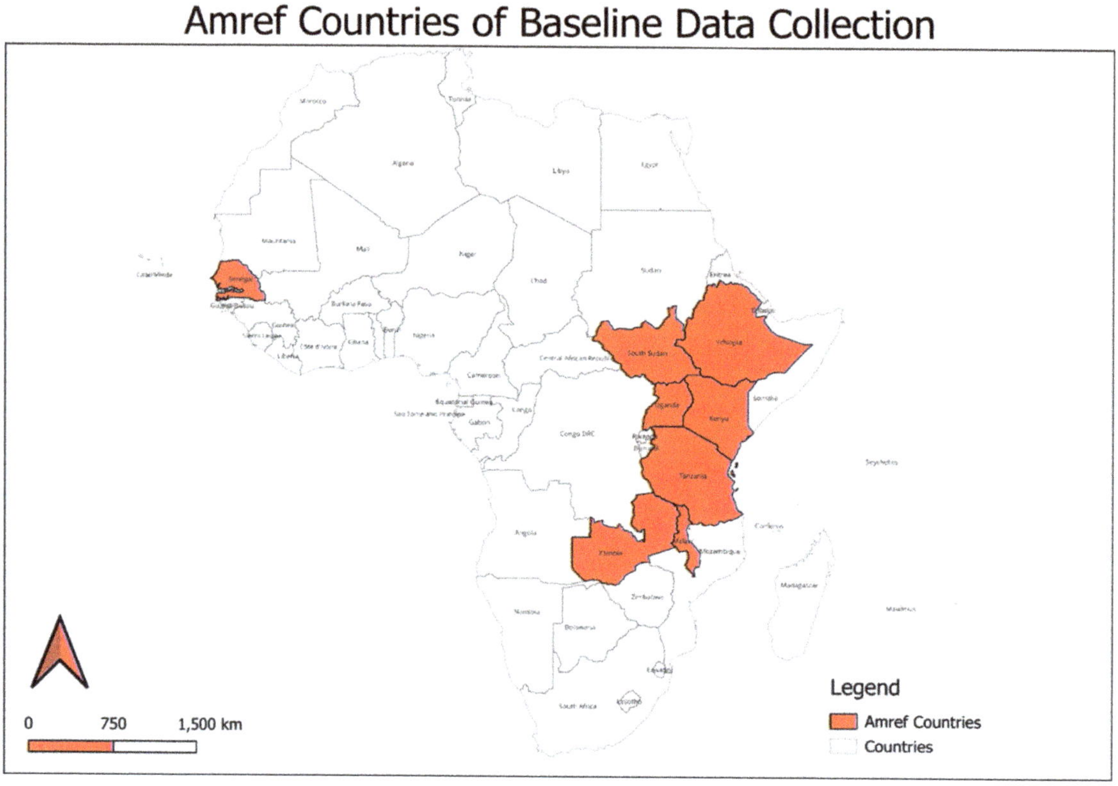

Figure 1. Amref Health Africa: implementing countries. Created using QGIS 3.34.

In Ethiopia, data was collected from four regional states—Oromia, Amhara, Afar, and the South Ethiopia regional states and Addis Ababa city administration. The country's health workforce heavily relies on Health Extension Workers (HEWs), who form the backbone of its primary healthcare system by delivering essential services at the community level, particularly in preventive and promotive care. This program has significantly enhanced access to basic healthcare in rural areas. Ethiopia prioritizes primary healthcare with a strong emphasis on disease prevention and community-based interventions [36,37]. However, challenges include a shortage of trained healthcare professionals, the uneven distribution of workers between urban and rural areas, limited professional-development opportunities, and a high population-to-health-worker ratio, all of which strain the system and impact job satisfaction and service delivery [38].

In Kenya, the study was conducted in eight counties—Nairobi, Narok, Vihiga, Siaya, Nyeri, West Pokot, Samburu, and Tharaka Nithi. These counties were purposively selected to represent diverse geographical settings, including urban, rural, arid, and semi-arid regions, and to address unique Primary Health Care (PHC) challenges and the presence of Amref Health Africa programs. Kenya operates a decentralized healthcare system, with county governments playing a central role in service delivery [39]. The country has a diverse health workforce, including doctors, nurses, clinical officers, and community health volunteers (CHVs), but faces inequitable distribution, particularly in rural and marginalized areas. A robust private-health sector creates competitive opportunities, often contributing to attrition in the public sector. Despite government investments in human resources for health, such as expanding training institutions and increasing healthcare worker training in rural areas, challenges remain in absorbing trained professionals into the workforce, leading to unemployment among qualified health workers [40].

In Uganda, data was collected from the five districts of Iganga, Mayuge, Bugiri, Namayinga, and Pader. Like Kenya, Uganda operates a decentralized health system with a strong focus on community-based healthcare delivery [39]. The country has made progress in addressing workforce shortages by scaling up training programs, particularly for front-line health workers, to improve the detection of, reporting of, and response to disease epidemics [41]. However, significant challenges persist, including widespread workforce shortages, high absenteeism rates, and limited access to essential medical supplies, all of which negatively impact job satisfaction [42]. To address these issues, Uganda has adopted task-shifting strategies, enabling community health workers (CHWs) to take on expanded roles in healthcare delivery [43,44].

Tanzania's health workforce emphasizes task sharing and integrating CHWs to address acute shortages of skilled professionals [43]. The government has prioritized workforce development in its national strategies, but challenges persist, particularly in rural areas. Issues such as low salaries, limited opportunities for promotion and career development, and inadequate training programs negatively affect workforce morale and retention [45]. While the decentralization of health services has improved community access, it has also increased administrative burdens on health workers. Data was collected from the nine regions of Morogoro, Tanga, Mara, Songwe, Lindi, Tabora, Singida, Kaskazini Unguja, and Kaskazini Pemba.

In Malawi, data was collected from six districts—Mchinji, Chitipa, Karonga, Salima, Mangochi, and Chikwawa. The country has one of the world's lowest health-worker densities, with critical shortages of skilled professionals such as doctors and nurses [46]. To address this, the government introduced initiatives like the Emergency Human Resources Program to increase workforce numbers and improve distribution. However, low salaries, heavy workloads, and limited access to essential equipment and supplies continue to undermine job satisfaction. International aid and partnerships, including support from the UK Department for International Development (DfID) and the Norwegian Agency for Development Cooperation (NORAD), play a vital role in training and retaining health workers [47].

In Zambia, data was collected from four provinces and districts—Central (Kabwe), Copperbelt (Kitwe), Luapula (Mwense), and Eastern (Sinda). The country's health workforce has grown due to increased investments in training institutions and partnerships with global-health initiatives. However, high attrition rates remain a challenge, particularly in rural and remote areas. Contributing factors include inadequate remuneration, limited career-advancement opportunities, and insufficient infrastructure. The introduction of community health assistants has been a significant innovation, extending care to underserved areas and alleviating the workload of formal health workers [48–50].

South Sudan faces some of the most severe health-workforce challenges globally due to conflict and limited infrastructure. The health workforce is small, with most of the health facilities functioning as a result of donor funding [51]. Frequent insecurity disrupts service delivery and deters workers from remaining in the profession [52]. Despite these challenges, there is growing international support to train health workers locally and build capacity for a resilient health system. Data was collected from five states and counties—Warrap

(Twic East, Tonj South), Western Bahr el Ghazal (Wau), Eastern (Kapoeta South), Central Equatoria (Juba and Kajokeji), and Western Equatoria (Yambio, Maridi, and Nzara).

In Senegal, data was collected from five districts: Kolda, Sédhiou, Goudomp, Matam, and Guédiawaye. The expanding health infrastructure in Senegal has been accompanied by a growing health workforce, which is attributed to reinforced training programs that built on the national training plan for health personnel that was established in 1996 [53]. The country has a strong tradition of community-based healthcare, with health posts and community health workers playing vital roles. However, disparities in workforce distribution and insufficient financial incentives remain significant barriers to achieving equitable health-service delivery. Recent investments in digital health have improved workforce efficiency and data management, though these initiatives are still in the early stages [54,55].

2.3. Study Respondents

The health-workforce data was collected from health facilities and community health workers present in the health facilities at the time of the survey. The study included healthcare workers who had worked in primary health facilities (health centers, dispensaries, health posts, and nursing homes) for more than one year. The facility in-charge and 2 healthcare workers per facility, i.e., nurses/midwives, the Clinical Officer, Medical Officer and admins, were interviewed. At the community level, Community Health Volunteers working within the catchment area of the facility targeted were interviewed.

2.4. Data Collection

The job-satisfaction assessment tool was adopted from a validated tool by Alpern et.al (2013) [56], originally developed for use in low-income healthcare settings. The tool was reviewed by staff from all the country offices to ensure contextual relevance and organization alignment. The survey data collection tool was organized into five dimensions: employee–employer relationships, remuneration and recognition, professional development, physical environment, and supportive supervision, to effectively assess job satisfaction and health among workers. The responses were measured on a 5-point Likert scale of 0: Not applicable, 1: Very dissatisfied, 2: Dissatisfied, 3: Neutral, 4: Satisfied, and 5: Very satisfied. Tools were collaboratively reviewed by countries and aligned to fit the context, and questions for each dimension were drafted from the existing literature and practice to ensure validity. The main tool in the English version was then translated to Kiswahili for Kenya and Tanzania, Arabic for South Sudan, Amharic for Ethiopia, French for Senegal, and Chichewa for Zambia and Malawi. Each country conducted standardized training sessions for research assistants and embarked on a pretest of tools to ensure reliability. Teams converged after the pretest exercise to discuss revisions required based on the pretest; updates were incorporated into the tools, including KoboCollect forms, before the actual data collection. Data collection continued simultaneously from November 2023 to January 2024 in all the countries using the KoboCollect tool, and the data was stored in secure Kobo servers. The data was then downloaded into Excel workbooks for cleaning and later uploaded into R version 4.2.3 (c) 2023, The R Foundation for Statistical Computing, for analysis. The satisfaction survey tool for health workers has been added as a Supplementary Material.

2.5. Sample-Size Determination

Each of the countries used a two-stage cluster sampling formula to compute the number of health facilities and health workers per facility to be interviewed. This method ensured a representative sample of health workers across diverse geographic and facility contexts, while accounting for the hierarchical structure of health systems.

The sample sizes were calculated using the formulae where the sample size (n) was calculated based on a 95% confidence interval (Z = 1.96) and a margin of error (MOE) of 0.05, adjusted for clustering using the design effect (DEFF). The DEFF accounted for variability at two levels: primary and secondary clusters. It is calculated as DEFF = 1 + (M1 − 1) × ICC1 + (M2ij − 1) × ICC2ij, where M1 was the average size of primary clusters (number of health workers per subcounty per 10,000 population), M2ij was the average number of health workers in a health facility (HF) within a subcounty, ICC1 was the intra-cluster correlation at the primary cluster level, and ICC2ij the intra-cluster correlation at the secondary cluster level. Each country adjusted its calculated sample size by 10% to account for potential non-responses.

$$n = \left[\frac{Z^2 \cdot \pi_1 \cdot \pi_{2ij} \cdot M_1 \cdot M_{2ij}}{MOE^2 \cdot DEFF} \right]$$

The study employed a two-stage cluster sampling design to select health facilities and health workers in each of the eight countries. This approach aimed to ensure a representative sample of health workers across various regions while accounting for the hierarchical structure of the data. The sampling procedure can be broken down as follows.

In the first stage, a list of eligible health facilities was compiled from each country's health-department database. The facilities were selected using a probability proportional to size (PPS) method to ensure that facilities with larger populations of health workers had a higher chance of being selected. This approach was applied to all health facilities within the defined geographic regions of each country, considering factors like urban vs. rural settings and facility type (e.g., hospitals, health centers).

In the second stage, within each selected health facility, purposive sampling was utilized to select health-facility incharges. Additionally, two health workers present at the facility during the day of the interview were randomly selected. However, in some cases, the total number of respondents per facility exceeded the straightforward ratio of 1 facility in-charge and 2 staff members. This discrepancy was due to purposeful oversampling to account for potential non-responses and to ensure sufficient representation of health workers across different cadres and demographics, enhancing the statistical robustness and generalizability of the findings. If some health workers were unavailable for interviews, additional staff were selected to maintain the desired sample size.

The health-worker sample was distributed equally across health-facilities samples, to obtain a probable number of persons to interview per facility. In smaller facilities with fewer staff than the required number, all available workers were interviewed. In contrast, larger facilities could support additional respondents, ensuring the sample targets were met. All of the targeted respondents participated in the survey, resulting in a 100% response rate. This comprehensive participation strengthened the reliability of the data and allowed for richer analysis of the factors influencing job satisfaction among primary healthcare workers.

Table 1 (referenced below) presents the number of health facilities and health workers interviewed in each country. The distribution of health-worker interviews across facilities was proportionally allocated to ensure representativeness.

Table 1. Sample size by country.

Sample Type	Ethiopia	Kenya	Tanzania	Malawi	South Sudan	Uganda	Senegal	Zambia	Total
Respondents	171	143	615	123	66	310	192	91	1711
Response Rate	100%	100%	100%	100%	100%	100%	100%	100%	100%

Table 1. *Cont.*

Sample Type	Ethiopia	Kenya	Tanzania	Malawi	South Sudan	Uganda	Senegal	Zambia	Total
% proportion of sample size against the total health workforce in the area of study	9.99%	8.36%	35.94%	7.19%	3.86%	18.12%	11.22%	5.32%	100.00%
Health Facilities	65	49	93	32	64	21	13	20	357

2.6. Data Analysis

For analysis, the quantitative data underwent univariate (descriptive) and bivariate (cross-tabulation) analysis, with the results presented in tables disaggregated by country, gender, and age categories. The data was grouped into five themes that spoke about different elements that make up job satisfaction. These themes were analyzed separately, but their results collectively formed overall job satisfaction. These were

1. Employer–Employee Relationship
   This component of job satisfaction was assessed by looking at factors such as the support received from the management, the evaluation of work based on a fair system of performance standards, and the extent to which the institutional rules in place made it easy to work;
2. Remuneration
   When evaluating remuneration as an aspect of job satisfaction, different components were considered. These included the pay being commensurate with the amount of work performed, the pay being commensurate with one's skills, the bonuses and allowances received, and whether the worker's efforts were being recognized;
3. Professional Development
   Job satisfaction as it relates to the professional development of health workers was examined by looking at the Training Opportunities for Professional Development that were available to the health workers, their satisfaction with the Space and Opportunities to Learn New Skills, and the Quality of Blended Training Received;
4. Physical Environment
   This was composed of factors like the Protection against Occupational Hazards, the Sufficiency of Work Equipment, the Safety of the Physical Environment, and satisfaction regarding the housing facilities/housing allowance provided;
5. Supportive Supervision
   Supportive supervision was analyzed by looking at the Coaching Received from the Direct Supervisor, the extent to which suggestions are heard by the supervisor, and the availability of the supervisor to answer work-related questions

3. Results

3.1. Demographic and Professional Characteristics

A total of 1711 health workers participated in the study, with representation from Tanzania (36%), Uganda (18%), Senegal (11%), Ethiopia (10%), Kenya (8%), Malawi (7%), Zambia (5%), and South Sudan (4%). The median length of service among the respondents was 8 years, with Zambia reporting the longest median at 11 years and Ethiopia the shortest at 7 years. Overall, the median facility service length was 4 years, with Zambia and Senegal having the highest at 6 years and Ethiopia and Malawi having the lowest at 3 years. Gender distribution revealed that women made up the majority of health workers in most countries, apart from Malawi and South Sudan. Overall, 59% of respondents were female, with Zambia exhibiting the highest proportion (72%), followed by Tanzania (64%), Senegal (60%), Kenya (59%), Uganda (58%), Ethiopia (55%), South Sudan (45%), and Malawi (43%). The median age of respondents was 36 years, with Zambia reporting the highest median at 42 years and Ethiopia reporting the lowest at 30 years. Community-based health workers made up 40% of the workforce, with the highest representation in Senegal (77%) and the lowest in Ethiopia (8.2%), while facility-based health workers accounted for the remaining 60%. See Table 2 for details.

Table 2. Characteristics of the health workforce.

Characteristic	Overall (n = 1711)	Ethiopia (n = 171.10%)	Kenya (n = 143.8%)	Malawi (n = 123.7%)	Senegal (n= 192.11%)	South Sudan (n = 66.4%)	Tanzania (n = 615.36%)	Uganda (n = 310.18%)	Zambia (n = 91.5%)
Length of Service (Years)									
Median (lower, upper years)	8 (4, 14)	7 (4, 10)	10 (6, 14)	8 (3, 16)	8 (5, 13)	8 (4, 14)	8 (3, 13)	10 (5, 16)	11 (5, 18)
Service Length in Facility (Years)									
Median (lower, upper years)	4 (2, 9)	3 (2, 5)	4 (2, 7)	3 (1, 6)	6 (3, 11)	4 (2, 6)	5 (2, 9)	5 (2, 13)	6 (4, 13)
Respondent Sex									
Female	1003 (59%)	93 (55%)	83 (59%)	52 (43%)	113 (60%)	29 (45%)	391 (64%)	177 (58%)	65 (72%)
Male	688 (41%)	77 (45%)	57 (41%)	69 (57%)	76 (40%)	36 (55%)	220 (36%)	128 (42%)	25 (28%)
Respondent Age (Years)									
Median (lower, upper years)	36 (30, 45)	30 (28, 35)	37 (32, 43)	37 (30, 45)	36 (30, 44)	35 (31, 46)	36 (30, 47)	37 (32, 47)	42 (32, 54)
Cadre									
Community-Based	684 (40%)	14 (8.2%)	42 (29%)	27 (22%)	140 (77%)	11 (17%)	254 (41%)	149 (49%)	47 (52%)
Facility-Based	1005 (60%)	156 (92%)	101 (71%)	95 (78%)	43 (23%)	52 (83%)	361 (59%)	153 (51%)	44 (48%)

3.2. *Job Satisfaction*

Satisfaction with the employer–employee relationship was highest in Zambia (80%) and lowest in Tanzania (16%). Remuneration satisfaction was notably higher in Senegal (63%) and was followed by Zambia (49%), but was extremely low in Malawi (9.8%) and Ethiopia (2.3%). Overall, 44% of the respondents reported being satisfied with their professional development, with Uganda leading (62%) and Ethiopia reporting the lowest satisfaction (29%). Satisfaction with the physical environment stood at 27% overall, with Uganda reporting the highest (40%) and Kenya the lowest (12%). Satisfaction with supervisory support was at 62%, with Zambia showing the highest satisfaction levels (73%) and Ethiopia the lowest (30%). See Table 3 below.

Table 3. Job satisfaction of health workforce.

Characteristic	Overall (n = 1711)	Ethiopia (n = 171.10%)	Kenya (n = 143.8%)	Malawi (n = 123.7%)	Senegal (n = 192.11%)	South Sudan (n = 66.4%)	Tanzania (n = 615.36%)	Uganda (n = 310.18%)	Zambia (n = 91.5%)
Employee–Employer Satisfaction									
Not Satisfactory	1004 (59%)	104 (61%)	57 (40%)	71 (58%)	107 (56%)	32 (48%)	510 (84%)	105 (34%)	18 (20%)
Satisfactory	693 (41%)	67 (39%)	85 (60%)	52 (42%)	83 (44%)	34 (52%)	94 (16%)	205 (66%)	73 (80%)

Table 3. *Cont.*

Characteristic	Overall (n = 1711)	Ethiopia (n = 171.10%)	Kenya (n = 143.8%)	Malawi (n = 123.7%)	Senegal (n = 192.11%)	South Sudan (n = 66.4%)	Tanzania (n = 615.36%)	Uganda (n = 310.18%)	Zambia (n = 91.5%)
Remuneration Satisfaction									
Not Satisfactory	1258 (74%)	167 (98%)	107 (75%)	111 (90%)	71 (37%)	55 (83%)	505 (82%)	196 (63%)	46 (51%)
Satisfactory	453 (26%)	4 (2.3%)	36 (25%)	12 (9.8%)	121 (63%)	11 (17%)	110 (18%)	114 (37%)	45 (49%)
Professional-Development Satisfaction									
Not Satisfactory	929 (56%)	121 (71%)	87 (61%)	74 (62%)	104 (56%)	30 (46%)	358 (61%)	117 (38%)	38 (42%)
Satisfactory	742 (44%)	49 (29%)	55 (39%)	46 (38%)	81 (44%)	35 (54%)	231 (39%)	193 (62%)	52 (58%)
Physical-Environment Satisfaction									
Not Satisfactory	1232 (73%)	141 (82%)	125 (88%)	97 (79%)	120 (66%)	46 (71%)	456 (74%)	185 (60%)	62 (68%)
Satisfactory	467 (27%)	30 (18%)	17 (12%)	26 (21%)	63 (34%)	19 (29%)	159 (26%)	124 (40%)	29 (32%)
Support Supervisory Satisfaction									
Not Satisfactory	647 (38%)	120 (70%)	43 (30%)	66 (54%)	75 (40%)	30 (45%)	195 (32%)	93 (30%)	25 (27%)
Satisfactory	1058 (62%)	51 (30%)	98 (70%)	56 (46%)	114 (60%)	36 (55%)	420 (68%)	217 (70%)	66 (73%)

3.3. Predictors of Employer–Employee Relationship Satisfaction

The multivariable analysis of employer–employee-relationship satisfaction revealed significant variations based on country, demographics, and job-related factors (Table 4). Health workers in Zambia showed the highest odds of satisfaction with their employer (OR = 4.97, 95% CI: 2.48–10.30, $p < 0.001$), followed by Uganda (OR = 2.17, 95% CI: 1.35–3.49, $p = 0.001$). Conversely, Tanzania struggles the most (OR = 0.17, 95% CI: 0.11–0.27, $p < 0.001$), indicating widespread dissatisfaction. Satisfaction was also associated with longer service duration. Health workers satisfied with their employer had a mean service duration of 11.1 years, compared to 9.7 years for those dissatisfied (OR = 1.03, 95% CI: 1.01–1.06, $p = 0.014$). Professional cadre influenced satisfaction, with facility-based workers being more likely to report satisfaction than community-based workers (OR = 3.49, 95% CI: 2.51–4.89, $p < 0.001$). Job attributes such as pay, professional growth opportunities, the physical environment, and supervisory support were strongly correlated with employer satisfaction. Workers satisfied with their pay were 74% more likely to be satisfied with their employer (OR = 1.74, 95% CI: 1.25–2.41, $p = 0.001$). Positive perceptions of professional development (OR = 2.24, 95% CI: 1.73–2.92, $p < 0.001$) and the workplace environment (OR = 1.98, 95% CI: 1.47–2.66, $p < 0.001$) significantly increased satisfaction. The strongest association was with supervisory support, where workers who felt supported were over three times more likely to be satisfied with their employer (OR = 3.34, 95% CI: 2.51–4.45, $p < 0.001$).

Table 4. Predictors of employer–employee-relationship satisfaction among health workforce in 8 African countries.

Health Workforce: Characteristics		OR (Univariable)	OR (Multivariable)
Country Name	Ethiopia	-	-
	Kenya	2.31 (1.47–3.66, $p < 0.001$)	1.60 (0.94–2.72, $p = 0.085$)
	Malawi	1.14 (0.71–1.82, $p = 0.594$)	0.99 (0.57–1.69, $p = 0.957$)
	Senegal	1.20 (0.79–1.84, $p = 0.386$)	1.05 (0.60–1.82, $p = 0.871$)
	South Sudan	1.65 (0.93–2.93, $p = 0.087$)	1.18 (0.60–2.33, $p = 0.632$)
	Tanzania	0.29 (0.20–0.42, $p < 0.001$)	0.17 (0.11–0.27, $p < 0.001$)
	Uganda	3.03 (2.06–4.48, $p < 0.001$)	2.17 (1.35–3.49, $p = 0.001$)
	Zambia	6.30 (3.52–11.74, $p < 0.001$)	4.97 (2.48–10.30, $p < 0.001$)

Table 4. *Cont.*

Health Workforce: Characteristics		OR (Univariable)	OR (Multivariable)
Length of Service (Years)	Mean (SD)	1.02 (1.01–1.03, $p = 0.001$)	1.03 (1.01–1.06, $p = 0.014$)
Service Length in Facility (Years)	Mean (SD)	1.01 (1.00–1.03, $p = 0.055$)	0.99 (0.96–1.02, $p = 0.469$)
Respondent Sex	Female Male	- 1.03 (0.84–1.26, $p = 0.772$)	- 1.09 (0.84–1.40, $p = 0.523$)
Respondent Age	Mean (SD)	1.01 (1.00–1.02, $p = 0.085$)	0.99 (0.97–1.01, $p = 0.314$)
Cadre	Community Based Facility Based	- 1.37 (1.12–1.67, $p = 0.002$)	- 3.49 (2.51–4.89, $p < 0.001$)
Renumeration Satisfaction	not satisfactory satisfactory	- 1.77 (1.42–2.20, $p < 0.001$)	- 1.74 (1.25–2.41, $p = 0.001$)
Professional Development Satisfaction	not satisfactory satisfactory	- 3.12 (2.55–3.83, $p < 0.001$)	- 2.24 (1.73–2.92, $p < 0.001$)
Physical Environment Satisfaction	not satisfactory satisfactory	- 2.03 (1.63–2.52, $p < 0.001$)	- 1.98 (1.47–2.66, $p < 0.001$)
Support Supervisory Satisfaction	not satisfactory satisfactory	- 3.22 (2.59–4.00, $p < 0.001$)	- 3.34 (2.51–4.45, $p < 0.001$)

OR = Odds Ratio, SD = Standard Deviation.

3.4. Predictors of Remuneration Satisfaction

Table 5 presents the predictors of remuneration satisfaction across the eight countries. Health workers in Senegal were the most satisfied with their pay (OR = 26.34, 95% CI: 10.04–90.98, $p < 0.001$), followed by those in Zambia (OR = 19.47, 95% CI: 6.98–69.82, $p < 0.001$). In contrast, only 2.3% of Ethiopian health workers reported satisfaction with their remuneration. Significant satisfaction levels were also observed in Kenya (OR = 8.49, 95% CI: 3.10–30.02, $p < 0.001$), Uganda (OR = 8.86, 95% CI: 3.46–30.13, $p < 0.001$), and Tanzania (OR = 4.98, 95% CI: 1.94–16.98, $p = 0.003$). While univariable analysis suggested an association between length of service and remuneration satisfaction (OR = 1.05, 95% CI: 1.03–1.07, $p < 0.001$), this was not significant in the multivariable model (OR = 1.02, 95% CI: 0.99–1.05, $p = 0.281$). Facility-based health workers were significantly less likely to be satisfied with their pay than community-based workers (OR = 0.20, 95% CI: 0.15–0.28, $p < 0.001$). Job attributes also played a critical role in remuneration satisfaction. Positive employer–employee relationships (OR = 1.64, 95% CI: 1.17–2.31, $p = 0.004$), professional-development opportunities (OR = 1.59, 95% CI: 1.18–2.15, $p = 0.002$), and a favorable physical environment (OR = 1.57, 95% CI: 1.16–2.12, $p = 0.003$) were all associated with higher remuneration satisfaction. However, supervisory support was not a significant predictor in the multivariable analysis (OR = 1.11, 95% CI: 0.80–1.56, $p = 0.525$).

Table 5. Predictors of renumeration satisfaction among health workforce in 8 African countries.

Health Workforce: Renumeration		OR (Univariable)	OR (Multivariable)
Country Name	Ethiopia Kenya Malawi Senegal South Sudan Tanzania Uganda Zambia	- 14.05 (5.43–47.95, $p < 0.001$) 4.51 (1.53–16.47, $p = 0.011$) 71.15 (28.55–238.32, $p < 0.001$) 8.35 (2.73–31.11, $p < 0.001$) 9.09 (3.75–29.99, $p < 0.001$) 24.28 (9.94–80.39, $p < 0.001$) 40.84 (15.59–140.80, $p < 0.001$)	- 8.49 (3.10–30.02, $p < 0.001$) 3.43 (1.12–12.88, $p = 0.043$) 26.34 (10.04–90.98, $p < 0.001$) 2.72 (0.71–11.50, $p = 0.149$) 4.98 (1.94–16.98, $p = 0.003$) 8.86 (3.46–30.13, $p < 0.001$) 19.47 (6.98–69.82, $p < 0.001$)
Length of Service (Years)	Mean (SD)	1.02 (1.01–1.03, $p = 0.005$)	1.00 (0.97–1.03, $p = 0.880$)

Table 5. *Cont.*

Health Workforce: Renumeration		OR (Univariable)	OR (Multivariable)
Service Length in Facility (Years)	Mean (SD)	1.05 (1.03–1.07, $p < 0.001$)	1.02 (0.99–1.05, $p = 0.281$)
Respondent Sex	Female Male	- 0.98 (0.78–1.22, $p = 0.836$)	- 1.17 (0.89–1.54, $p = 0.268$)
Respondent Age	Mean (SD)	1.02 (1.01–1.03, $p < 0.001$)	0.99 (0.97–1.00, $p = 0.141$)
Cadre	Community Based Facility Based	- 0.15 (0.12–0.20, $p < 0.001$)	- 0.20 (0.15–0.28, $p < 0.001$)
Employee–Employer Satisfaction	not satisfactory satisfactory	- 1.77 (1.42–2.20, $p < 0.001$)	- 1.64 (1.17–2.31, $p = 0.004$)
Professional Development Satisfaction	not satisfactory satisfactory	- 2.28 (1.83–2.85, $p < 0.001$)	- 1.59 (1.18–2.15, $p = 0.002$)
Physical Environment Satisfaction	not satisfactory satisfactory	- 2.65 (2.10–3.33, $p < 0.001$)	- 1.57 (1.16–2.12, $p = 0.003$)
Support Supervisory Satisfaction	not satisfactory satisfactory	- 1.87 (1.48–2.37, $p < 0.001$)	- 1.11 (0.80–1.56, $p = 0.525$)

OR = Odds Ratio, SD = Standard Deviation.

3.5. Predictors of Health-Worker Satisfaction with Professional Development

Table 6 outlines the predictors of health-worker satisfaction with professional development. Health workers satisfied with employer–employee relationships were significantly more likely to be satisfied with their professional development (OR = 2.20, 95% CI: 1.69–2.85, $p < 0.001$). Satisfaction with remuneration (OR = 1.59, 95% CI: 1.19–2.13, $p = 0.002$), the physical environment (OR = 1.71, 95% CI: 1.32–2.22, $p < 0.001$), and supervisory support (OR = 3.58, 95% CI: 2.78–4.62, $p < 0.001$) were also strong predictors. While satisfaction varied by country, it was not a significant predictor after adjusting for other factors. Although health workers in Uganda and South Sudan reported higher satisfaction, these findings were not statistically significant in the multivariable analysis. Demographic factors such as sex, age, and professional cadre had no significant impact, nor did facility tenure or total years of service.

Table 6. Predictors of professional-development satisfaction among health workforce in 8 African countries.

Health Workforce: Professional Development		OR (Univariable)	OR (Multivariable)
Country Name	Ethiopia Kenya Malawi Senegal South Sudan Tanzania Uganda Zambia	- 1.56 (0.97–2.51, $p = 0.065$) 1.54 (0.93–2.52, $p = 0.090$) 1.92 (1.24–3.00, $p = 0.004$) 2.88 (1.60–5.23, $p < 0.001$) 1.59 (1.11–2.32, $p = 0.014$) 4.07 (2.74–6.14, $p < 0.001$) 3.38 (1.99–5.80, $p < 0.001$)	- 0.71 (0.41–1.22, $p = 0.218$) 1.11 (0.63–1.94, $p = 0.716$) 0.93 (0.54–1.61, $p = 0.796$) 1.97 (0.99–3.93, $p = 0.053$) 0.99 (0.64–1.55, $p = 0.975$) 1.52 (0.95–2.46, $p = 0.085$) 0.96 (0.51–1.81, $p = 0.901$)
Length of Service (Years)	Mean (SD)	1.02 (1.01–1.03, $p = 0.001$)	1.01 (0.99–1.04, $p = 0.297$)
Service Length in Facility (Years)	Mean (SD)	1.03 (1.01–1.04, $p < 0.001$)	0.98 (0.96–1.01, $p = 0.146$)
Respondent Sex	Female Male	- 0.95 (0.78–1.16, $p = 0.621$)	- 0.99 (0.78–1.24, $p = 0.916$)
Respondent Age	Mean (SD)	1.02 (1.01–1.03, $p < 0.001$)	1.01 (0.99–1.03, $p = 0.254$)
Cadre	Community Based Facility Based	- 0.70 (0.58–0.85, $p < 0.001$)	- 0.88 (0.66–1.16, $p = 0.359$)

Table 6. *Cont.*

Health Workforce: Professional Development		OR (Univariable)	OR (Multivariable)
Employee–Employer Satisfaction	not satisfactory	-	-
	satisfactory	3.12 (2.55–3.83, $p < 0.001$)	2.20 (1.69–2.85, $p < 0.001$)
Remuneration Satisfaction	not satisfactory	-	-
	satisfactory	2.28 (1.83–2.85, $p < 0.001$)	1.59 (1.19–2.13, $p = 0.002$)
Physical-Environment Satisfaction	not satisfactory	-	-
	satisfactory	2.69 (2.16–3.36, $p < 0.001$)	1.71 (1.32–2.22, $p < 0.001$)
Support Supervisory Satisfaction	not satisfactory	-	-
	satisfactory	4.63 (3.72–5.80, $p < 0.001$)	3.58 (2.78–4.62, $p < 0.001$)

OR = Odds Ratio, SD = Standard Deviation.

3.6. Predictors of Physical-Environment Satisfaction

The predictors of physical-environment satisfaction are presented in Table 7. Satisfaction with the physical environment was significantly influenced by employer–employee relationships (OR = 1.96, 95% CI: 1.46–2.64, $p < 0.001$), remuneration satisfaction (OR = 1.59, 95% CI: 1.18–2.14, $p = 0.002$), professional-development satisfaction (OR = 1.68, 95% CI: 1.29–2.19, $p < 0.001$), and supervisory support (OR = 2.14, 95% CI: 1.59–2.91, $p < 0.001$). Healthcare workers in Kenya (OR = 0.26, 95% CI: 0.13–0.53, $p < 0.001$) and Zambia (OR = 0.49, 95% CI: 0.24–0.99, $p = 0.046$) were significantly less likely to report satisfaction with their physical environment compared to Ethiopian workers.

Table 7. Predictors of physical-environment satisfaction among health workforce in 8 African countries.

Health Workforce:		OR (Univariable)	OR (Multivariable)
Country Name	Ethiopia	-	-
	Kenya	0.64 (0.33–1.20, $p = 0.172$)	0.26 (0.13–0.53, $p < 0.001$)
	Malawi	1.26 (0.70–2.26, $p = 0.439$)	0.85 (0.44–1.62, $p = 0.622$)
	Senegal	2.47 (1.51–4.10, $p < 0.001$)	0.61 (0.33–1.11, $p = 0.100$)
	South Sudan	1.94 (0.99–3.76, $p = 0.050$)	1.10 (0.51–2.36, $p = 0.800$)
	Tanzania	1.64 (1.08–2.57, $p = 0.026$)	0.84 (0.51–1.41, $p = 0.503$)
	Uganda	3.15 (2.02–5.03, $p < 0.001$)	0.82 (0.48–1.42, $p = 0.478$)
	Zambia	2.20 (1.22–3.98, $p = 0.009$)	0.49 (0.24–0.99, $p = 0.046$)
Length of Service (Years)	Mean (SD)	1.01 (1.00–1.03, $p = 0.033$)	0.99 (0.96–1.02, $p = 0.510$)
Service Length in Facility (Years)	Mean (SD)	1.04 (1.03–1.06, $p < 0.001$)	1.02 (0.99–1.05, $p = 0.175$)
Respondent Sex	Female	-	-
	Male	0.89 (0.71–1.10, $p = 0.282$)	0.84 (0.65–1.08, $p = 0.171$)
Respondent Age	Mean (SD)	1.02 (1.01–1.03, $p < 0.001$)	0.99 (0.98–1.01, $p = 0.444$)
Cadre	Community Based	-	-
	Facility Based	0.29 (0.23–0.36, $p < 0.001$)	0.31 (0.23–0.41, $p < 0.001$)
Employee–Employer Satisfaction	not satisfactory	-	-
	satisfactory	2.03 (1.63–2.52, $p < 0.001$)	1.96 (1.46–2.64, $p < 0.001$)
Renumeration Satisfaction	not satisfactory	-	-
	satisfactory	2.65 (2.10–3.33, $p < 0.001$)	1.59 (1.18–2.14, $p = 0.002$)
Professional-Development Satisfaction	not satisfactory	-	-
	satisfactory	2.69 (2.16–3.36, $p < 0.001$)	1.68 (1.29–2.19, $p < 0.001$)
Support Supervisory Satisfaction	not satisfactory	-	-
	satisfactory	3.06 (2.39–3.95, $p < 0.001$)	2.14 (1.59–2.91, $p < 0.001$)

OR = Odds Ratio, SD = Standard Deviation.

Interestingly, while the length of service did not emerge as a significant predictor, facility-based workers were significantly less likely to report satisfaction with the physical environment compared to community-based workers (OR = 0.31, 95% CI: 0.23–0.41, $p < 0.001$).

3.7. Predictors of Supportive Supervision Satisfaction

The predictors of satisfaction with supportive supervision are summarized in Table 8. Satisfaction was most strongly associated with remuneration (OR = 2.39, 95% CI: 1.77–3.22, $p < 0.001$) and employer–employee relationships (OR = 2.51, 95% CI: 1.90–3.30, $p < 0.001$). Similarly, satisfaction with professional development (OR = 1.95, 95% CI: 1.41–2.68, $p < 0.001$) and the physical environment (OR = 2.10, 95% CI: 1.59–2.76, $p < 0.001$) were significant predictors of supportive supervision satisfaction. Tanzania (OR = 6.53, 95% CI: 4.19–10.33, $p < 0.001$) and Kenya (OR= 5.02, 95% CI: 2.88–8.89, $p < 0.001$) showed the highest and most significant levels of satisfaction with supervision, while health workers in Malawi (OR =1.86, 95% CI: 1.05–3.29, $p = 0.032$) were significantly less likely to report satisfaction.

Table 8. Predictors of supportive supervision satisfaction among the health workforce in 8 African countries.

Health Workforce:		OR (Univariable)	OR (Multivariable)
Country Name	Ethiopia	-	-
	Kenya	5.36 (3.32–8.79, $p < 0.001$)	5.02 (2.88–8.89, $p < 0.001$)
	Malawi	2.00 (1.23–3.25, $p = 0.005$)	1.86 (1.05–3.29, $p = 0.032$)
	Senegal	3.58 (2.32–5.58, $p < 0.001$)	2.78 (1.58–4.95, $p < 0.001$)
	South Sudan	2.82 (1.58–5.10, $p = 0.001$)	1.87 (0.93–3.80, $p = 0.081$)
	Tanzania	5.07 (3.52–7.38, $p < 0.001$)	6.53 (4.19–10.33, $p < 0.001$)
	Uganda	5.49 (3.67–8.31, $p < 0.001$)	3.12 (1.91–5.16, $p < 0.001$)
	Zambia	6.21 (3.57–11.09, $p < 0.001$)	3.03 (1.56–6.03, $p = 0.001$)
Length of Service (Years)	Mean (SD)	1.02 (1.01–1.03, $p = 0.001$)	0.99 (0.97–1.02, $p = 0.619$)
Service Length in Facility (Years)	Mean (SD)	1.04 (1.03–1.06, $p < 0.001$)	1.04 (1.01–1.07, $p = 0.003$)
Respondent Sex	Female	-	-
	Male	0.86 (0.70–1.05, $p = 0.135$)	0.89 (0.70–1.13, $p = 0.326$)
Respondent Age	Mean (SD)	1.02 (1.01–1.03, $p < 0.001$)	1.00 (0.98–1.01, $p = 0.606$)
Cadre	Community Based	-	-
	Facility Based	0.67 (0.55–0.82, $p < 0.001$)	1.08 (0.80–1.46, $p = 0.601$)
Employee–Employer Satisfaction	not satisfactory	-	-
	satisfactory	3.22 (2.59–4.00, $p < 0.001$)	3.10 (2.34–4.11, $p < 0.001$)
Remuneration Satisfaction	not satisfactory	-	-
	satisfactory	1.87 (1.48–2.37, $p < 0.001$)	1.15 (0.83–1.60, $p = 0.410$)
Professional-Development Satisfaction	not satisfactory	-	-
	satisfactory	4.63 (3.72–5.80, $p < 0.001$)	3.55 (2.76–4.59, $p < 0.001$)
Physical-Environment Satisfaction	not satisfactory	-	-
	satisfactory	3.06 (2.39–3.95, $p < 0.001$)	2.12 (1.57–2.86, $p < 0.001$)

OR = Odds Ratio, SD = Standard Deviation.

4. Discussion

This study offers insights into the demographic and professional characteristics of health workers across eight African countries, highlighting variations in workforce composition, tenure, and gender distribution. Tanzania had the largest representation (36%), followed by Uganda (18%) and Senegal (11%), while Zambia (5%) and South Sudan (4%) had the smallest, reflecting differences in workforce distribution and study participation. The median length of service was 8 years, with Zambia reporting the longest at 11 years and Ethiopia the shortest at 7 years. Zambia and Senegal had the longest median facility-service duration (6 years), suggesting a relatively stable workforce, whereas Ethiopia and Malawi had the shortest (3 years), potentially indicating higher turnover or workforce mobility.

The average length of service for healthcare workers in Sub-Saharan Africa (SSA) is significantly shorter compared to high-income regions, primarily due to high attrition rates driven by migration, burnout, and poor working conditions. Studies suggest that many doctors and nurses leave their positions within 5–10 years, with some departing even sooner for better opportunities abroad [57–59]. For instance, the World Health Organisation (WHO) reports that 55% of African-trained doctors emigrate to wealthier nations, particularly to Europe, North America, and the Gulf states, within a few years of qualification [60]. Nurses and midwives tend to stay slightly longer, averaging 5–10 years, but these roles still face high turnover due to low wages and heavy workloads [57,61,62]. Community health workers (CHWs), who play a crucial role in rural healthcare, often have even shorter tenures (2–5 years) because of informal employment structures and inadequate compensation [63].

The high turnover in some countries could point to job dissatisfaction, poor working conditions, or a lack of career-growth opportunities. Countries such as Zambia and Uganda, which showed longer service duration, may do so because of better retention policies, but this could also indicate fewer opportunities for mobility or promotion. While the findings suggest that health workers have multiple years of service, sub-Saharan Africa is faced with challenges such as corruption, poor working conditions, and a sub-optimal use of time, which end up affecting overall healthcare delivery [64].

Women comprised the majority of health workers in all countries except Malawi and South Sudan. Overall, 59% of respondents were female, with the highest proportion in Zambia (72%), whereas Malawi (43%) and South Sudan (45%) have a more balanced or male-dominated workforce. Such variations may have implications for gender-sensitive health services, particularly in maternal and child-health programs, where female health workers often play a crucial role. The predominance of female health workers aligns with global trends, particularly in nursing and community health roles where women make up 70% of the workforce [65].

The median age of health workers was 36 years, with Zambia having the oldest median at 42 years and Ethiopia the youngest at 30 years. The relatively older workforce in Zambia suggests a more experienced health sector, whereas Ethiopia's younger workforce could indicate recent recruitment efforts or a higher attrition of older health professionals. However, Africa's general population is notably young, with a median age of about 20 years. This youthful demographic suggests that the health workforce may also be relatively young, which calls for in-service training, mentorship, and career-progression opportunities to improve care [66].

This study assessed job satisfaction among 1711 health workers across eight sub-Saharan African countries, Ethiopia, Kenya, Malawi, Senegal, South Sudan, Tanzania, Uganda, and Zambia, focusing on five dimensions: employer–employee relationships, remuneration and recognition, professional development, the physical work environment, and supportive supervision. The cross-country differences in health-worker job satisfaction observed in this study reflect broader structural, policy, and contextual factors that influence health systems across sub-Saharan Africa. For instance, Zambia's relatively high satisfaction levels across multiple domains, including employer–employee relationships and supportive supervision, may be attributed to its ongoing investments in health-workforce governance and human-resource management. Studies have shown that the implementation of supportive supervision frameworks and performance-management systems in Zambia has contributed to improved health-worker morale and retention [67,68]. In contrast, Tanzania and Ethiopia exhibited some of the lowest satisfaction levels, particularly in employer–employee relations and remuneration. Previous studies in Tanzania have highlighted systemic issues such as unclear promotion structures, delayed salaries, and insufficient recognition, which diminish health-worker motivation [69]. Similarly, in Ethiopia, chronic underinvestment in human resources and limited professional-development opportunities in rural areas have been linked to dissatisfaction and workforce attrition [70,71].

These findings align with previous research highlighting the critical role of remuneration, professional development, and working conditions in health-worker satisfaction.

Studies in Uganda and Zambia identified employer–employee relationships and supervisory support as key satisfaction drivers [72]. Tanzania reported significantly lower satisfaction at 16%, indicating potential challenges in employer engagement, communication, or workplace policies [13]. A similar study in Kenya, Uganda, and Zambia identified employer–employee relationships and supervisory support as key satisfaction drivers [73]. Positive employer–employee relationships foster a sense of workplace belonging and trust, which directly influences satisfaction with the physical work environment [74], leading to a more positive supervisory experience [16]. Additionally, the existing literature emphasizes the importance of supportive work environments, fair compensation, and effective supervision in enhancing job satisfaction among healthcare professionals [30].

The high satisfaction with remuneration observed in Senegal aligns with findings from evaluations of its performance-based financing (PBF) programs, which have introduced financial incentives and improved accountability in health facilities [75]. The low satisfaction with physical work environments in Kenya contrasts with its relatively well-resourced urban health facilities. This, however, suggests persistent inequalities in health infrastructure in urban and rural areas, as reported in studies examining health-worker experiences in county-level facilities [76]. Job attributes such as pay, professional-growth opportunities, the physical environment, and supervisory support were strongly correlated with employer satisfaction. This corroborates findings from a similar study conducted in Ethiopia, which reported salary and incentives, benefit packages, recognition by management, patient appreciation, the working environment, developmental opportunities, better management, clear communication, and staff working relationships as strong predictors of job satisfaction [77].

Health-worker satisfaction with remuneration in Africa varies across regions and is influenced by multiple factors. A study conducted in Ethiopia documented that despite governmental efforts to enhance health infrastructure and workforce numbers, national health services often struggle to attract and retain health workers. This challenge is partly due to inadequate remuneration and insufficient attention to incentives and motivation, leading to decreased productivity and increased turnover among health professionals [77]. Facility-based health workers were significantly less satisfied with their remuneration compared to community-based workers. This could be due to differences in workload, compensation models, or perceived fairness in pay structures, such as working conditions, resource availability, and management practices. The findings are similar to a study [78] which consistently identified poor remuneration, limited career growth, and inadequate working conditions as major drivers of dissatisfaction among health workers in low-resource settings. These results align with previous studies emphasizing the role of financial incentives and workplace relationships in enhancing supervisory satisfaction [30]. Additionally, a study in Uganda and Zambia has demonstrated that satisfaction with pay and management quality significantly influences job satisfaction and retention [79].

Uganda's lead in professional-development satisfaction is supported by evidence of targeted training programs and continuous professional education supported by the government and partners [75]. This aligns with findings from Namazzi who documented increased training coverage and mentoring in maternal and child-health programs. Conversely, Malawi's low scores on remuneration and recognition reflect constraints associated with wage freezes and heavy reliance on donor-funded vertical programs, which often bypass national HRH priorities [80].

These cross-country comparisons emphasize that while some countries have adopted effective workforce-strengthening strategies, others face persistent gaps in management, supervision, and support systems. These differences underscore the need for tailored health workforce policies that are responsive to national contexts, as also emphasized in the WHO's Global Strategy on Human Resources for Health [33]. Job satisfaction levels among health workers varied significantly across the eight countries studied, reflecting the influence of broader systemic, economic, and institutional differences. The higher satisfaction scores in Zambia and Senegal may reflect relatively better remuneration systems, stronger supervisory structures, or more coordinated health-workforce strategies, while lower satisfaction in Ethiopia and Malawi may stem from chronic health-system underfunding, limited professional growth, and inadequate infrastructure—patterns consistent with previous findings in low-resource settings [30,81,82]. These disparities mirror structural health-system differences that are also evident when comparing sub-Saharan Africa to high-income countries. For instance, in many OECD countries, job satisfaction among health workers tends to be higher due to better salaries, stronger professional-development pathways, safer working environments, and more participatory management practices [83,84].

In contrast to sub-Saharan Africa, where dissatisfaction is often rooted in resource scarcity and systemic weaknesses, studies from countries such as Sweden, the Netherlands, and Canada point to job satisfaction being influenced more by workload balance, autonomy, and opportunities for innovation [35,85]. Moreover, the presence of robust health-worker unions and stronger policy mechanisms for staff well-being and accountability in high-income countries contributes to greater professional agency and morale. These comparative insights highlight the importance of tailoring health-workforce strategies to local contexts while learning from successful models of governance, training, and incentives employed in more developed systems.

Organizations that prioritize career development contribute positively to health workers' satisfaction, as documented by Essex County Council in the UK, where emphasis on the career progression of its social workers led to improved morale and retention [86]. Similarly, a meta-analysis in Ethiopia identified salary, recognition, professional development, and supportive supervision as strong predictors of job satisfaction. The observed country-specific variations underscore the necessity for tailored interventions, as highlighted in studies comparing job satisfaction across different African countries.

Although most studies conducted focus on specific countries, this study, however, adds to the evidence by providing multi-country comparative data using a standardized methodology, allowing for more nuanced cross-national analysis within the sub-Saharan African context. Strengths of the study include its large, multi-country sample (n = 1711), use of a standardized data-collection tool, and a robust sampling methodology, which increase the generalizability and reliability of findings across diverse health systems. The study also assessed multiple facets of job satisfaction through multivariable regression analysis, which provided valuable insights into predictors of job satisfaction, providing a holistic view of job satisfaction in SSA countries.

Limitations of the study include potential response bias due to self-reported data and variability in the interpretation of satisfaction scales. Furthermore, although efforts were made to include a representative sample, oversampling in some facilities and reliance on availability during data collection may have introduced selection bias. The cross-sectional design also limits causal inferences, and differences in healthcare systems across countries may affect comparability [72]. Lastly, the study did not account for the impact of external factors like political instability or economic conditions, which could influence job satisfaction. The cross-sectional design restricts causal inference between predictors and satisfaction. Self-reported responses may be influenced by social desirability or cultural biases in interpreting Likert-scale items [87,88]. Furthermore, the study did not account for facility-level or regional health-system factors, such as staffing ratios, management style, or workload, which may independently affect satisfaction [89]. Future research using longitudinal, mixed-methods, or multilevel designs could provide more nuanced and generalizable evidence to inform reforms in health-worker motivation and retention.

The study provides critical, actionable insights for health-workforce strengthening in sub-Saharan Africa, grounded in Herzberg's Two-Factor Theory of Motivation. According to the theory, job satisfaction is influenced by two categories of factors: motivators (e.g., recognition, professional development, meaningful work) and hygiene factors (e.g., pay, supervision, working conditions). This study demonstrates that both sets of factors are significantly associated with health-worker satisfaction.

Key findings—such as the strong association between supervisory support, remuneration, employer–employee relationships, and job satisfaction—highlight the need for strategic investment in both intrinsic motivators and extrinsic conditions. In particular, supportive supervision emerged as the most powerful predictor of satisfaction (OR = 3.34), underscoring the importance of strengthening leadership and accountability mechanisms within health systems.

The study provides critical evidence to guide health-workforce interventions in sub-Saharan Africa. Policymakers and health-system planners should prioritize improving employer–employee relationships, investing in fair and transparent remuneration systems, enhancing supervision structures, and upgrading physical work environments. The country-specific variations underscore the need for localized strategies rather than generic approaches. Improving employer–employee relationships, ensuring fair remuneration, enhancing professional development opportunities, and providing supportive supervision are vital for boosting health-worker satisfaction and retention. These findings can serve as a baseline for evaluating the effectiveness of workforce reforms and informing donor investments in health-workforce strengthening.

5. Conclusions

This study provides compelling evidence that job satisfaction among health workers in sub-Saharan Africa is shaped by a complex interplay of factors, including employer–employee relationships, remuneration, professional-development opportunities, physical working conditions, and supportive supervision. Significant cross-country variations were observed, underscoring the critical need for context-specific workforce strategies. Countries such as Zambia and Senegal demonstrated comparatively higher levels of satisfaction across several domains, including remuneration and supervisory support, whereas Ethiopia and Tanzania consistently reported the lowest satisfaction, particularly with working conditions and managerial relationships.

The findings reinforce the importance of Herzberg's Two-Factor Theory, where both hygiene factors (e.g., pay, work environment) and motivators (e.g., recognition, advancement) must be addressed to enhance satisfaction and reduce turnover. The strong association between supervisory support and overall satisfaction highlights the value of effective management practices in motivating and retaining staff.

Moreover, the study reveals meaningful workforce dynamics, including gender imbalances, varied lengths of service, and differing distributions between facility- and community-based workers, which can influence satisfaction and performance. For instance, Zambia's longer service duration may point to better retention practices, while Ethiopia's lower tenure suggests a need to investigate and address drivers of early attrition.

To strengthen health systems across the region, targeted interventions should focus on building supportive supervision structures, ensuring fair and transparent compensation systems, fostering professional-growth opportunities, and improving physical working environments. Given the diversity across countries, one-size-fits-all solutions are unlikely to succeed. Policymakers and development partners must prioritize tailored approaches that reflect the unique health system contexts, labor-market dynamics, and demographic realities of each country.

Finally, the study serves as an important baseline for measuring progress and guiding health workforce reform. It offers actionable evidence for governments, donors, and implementers aiming to build a resilient, motivated health workforce—one that is essential for delivering quality care, reducing health inequities, and achieving broader health and development goals in sub-Saharan Africa.

Supplementary Materials: The following supporting information can be downloaded at: https://www.mdpi.com/article/10.3390/ijerph22071108/s1, Table S1: CS_02 SATISFACTION SURVEY FOR HEALTH WORKERS (INDICATOR 2.1).

Author Contributions: Conceptualization, S.M., Y.O. and M.J.; Data curation, S.M., L.O., B.A., M.J. and R.K.; Formal analysis, L.O., B.A. and R.K.; Investigation, S.M. and M.J.; Methodology, S.M., Y.O. and M.J.; Software, S.M., Y.O. and M.J.; Validation, S.M., L.O., M.J., B.A. and R.K.; Writing—original draft, S.M., Y.O., S.K., L.O., R.Z.M., B.A., M.J., I.G. and R.K.; Writing—review and editing, S.M., Y.O., S.K., L.O., R.Z.M., B.A., M.J., L.N., I.G., R.K., J.K., T.S. and G.K. All authors have read and agreed to the published version of the manuscript.

Funding: This research received no external funding and no specific grant from any funding agency in the public, commercial, or not-for-profit sectors. The research was funded by Amref Health Africa.

Institutional Review Board Statement: The countries were governed by approved research protocols that were approved by local ethics committees. Five countries received ethical approval: Ethiopia and Kenya were approved by the Amref Ethics and Scientific Review Committee (ESRC), ESRC P1580/2023 on 21 November 2023. Tanzania was approved by the National Institute for Medical Research, NIMR/HQ/R.8a/Vol.IX/4440 on 27 October 2023 and by the Zanzibar Health Research Institute, ZAHREC/04/PR/NOV/2023/35 on 17 November 2023. Zambia was approved by Eres Converge, an independent ethics board, 2023-Nov-001 on 28 November 2023 and the National Health Research Authority (NHRA) on 27 November 2023. Uganda was approved by the Uganda Christian University Review and Ethics Committee, UCUREC-2023-699 on 7 November 2023. South Sudan, Malawi, and West Africa received a waiver for a full review of their proposals from Ethics Boards because, being evaluations, they did not meet standards to undergo ethical approval according to the country standard (waiver letter from Malawi is attached for reference).

Informed Consent Statement: The researchers obtained informed consent from all participants before they participated. The participants were informed that they were free to end their involvement in the interview at any time. They were also assured that withdrawal from the study would not affect in any way the intended support from Amref Health Africa. To protect confidentiality, records contained no names or other personal identifiers. Interviews were also conducted in private to ensure there were no other people around to listen to the interviews. Care was also taken not to raise expectations that the participants or their family or community would receive material benefits such as money because of their participation. Consent for publication is not applicable.

Data Availability Statement: Data is available upon reasonable request.

Acknowledgments: We extend our sincere gratitude to the Amref Health Africa leadership and management for the crucial role they played in the successful undertaking of this survey. Without your approval and financing, this undertaking would not have been possible. We also acknowledge the special role that was played by the countries' teams and focal persons in ensuring the smooth running of the survey and the end-to-end delivery of a successful study. We deeply appreciate the effort you put into ensuring that the survey was conducted successfully. Our deepest gratitude goes to all the participants from the different countries who sacrificed their time to take part in the survey and to give valuable feedback and responses to the questions we raised. We also appreciate the research assistants who diligently took the participants through the survey with great patience and skill to enable us have quality data that has helped in the writing of the paper.

Conflicts of Interest: The authors declare that there are no conflicts of interest regarding the publication of this paper. All authors have contributed significantly to the creation of this manuscript and have read and approved the final version submitted. There are no financial or personal relationships with other people or organizations that could inappropriately influence our findings.

Abbreviations

The following abbreviations are used in this manuscript:

LMICs	Low- and Middle-Income Countries
PHC	Primary Health Care
UHC	Universal Health Coverage
HEWs	Health Extension Workers
CHVs	Community Health Volunteers
CHWs	Community Health Workers
DfID	Department for International Development
NORAD	Norwegian Agency for Development Cooperation
DHS	Demographic and Health Survey
DHIS	District Health Information System

References

1. Ivancevich, J.M.; Konopaske, R.; Matteson, M.T. *Organizational, Behavior & Management*, 10th ed.; McGraw Hill Higher Education: New York, NY, USA, 2014.
2. Gazi, M.A.I.; Yusof, M.F.; Islam, M.A.; Amin, M.B.; Senathirajah, A.R.B.S. Analyzing the impact of employee job satisfaction on their job behavior in the industrial setting: An analysis from the perspective of job performance. *J. Open Innov. Technol. Mark. Complex.* **2024**, *10*, 100427. [CrossRef]
3. Lu, Y.; Hu, X.-M.; Huang, X.-L.; Zhuang, X.-D.; Guo, P.; Feng, L.-F.; Hu, W.; Chen, L.; Hao, Y.-T. Job satisfaction and associated factors among healthcare staff: A cross-sectional study in Guangdong Province, China. *BMJ Open* **2016**, *6*, e011388. [CrossRef] [PubMed]
4. Toh, S.G.; Ang, E.; Devi, M.K. Systematic review on the relationship between the nursing shortage and job satisfaction, stress and burnout levels among nurses in oncology/haematology settings. *Int. J. Evid. Based Healthc.* **2012**, *10*, 126–141. [CrossRef]
5. Primary Health Care. Available online: https://www.who.int/health-topics/primary-health-care#tab=tab_1 (accessed on 18 March 2025).
6. Diakos, G.; Koupidis, S.; Dounias, G. Measurement of job satisfaction among healthcare workers during the COVID-19 pandemic: A cross-sectional study. *Med. Int.* **2022**, *3*, 2. [CrossRef] [PubMed]
7. Lu, H.; Barriball, K.L.; Zhang, X.; While, A.E. Job satisfaction among hospital nurses revisited: A systematic review. *Int. J. Nurs. Stud.* **2012**, *49*, 1017–1038. [CrossRef] [PubMed]
8. Aiken, L.H.; Clarke, S.P.; Sloane, D.M.; Sochalski, J.; Silber, J.H. Hospital Nurse Staffing and Patient Mortality, Nurse Burnout, and Job Dissatisfaction. *JAMA* **2002**, *288*, 1987–1993. [CrossRef]
9. State of the Global Workplace Report—Gallup. Available online: https://www.gallup.com/workplace/349484/state-of-the-global-workplace.aspx (accessed on 18 March 2025).
10. Afulani, P.A.; Nutor, J.J.; Agbadi, P.; Gyamerah, A.O.; Musana, J.; Aborigo, R.A.; Odiase, O.; Getahun, M.; Ongeri, L.; Malechi, H.; et al. Job satisfaction among healthcare workers in Ghana and Kenya during the COVID-19 pandemic: Role of perceived preparedness, stress, and burnout. *PLOS Glob. Public Health* **2021**, *1*, e0000022. [CrossRef]
11. Second Round of the National Pulse Survey on Continuity of Essential Health Services During the COVID-19 Pandemic: January-March 2021: Interim Report, 22 April 2021. Available online: https://iris.who.int/handle/10665/340937 (accessed on 18 March 2025).
12. Frenk, J.; Chen, L.; Bhutta, Z.A.; Cohen, J.; Crisp, N.; Evans, T.; Fineberg, H.; Garcia, P.; Ke, Y.; Kelly, P.; et al. Health professionals for a new century: Ttransforming education to strengthen health systems in an interdependent world. *Lancet* **2010**, *376*, 1923–1958. [CrossRef]
13. Blaauw, D.; Ditlopo, P.; Maseko, F.; Chirwa, M.; Mwisongo, A.; Bidwell, P.; Thomas, S.; Normand, C. Comparing the job satisfaction and intention to leave of different categories of health workers in Tanzania, Malawi, and South Africa. *Glob. Health Action.* **2013**, *6*, 19287. [CrossRef]
14. Jaeger, F.N.; Bechir, M.; Harouna, M.; Moto, D.D.; Utzinger, J. Challenges and opportunities for healthcare workers in a rural district of Chad. *BMC Health Serv. Res.* **2018**, *18*, 7. [CrossRef]

15. Moyo, E.; Dzobo, M.; Moyo, P.; Murewanhema, G.; Chitungo, I.; Dzinamarira, T. Burnout among healthcare workers during public health emergencies in sub-Saharan Africa: Contributing factors, effects, and prevention measures. *Hum. Factors Healthc.* **2023**, *3*, 100039. [CrossRef]
16. Mathauer, I.; Imhoff, I. Health worker motivation in Africa: The role of non-financial incentives and human resource management tools. *Hum. Resour. Health* **2006**, *4*, 24. [CrossRef]
17. World Development Indicators | DataBank. Available online: https://databank.worldbank.org/reports.aspx?source=2&country=ARE (accessed on 18 March 2025).
18. World Health Statistics 2023. Available online: https://www.who.int/publications/b/69040 (accessed on 18 March 2025).
19. Human Development Report 2023-24 | Human Development Reports. Available online: https://hdr.undp.org/content/human-development-report-2023-24 (accessed on 18 March 2025).
20. World Health Organization. *Health Sector Transformation Plan II*; World Health Organization: Geneva, Switzerland, 2021.
21. World Health Organization. *Kenya Health Sector Strategic Plan*; World Health Organization: Geneva, Switzerland, 2018.
22. Food and Agriculture Organization. *Government of the Republic of Malawi Health Sector Strategic Plan II 2 Acknowledgements*; Food and Agriculture Organization: Rome, Italy, 2022.
23. Ministry of Health Senegal. Plan National de Développement Sanitaire et Social 2019–2028. 2021. Available online: https://www.sante.gouv.sn/sites/default/files/1%20MSAS%20PNDSS%202019%202028%20Version%20Finale.pdf (accessed on 18 March 2025).
24. South Sudan Humanitarian Needs Overview 2023 (November 2022) | OCHA. Available online: https://www.unocha.org/publications/report/south-sudan/south-sudan-humanitarian-needs-overview-2023-november-2022 (accessed on 18 March 2025).
25. Ministry of Health South_Sudan_National_Health_Policy_2016_to_2026. Available online: https://extranet.who.int/countryplanningcycles/sites/default/files/planning_cycle_repository/south_sudan/south_sudan_national_health_policy_2016_to_2025_2.pdf (accessed on 18 March 2025).
26. United Republic of Tanzania. Ministry of Health, Community Development, Gender, Elderly and Children. Health Sector Strategic Plan Leaving No One Behind. 2021. Available online: https://www.moh.go.tz/storage/app/uploads/public/672/630/145/6726301451e92438381140.pdf (accessed on 18 March 2025).
27. Ministry of Health Uganda. Health Sector Development Plan 2020/21–2024/25. 2021. Available online: https://library.health.go.ug/monitoring-and-evaluation/work-plans/health-sector-development-plan-201516-201920 (accessed on 18 March 2025).
28. Ministry of Health Zambia. National Health Strategic Plan 2022–2026 "Towards Attainment of Quality Universal Health Coverage Through Decentralisation". Available online: https://endmalaria.org.zm/wp-content/uploads/2023/11/National-Health-Stratergic-Plan-for-Zambia-2022-to-2026-revised-February-2023.pdf (accessed on 18 March 2025).
29. Campbell, J.; Dussault, G.; Buchan, J.; Pozo-Martin, F.; Guerra Arias, M.; Leone, C.; Siyam, A.; Cometto, G. *A Universal Truth: No Health Without a Workforce*; World Health Organization: Geneva, Switzerland, 2013.
30. Willis-Shattuck, M.; Bidwell, P.; Thomas, S.; Wyness, L.; Blaauw, D.; Ditlopo, P. Motivation and retention of health workers in developing countries: A systematic review. *BMC Health Serv. Res.* **2008**, *8*, 247. [CrossRef]
31. Republic of Kenya Ministry of Health. Kenya Health Strategic Plan. Available online: https://www.health.go.ke/sites/default/files/2024-10/DRAFT%20STRATEGIC%20PLAN%202023-2027%20SDPH&PS%20Sept%2027-4.pdf (accessed on 18 March 2025).
32. Human Resources for Health Strategic Plan 2020–2030 MOH Knowledge Management Portal. Available online: https://library.health.go.ug/human-resources-health/human-resources-health-strategic-plan-2020-2030 (accessed on 18 March 2025).
33. Global Strategy on Human Resources for Health: Workforce 2030. Available online: https://www.who.int/publications/i/item/9789241511131 (accessed on 18 March 2025).
34. Kruk, M.E.; Gage, A.D.; Arsenault, C.; Jordan, K.; Leslie, H.H.; Roder-DeWan, S.; Adeyi, O.; Barker, P.; Daelmans, B.; Doubova, S.V.; et al. High-quality health systems in the Sustainable Development Goals era: Time for a revolution. *Lancet Glob. Health* **2018**, *6*, e1196–e1252. [CrossRef] [PubMed]
35. Shields, M.A.; Ward, M. Improving nurse retention in the National Health Service in England: The impact of job satisfaction on intentions to quit. *J. Health Econ.* **2001**, *20*, 677–701. [CrossRef] [PubMed]
36. The Health Workforce in Ethiopia by World Bank Staff (Ebook). Available online: https://documents1.worldbank.org/curated/en/433741468250204395/pdf/662180PUB0EPI00pia0health0workforse.pdf (accessed on 18 March 2025).
37. Ethiopian Community Health Worker Programs. Available online: https://chwcentral.org/ethiopian-community-health-worker-programs/ (accessed on 18 March 2025).
38. Hilo, A.A.; McPeak, J. Addressing concerns of access and distribution of health workforce: A discrete choice experiment to develop rural attraction and retention strategies in southwestern Ethiopia. *BMC Health Serv. Res.* **2024**, *24*, 1603. [CrossRef] [PubMed]
39. Bossert, T.J.; Beauvais, J.C. Decentralization of health systems in Ghana, Zambia, Uganda and the Philippines: A comparative analysis of decision space. *Health Policy Plan.* **2002**, *17*, 14–31. [CrossRef]

40. Okoroafor, S.C.; Kwesiga, B.; Ogato, J.; Gura, Z.; Gondi, J.; Jumba, N.; Ogumbo, T.; Monyoncho, M.; Wamae, A.; Wanyee, M.; et al. Investing in the health workforce in Kenya: Trends in size, composition and distribution from a descriptive health labour market analysis. *BMJ Glob. Health* **2022**, *7*, e009748. [CrossRef]
41. Facilitator Guide—Integrated Disease Surveillance and Response District Level Training Course | WHO | Regional Office for Africa. Available online: https://www.afro.who.int/publications/facilitator-guide-integrated-disease-surveillance-and-response-district-level-training (accessed on 18 March 2025).
42. Mukasa, M.N.; Bahar, O.S.; Ssewamala, F.M.; KirkBride, G.; Kivumbi, A.; Namuwonge, F.; Damulira, C. Examining the organizational factors that affect health workers' attendance: Findings from southwestern Uganda. *Int. J. Health Plan. Manag.* **2019**, *34*, 644–656. [CrossRef]
43. Okoroafor, S.C.; Christmals, C.D. Task Shifting and Task Sharing Implementation in Africa: A Scoping Review on Rationale and Scope. *Healthcare* **2023**, *11*, 1200. [CrossRef]
44. Dambisya, Y.M.; Matinhure, S. Policy and programmatic implications of task shifting in Uganda: A case study. *BMC Health Serv. Res.* **2012**, *12*, 61. [CrossRef] [PubMed]
45. Njunwa, K.M. Employee's Motivation in Rural Local Governments in Tanzania: Empirical Evidence from Morogoro District Council. *J. Public Adm. Gov.* **2017**, *7*, 224–237. [CrossRef]
46. Malawi-Harmonized Health Facility Assessment: 2018–2019 Report (Vol. 1 of 4): Main Report. Available online: https://documents.worldbank.org/en/publication/documents-reports/documentdetail/417871611550272923/417871611550272923 (accessed on 18 March 2025).
47. Article: The Emigration of Health-Care Workers: Ma. | Migrationpolicy.org. Available online: https://www.migrationpolicy.org/article/emigration-health-care-workers-malawi%E2%80%99s-recurring-challenges (accessed on 18 March 2025).
48. Prust, M.L.; Kamanga, A.; Ngosa, L.; McKay, C.; Muzongwe, C.M.; Mukubani, M.T.; Chihinga, R.; Misapa, R.; Broek, J.W.v.D.; Wilmink, N. Assessment of interventions to attract and retain health workers in rural Zambia: A discrete choice experiment. *Hum. Resour. Health* **2019**, *17*, 26. [CrossRef]
49. Gow, J.; George, G.; Mwamba, S.; Ingombe, L.; Mutinta, G. An evaluation of the effectiveness of the Zambian Health Worker Retention Scheme (ZHWRS) for rural areas. *Afr. Health Sci.* **2013**, *13*, 800–807. [CrossRef] [PubMed]
50. Goma, F.M.; Murphy, G.T.; MacKenzie, A.; Libetwa, M.; Nzala, S.H.; Mbwili-Muleya, C.; Rigby, J.; Gough, A. Evaluation of recruitment and retention strategies for health workers in rural Zambia. *Hum. Resour. Health* **2014**, *12*, S1. [CrossRef]
51. Health Workforce. Available online: https://www.who.int/health-topics/health-workforce#tab=tab_1 (accessed on 18 March 2025).
52. Deteriorating Humanitarian Situation in South Sudan, Rising Attacks on Aid Workers 'Worrying' Special Representative Tells Security Council | Meetings Coverage and Press Releases. Available online: https://press.un.org/en/2021/sc14636.doc.htm (accessed on 18 March 2025).
53. How did Senegal implement? | Exemplars in Global Health. Available online: https://www.exemplars.health/topics/under-five-mortality/senegal/how-did-senegal-implement (accessed on 18 March 2025).
54. Peretti-Watel, P.; Cortaredona, S.; Ly, E.Y.; Seror, V.; Ndiaye, S.; Gaye, I.; Fall, M. Determinants of childhood immunizations in Senegal: Adding previous shots to sociodemographic background. *Hum. Vaccin. Immunother.* **2020**, *16*, 363–370. [CrossRef] [PubMed]
55. Zurn, P.; Codjia, L.; Sall, F.L.; Braichet, J.M. How to recruit and retain health workers in underserved areas: The senegalese experience. *Bull. World Health Organ.* **2010**, *88*, 386–389. [CrossRef] [PubMed]
56. Alpern, R.; Canavan, M.E.; Thompson, J.T.; McNatt, Z.; Tatek, D.; Lindfield, T.; Bradley, E.H.; Tu, Y.-K. Development of a Brief Instrument for Assessing Healthcare Employee Satisfaction in a Low-Income Setting. *PLoS ONE* **2013**, *8*, e79053. [CrossRef] [PubMed]
57. Ayalew, E.; Workineh, Y.; Semachew, A.; Woldgiorgies, T.; Kerie, S.; Gedamu, H.; Zeleke, B. Nurses' intention to leave their job in sub-Saharan Africa: A systematic review and meta-analysis. *Heliyon* **2021**, *7*, e07382. [CrossRef]
58. Sheffel, A.; Andrews, K.G.; Conner, R.; Di Giorgio, L.; Evans, D.K.; Gatti, R.; Lindelow, M.; Sharma, J.; Svensson, J.; Wane, W.; et al. Human resource challenges in health systems: Evidence from 10 African countries. *Health Policy Plan.* **2024**, *39*, 693–709. [CrossRef]
59. Lantz, B.; Fagefors, C. Assessing factors associated with nurses leaving the profession: A secondary analysis of cross-sectional data. *Int. J. Nurs. Stud. Adv.* **2025**, *8*, 100315. [CrossRef] [PubMed]
60. Atlas of African Health Statistics 2022: Health Situation Analysis of the WHO African Region—Country Profiles | WHO | Regional Office for Africa. Available online: https://iris.who.int/bitstream/handle/10665/364837/9789290234852-eng.pdf?sequence=3&isAllowed=y (accessed on 18 March 2025).
61. Worku, N.; Feleke, A.; Debie, A.; Nigusie, A. Magnitude of intention to leave and associated factors among health workers working at primary hospitals of North Gondar Zone, Northwest Ethiopia: Mixed methods. *Biomed. Res. Int.* **2019**, *2019*, 7092964. [CrossRef] [PubMed]

62. Hynes, L.; Geraghty, S.; McChlery, S.; Smyth, A.; Brar, R.; Clark-Burg, K. Nurses' and midwives' job satisfaction and retention during COVID-19: A scoping review. *BMC Nurs.* **2025**, *24*, 299. [CrossRef]
63. Kok, M.C.; Dieleman, M.; Taegtmeyer, M.; Broerse, J.E.; Kane, S.S.; Ormel, H.; Tijm, M.M.; de Koning, K.A. Which intervention design factors influence performance of community health workers in low- and middle-income countries? A systematic review. *Health Policy Plan.* **2015**, *30*, 1207–1227. [CrossRef] [PubMed]
64. Anyangwe, S.C.E.; Mtonga, C. Inequities in the Global Health Workforce: The Greatest Impediment to Health in Sub-Saharan Africa. *Int. J. Environ. Res. Public. Health* **2007**, *4*, 93–100. [CrossRef]
65. World Health Organization. Delivered by women, led by men: A gender and equity analysis of the global health and social workforce. *Hum. Resour. Health Obs. Ser.* **2019**, *24*, 1–60.
66. Daniels, B.; Chang, A.Y.; Gatti, R.; Das, J. The medical competence of health care providers in sub-Saharan Africa: Evidence from 16 127 providers across 11 countries. *Health Aff. Sch.* **2024**, *2*, qxae066. [CrossRef]
67. Zulu, J.M.; Kinsman, J.; Michelo, C.; Hurtig, A.K. Developing the national community health assistant strategy in Zambia: A policy analysis. *Health Res. Policy Syst.* **2013**, *11*, 24. [CrossRef]
68. Zambia National Health Strategic Plan 2017–2021. Available online: https://extranet.who.int/countryplanningcycles/sites/default/files/planning_cycle_repository/zambia/zambianhsp.pdf (accessed on 18 March 2025).
69. Manongi, R.N.; Marchant, T.C.; Bygbjerg, I.C. Human Resources for Health Improving motivation among primary health care workers in Tanzania: A health worker perspective. *Hum. Resour. Health* **2006**, *4*, 6–7. [CrossRef]
70. Assefa, T.; Mariam, D.H.; Mekonnen, W.; Derbew, M. Health system's response for physician workforce shortages and the upcoming crisis in Ethiopia: A grounded theory research. *Hum. Resour. Health* **2017**, *15*, 86. [CrossRef]
71. Michael, Y.; Jira, C.; Girma, B.; Tushune, K. Health workforce deployment, attrition and density in East Wollega Zone, Western Ethiopia. *Ethiop. J. Health Sci.* **2011**, *20*, 15–23. [CrossRef]
72. Kim, M.K.; Arsenault, C.; Atuyambe, L.M.; Kruk, M.E. Predictors of job satisfaction and intention to stay in the job among health-care providers in Uganda and Zambia. *Int. J. Qual. Health Care* **2021**, *33*, mzab128. [CrossRef]
73. Ojakaa, D.; Olango, S.; Jarvis, J. Factors affecting motivation and retention of primary health care workers in three disparate regions in Kenya. *Hum. Resour. Health* **2014**, *12*, 33. [CrossRef] [PubMed]
74. Dieleman, M.; Gerretsen, B.; van der Wilt, G.J. Human resource management interventions to improve health workers' performance in low and middle income countries: A realist review. *Health Res. Policy Syst.* **2009**, *7*, 7. [CrossRef] [PubMed]
75. Fretheim, A.; Witter, S.; Lindahl, A.K.; Olsen, I.T. Performance-based financing in low- and middle-income countries: Still more questions than answers. *Bull. World Health Organ.* **2012**, *90*, 559. [CrossRef]
76. Waithaka, D.; Kagwanja, N.; Nzinga, J.; Tsofa, B.; Leli, H.; Mataza, C.; Nyaguara, A.; Bejon, P.; Gilson, L.; Barasa, E.; et al. Prolonged health worker strikes in Kenya- perspectives and experiences of frontline health managers and local communities in Kilifi County. *Int. J. Equity Health* **2020**, *19*, 23. [CrossRef]
77. Deriba, B.K.; Sinke, S.O.; Ereso, B.M.; Badacho, A.S. Health professionals' job satisfaction and associated factors at public health centers in West Ethiopia. *Hum. Resour. Health* **2017**, *15*, 36. [CrossRef] [PubMed]
78. Merga, H.; Fufa, T. Impacts of working environment and benefits packages on the health professionals' job satisfaction in selected public health facilities in eastern Ethiopia: Using principal component analysis. *BMC Health Serv. Res.* **2019**, *19*, 494. [CrossRef] [PubMed]
79. Abate, H.K.; Mekonnen, C.K. Job satisfaction and associated factors among health care professionals working in public health facilities in ethiopia: A systematic review. *J. Multidiscip. Healthc.* **2021**, *2021*, 821–830. [CrossRef]
80. Ekirapa-Kiracho, E.; Namazzi, G.; Tetui, M.; Mutebi, A.; Waiswa, P.; Oo, H.; Peters, D.H.; George, A.S. Unlocking community capabilities for improving maternal and newborn health: Participatory action research to improve birth preparedness, health facility access, and newborn care in rural Uganda. *BMC Health Serv. Res.* **2016**, *16*, 638. [CrossRef]
81. Dieleman, M.; Toonen, J.; Touré, H.; Martineau, T. The match between motivation and performance management of health sector workers in Mali. *Hum. Resour. Health* **2006**, *4*, 2. [CrossRef] [PubMed]
82. WHO. (223). Global Health Workforce Statistics Database. Available online: https://www.who.int/data/gho/data/themes/topics/health-workforce (accessed on 18 March 2025).
83. Health at a Glance 2023 | OECD. Available online: https://www.oecd.org/en/publications/health-at-a-glance-2023_7a7afb35-en.html (accessed on 18 March 2025).
84. Global Evidence on Inequities in Rural Health Protection. New Data. Available online: https://paperzz.com/doc/8431629/global-evidence-on-inequities-in-rural-health-protection (accessed on 18 March 2025).
85. Van Der Heijden, B.; Mahoney, C.B.; Xu, Y. Impact of job demands and resources on nurses' burnout and occupational turnover intention towards an age-moderated mediation model for the nursing profession. *Int. J. Environ. Res. Public Health* **2019**, *16*, 2011. [CrossRef] [PubMed]
86. 'There's a Commitment to Progression That's Led from the Top': How Essex Made Career Development A Priority for Its Social Workers | Social Care Careers in Essex. Available online: https://linkcafe.co.uk/theres-a-commitment-to-progression-thats-led-

from-the-top-how-essex-made-career-development-a-priority-for-its-social-workers-social-care-careers-in-essex/ (accessed on 18 March 2025).

87. Harzing, A.W. Response styles in cross-national survey research: A 26-country study. *Int. J. Cross Cult. Manag.* **2006**, *6*, 243–266. [CrossRef]
88. Podsakoff, P.M.; MacKenzie, S.B.; Lee, J.Y.; Podsakoff, N.P. Common Method Biases in Behavioral Research: A Critical Review of the Literature and Recommended Remedies. *J. Appl. Psychol.* **2003**, *88*, 879–903. [CrossRef]
89. Franco, L.M.; Bennett, S.; Kanfer, R. Health sector reform and public sector health worker motivation: A conceptual framework. *Soc. Sci. Med.* **2002**, *54*, 1255–1266. [CrossRef]

International Journal of
Environmental Research and Public Health

MDPI

Article

Forecasting the Regional Demand for Medical Workers in Kazakhstan: The Functional Principal Component Analysis Approach

Berik Koichubekov [1,*], Bauyrzhan Omarkulov [2], Nazgul Omarbekova [1], Khamida Abdikadirova [3], Azamat Kharin [1] and Alisher Amirbek [2]

1 Department of Informatics and Biostatistics, Karaganda Medical University, Gogol St. 40, Karaganda 100008, Kazakhstan; omarbekova@qmu.kz (N.O.); harin@qmu.kz (A.K.)
2 Department of Family Medicine, Karaganda Medical University, Gogol St. 40, Karaganda 100008, Kazakhstan; omarkulov@qmu.kz (B.O.); amirbek@qmu.kz (A.A.)
3 Department of Physiology, Karaganda Medical University, Gogol St. 40, Karaganda 100008, Kazakhstan; abdikadirova@qmu.kz
* Correspondence: koychubekov@qmu.kz; Tel.:+77-017641381

Abstract

The distribution of the health workforce affects the availability of health service delivery to the public. In practice, the demographic and geographic maldistribution of the health workforce is a long-standing national crisis. In this study, we present an approach based on Functional Principal Component Analysis (FPCA) of data to identify patterns in the availability of health workers across different regions of Kazakhstan in order to forecast their needs up to 2033. FPCA was applied to the data to reduce dimensionality and capture common patterns across regions. To evaluate the forecasting performance of the model, we employed rolling origin cross-validation with an expanding window. The resulting scores were forecasted one year ahead using Autoregressive Integrated Moving Average (ARIMA) and Long Short-Term Memory (LSTM) methods. LSTM showed higher accuracy compared to ARIMA. The use of the FPCA method allowed us to identify national and regional trends in the dynamics of the number of doctors. We identified regions with different growth rates, highlighting where the most and least intensive growth is taking place. Based on the FPSA, we have predicted the need for doctors in each region in the period up to 2033. Our results show that the FPCA can serve as a significant tool for analyzing the situation relating to human resources in healthcare and be used for an approximate assessment of future needs for medical personnel.

Keywords: public health; healthcare workforce; FPCA; forecasting; time series

1. Introduction

Healthcare workers play a central role in healthcare systems. This is evidenced by the COVID-19 pandemic worldwide, during which the most common reason for disruptions in the provision of essential health services was staff shortages [1].

The distribution of the health workforce affects the availability and accessibility of health service delivery to the public. The ideal distribution is presented as a fair distribution and availability of the health workforce across the population, regardless of geographic location. In practice, the demographic and geographic maldistribution of the health workforce is a long-standing national crisis.

In Kazakhstan, as elsewhere in the world, there are problems with staffing of healthcare organizations. One of the pressing issues is the shortage of medical personnel, especially in primary health care. According to government agencies, in 2023 the shortage of doctors in healthcare institutions amounted to 4864 full-time positions. Doctors bear a high workload, as evidenced by the underemployment rate of doctors, which stands at 1.4. An additional factor complicating the situation is the large proportion of people of retirement and pre-retirement age—9.5 thousand and 2.5 thousand people, respectively. Another serious problem is the uneven distribution of medical personnel, concentrated mainly in large cities, while economically underdeveloped regions and rural areas experience a shortage of qualified medical specialists of various profiles.

The Ministry of Health is actively introducing new human resource planning methods that consider the socio-economic, demographic, sanitary, and epidemiological characteristics of the regions. However, improving the system of planning and forecasting the provision of medical workers remains an urgent task [2,3].

This study attempts to mathematically model the annual needs of various regions of Kazakhstan for doctors (including general practitioners and specialists) up to 2033, based on Functional Principal Component Analysis (FPCA). The initial data for this analysis relate to the provision of doctors in 16 regions of Kazakhstan from 2000 to 2024.

FPCA is a statistical method that extends classical Principal Component Analysis (PCA) to functional data, such as curves or functions (e.g., time series or trajectories). FPCA reduces the dimensionality of functional data by identifying the main directions of variability (principal components) in the function space. FPCA provides a compact representation of complex functional data and highlights their key features [4,5]. Many real problems have been solved based on this method, including modeling the curvature of the human cornea [6], analyses of set of density curves where the argument variable is the logarithm of income [7], and fMRI scanning of regions of the central nervous system [8]. Other different applications of Principal Component Analysis to functional data have been developed, including modeling child and adolescent growth [9] and mortality and fertility rates [10], and identifying species from bloodstains [11]. The Principal Component Analysis method has been successfully applied to spatial anisotropy [12], interpreting lactate curves [13], analyzing kinematic data [14], and gene classification [15], exploring the major source of variations in glomerular filtration rate curves [16], and estimating mean and covariance for functional snippets [17]. Using this methodology, growth trajectories were determined to distinguish children with normal growth from those with poor growth [18]. In [19], the method is applied to data from participants in a family study of mood spectrum disorders to characterize differences in daytime mood patterns in individuals with major subtypes of mood disorders.

The FPCA approach was shown to provide a better estimate compared to other conventional methods to handle longitudinal data in biomedical applications [20–25].

Some works in the field of medicine and related sciences include the application of FPCA for the analysis of wastewater data to assess psychoactive substance use across 42 European cities. FPCA identified weekly temporal patterns of drug consumption, such as ecstasy (MDMA), using Fourier and B-spline basis functions. The method demonstrated high stability and robustness to missing data compared to traditional PCA and wavelet-based PCA [26]. A similar 2020 study examined the weekly consumption patterns of six different drugs in 17 Italian cities. FPCA extracted key functional principal components (FPCs), enabling a more accurate description of consumption dynamics [27].

In another study, FPCA was applied to analyze the logarithmic mortality rates of French males over 200 years. While not strictly medical, the B-spline-based methodology highlights FPCA's potential for handling longitudinal medical data, such as vital signs or disease trajectories [28]. In related fields, FPCA has been used to analyze biomedical signals, such as electrocardiograms (ECG) and electroencephalograms (EEG). For instance, one study [29] employed FPCA to identify characteristic patterns in EEG data for epilepsy, improving diagnosis and patient monitoring.

FPCA has been used to study functional data in medical research, such as recovery trajectories after surgery. The method isolated key components of variability, simplifying the interpretation of complex time series [30]. Another study [31] used FPCA to analyze glucose changes in patients with diabetes to identify individual metabolic patterns and improve personalized treatment approaches.

Currently, there is no single ideal tool for planning human resources for medicine. Rather, there are several approaches, including modeling based on needs, demand, and supply, which apply various methods, such as regression models, simulation modeling, Markov chains, and others. In recent years, methods based on machine learning have been intensively developed. Each of these methods has its own advantages and disadvantages.

In our research, the FPCA method is used to analyze and forecast the needs of doctors in different regions of one healthcare system because it allows us to:

- Identify subtle changes in regional patterns: the method can capture how the number of doctors in certain regions changes over time, including nonlinear trends that traditional models may miss.
- Analyze regional shifts: the method allows you to track how the "peaks" in the number of doctors shift across regions (for example, from economically less developed regions to oil-rich regions or the capital), which may be due to an improvement in/worsening of the epidemiological situation or attractiveness. The method makes it possible to understand in which regions key changes are occurring.
- Simulate long-term and short-term trends simultaneously: the functional approach includes high-order principal components, making it possible to capture complex time dynamics, such as slowdowns/accelerations or periodic fluctuations in the number of doctors associated with various reasons.
- Analyze structural changes: the method can identify both general trends (for example, a general increase in the number of doctors in the Republic) and regional changes in individual regions.

The method supports coherent forecasting, where forecasts for different regions do not lead to unrealistic discrepancies or intersections. This helps the regulator create more plausible scenarios when planning human resources.

2. Materials and Methods

2.1. Data Sources

The dataset includes statistical data concerning Kazakhstan doctor counts by regions and by years in the period 2000–2024. The data for 2019 and 2020 were adjusted due to an unexplained decline in doctor counts in 2019, potentially reflecting reporting errors, followed by a correction in 2020. Interpolation between 2018 and 2021 values, along with manual adjustments for Region 8 (e.g., 1834 to 2090 in 2019), were applied to ensure data consistency.

These data were sourced from the Kazakhstan Bureau of National Statistics. According to the "Conditions for the use of official statistical information", users without a concluded contract with the Bureau of National Statistics of the Agency on Strategic Planning and Reforms of the Republic of Kazakhstan may freely use official statistical information (including repeatedly) without charge, indefinitely, and without limitations with respect to the territory of use. This includes the rights to copy, publish, distribute with reference to the source, modify, and combine with other information, as well as use of the data for the creation of program products and applications (https://stat.gov.kz/en/description/, accessed on 1 October 2024).

Until 2017, Kazakhstan was divided into 16 first-level administrative-territorial units: 14 regions and 2 cities of republican significance. Subsequently, some of the larger entities were divided, and there are currently 20 of them. To ensure that the time series included a sufficient number of dimensions, we used the previous administrative division into 16 regions, as presented in Figure 1. The regions were ranked by decreasing population size in 2000 and assigned codes from 1 to 16.

Code	Region	Population in 2000 year
1	South Kazakhstan	2,005,023
2	Almaty city	1,557,141
3	East Kazakhstan	1,516,785
4	Karaganda	1,390,454
5	Almaty province	1,130,439
6	Kostanay	988,787
7	Jambyl	986,144
8	Akmola	799,179
9	Pavlodar	790,774
10	North Kazakhstan	713,628
11	Aktobe	677,715
12	West Kazakhstan	609,161
13	Kyzylorda	598,526
14	Atyrau	441,692
15	Astana city	380,990
16	Mangystau	315,203

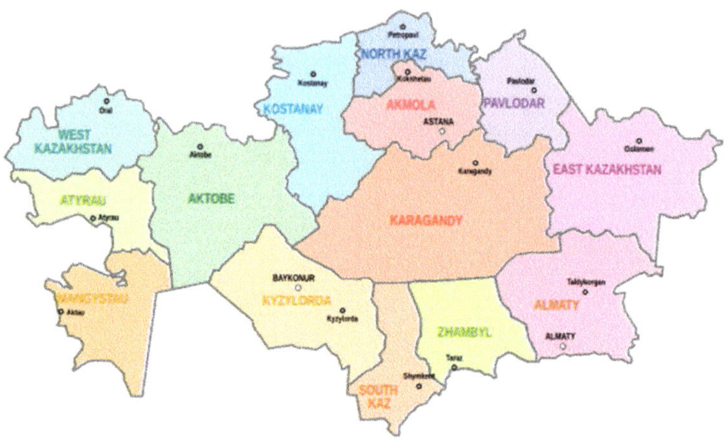

Figure 1. Kazakhstan regions encoding.

As a result, the data set included observations from 2000 to 2024 in 16 regions of Kazakhstan. The real and corrected data set is presented in Supplementary File S1.

2.2. Model Implementation

Functional Principal Component Analysis (FPCA) was applied to the data to reduce dimensionality and capture common patterns across regions.

The following assumptions are required to apply FPCA:

1. The data can be represented as functional dependencies (regional and time profiles of doctor availability), which makes FPCA a suitable method.
2. The data are pre-smoothed using orthogonal functions to represent them in functional form.
3. It is assumed that a significant part of the variance in the data is explained by several principal components.
4. The principal components can be interpreted in terms of national trends and regional features in the dynamics of the number of doctors.
5. FPCA is similar to PCA and EFA, but is designed for functional data, which makes it the best choice in this case.
6. The suitability of the method is also confirmed by the high accuracy of fitting and testing.

Let $y_t(x)$ be the observed doctor counts of region x in year t. It is assumed that it is realization of a smooth function $f_t(x)$ plus an observational error

$$y_t(x) = f_t(x) + \epsilon_t(x) \tag{1}$$

The time-dependent smooth function $f_t(x)$ is decomposed as

$$f_t(x) = \mu(x) + \sum_{j=1}^{J} \beta_j(x)\kappa_j(t) + e_t(x) \quad (2)$$

where:

$\mu(x)$ is the mean function of doctors counting for region x over time;

$\beta_j(x)$ is the set of orthonormal basis functions;

$\kappa_{j},(t)$ is the set of time-varying coefficients (scores); and

$e_t(x)$ is the error term.

We used automatic extraction orthonormal basis functions directly from the data through FPCA. This ensures that the basis functions are adapted to the underlying structure of the mortality data (package *ftsa* in R4.4.2).

The modeling process consists of several steps:

1. Set the $\mu(x)$ as the meaning of the $f_t(x)$ across the years.
2. Find $\beta_j(x)$ and $\kappa_j(t)$ through a Principal Component Analysis and choose number J of them for the model.
3. Choose a time series model for each of the $\kappa_j(t)$.
4. Forecast as follows: assume the last year observed is $t = T$. The time series model for the $\kappa_j(t)$ provides us with h-step forecasts $\hat{\kappa}_j(T+h)$, which in turn give us the h-step forecasts

$$\hat{y}_{T+h}(x) = \hat{f}_{T+h}(x) = \hat{\mu}(x) + \sum_{j=1}^{J} \hat{\kappa}_j(T+h)\beta_j(x) \quad (3)$$

Two methods were used to forecast principal components scores:

ARIMA with automatic stationarity checking and best parameters selection [32].

LSTM model with a single LSTM layer (50 units), a dropout layer (0.2), and a dense output layer [33].

The choice of 50 units in the single LSTM layer of the model was determined based on a balance between model complexity and computational efficiency, tailored to the characteristics of the dataset and the forecasting task. The dataset, while informative, is relatively small in terms of temporal depth (25 data points per region), which imposes limitations on the capacity of the model to learn complex patterns without risking overfitting.

A moderate number of units, for instance 50, was selected to ensure the LSTM layer had sufficient capacity to capture the underlying temporal dependencies and trends while avoiding excessive parameterization that could lead to overfitting on this limited dataset. This choice aligns with empirical guidelines in time series forecasting with LSTM models, where the number of units is often set between 20 and 100 for small to medium-sized datasets, depending on the complexity of the patterns and the length of the input sequence (in this case, a look-back period of 3 years).

Preliminary experiments with alternative configurations (e.g., 30 and 100 units) were conducted during the model development. A model with 30 units showed insufficient capacity to capture the nuances of the trends, resulting in higher mean absolute percentage error (MAPE) values (approximately 4–5% on cross-validation). Conversely, a model with 100 units exhibited signs of overfitting, with MAPE improving on the training set but degrading on the validation set (MAPE > 4% on cross-validation for 2017–2024). The 50-unit configuration achieved a robust balance, yielding an average MAPE of 3.19% across regions during cross-validation, indicating a good generalization performance given the data constraints.

Additionally, the inclusion of a dropout layer (0.2) further regularized the model, mitigating the risk of overfitting associated with the 50 units. This architecture was deemed sufficient for the study's objective of generating reliable forecasts for the number of doctors, as validated by the cross-validation results and the consistency of the predicted scores with historical trends.

The 50-unit single-layer LSTM was a practical and effective choice for this study given the dataset size and computational resources available.

The Adam optimizer was used with default settings (learning rate of 0.001), providing efficient and stable weight updates based on gradient descent. Preliminary tests with alternative optimizers (e.g., RMSprop) were conducted, but Adam demonstrated superior stability for the 25-year time series (2000–2024).

Mean squared error (MSE) was employed as the loss function, suitable for the regression task of forecasting the scores. MSE was selected due to its sensitivity to large deviations, which is critical for accurate predictions of doctor numbers where errors can have significant practical implications.

To ascertain the statistical significance of the FPCA–LSTM combination, a permutation test was implemented with 50 iterations. This involved randomly permuting the FPCA scores, retraining the LSTM model, and recomputing MAPE, allowing for the estimation of a p-value through comparison with the original MAPE distribution.

2.3. Model Validity

To evaluate the forecasting performance of the model, we employed rolling origin cross-validation with an expanding window [34]. The training set initially spanned the years 2000–2015 to forecast 2016, and with each subsequent fold, the training set was expanded by one year, up to 2000–2023 for forecasting 2024. For each fold, FPCA was performed on the training data. The resulting scores were forecasted one year ahead using ARIMA or LSTM. The forecasted scores were used to reconstruct the log-transformed number of doctors via the FPCA basis. The log-transformed forecasts were exponentiated to obtain the final forecasts.

This approach ensured that the temporal structure of the data was preserved while providing a robust assessment of the model's predictive accuracy.

Model accuracy was evaluated using Absolute Percentage Error (APE):

$$APE = \left| \frac{A_t - F_t}{A_t} \right| \times 100\% \quad (4)$$

where A_t is the actual data, F_t is the forecast data at time t, and n is the number of forecast years.

Mean Absolute Percentage Error (MAPE)

$$MAPE = \frac{1}{n} \sum_{t=1}^{n} \left| \frac{A_t - F_t}{A_t} \right| \times 100\% \quad (5)$$

All the analysis in this study is performed using R.

2.4. Final Forecast for 2025–2033

The entire dataset (2000–2024) was used as the training period for the final forecast: FPCA was applied to the full log-transformed data, followed by forecasting of scores for 2025–2033. Monte Carlo Dropout was applied by performing 100 forward passes with Dropout enabled during inference. The key points for choosing the parameters were:

- Bayesian Approximation: MC Dropout mimics Bayesian inference by sampling sub-networks, enabling uncertainty quantification.
- Number of Passes: 100 passes balance computational cost and stable variance estimation, based on empirical guidelines.

- Practical Benefits: improves robustness, quantifies uncertainty, and supports decision-making, especially for regions with variable prediction accuracy.
- Implementation: dropout was re-enabled during inference, with predictions averaged over 100 samples.

The 95% confidence intervals were calculated for the reconstructed number of doctors.

3. Results

3.1. FPCA Decomposition of Region- and Time-Specific Doctor Counts

According to the FPCA results, the contribution of the first component is 94.7%, while for the second component it is 2% and for the third it is 1.3%.

The graphs in Figure 2 characterize national and regional trends in the doctor count by region (principal components β1, β2, β3) and by year (scores k1t, k2t, k3t).

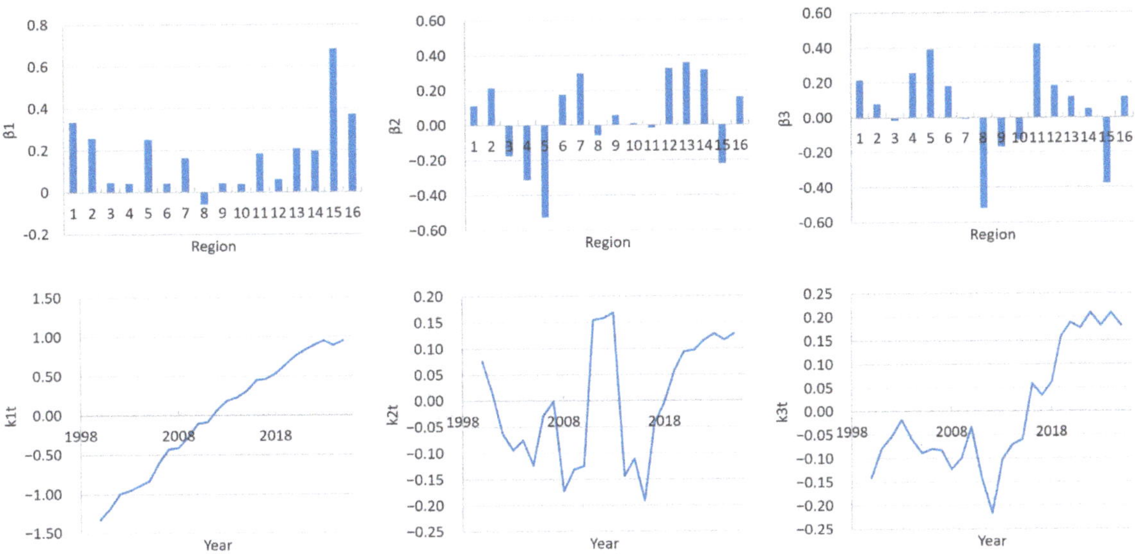

Figure 2. FPCA parameters.

The first principal component β1 within the FPCA framework represents the direction of maximum variation in the data, accounting for 94.7% of the total variance. In the context of our study, which analyzes the number of doctors (including general practitioners and specialists) across 16 regions from 2000 to 2024, β1 likely reflects the overarching long-term trend in doctor counts, dominating over regional or temporal fluctuations. This may be attributed to factors such as the overall growth of the medical workforce, driven by demographic changes, healthcare development, or national physician training programs.

In recent years, there has been a tendency towards an increase in the number of doctors in the Republic. The FPSA results also bear this out. For all regions except Region 8, the β1 values are positive, and the score k1t shows almost linear growth over the period 2000–2024 (Figure 2). The contribution of the first component (β1*k1t) of each region to the overall dynamics is presented in the graph in Figure 3. We have chosen to present this graph primarily to show the characteristics of regions 1, 8, 15, and 16 compared to other regions. Readers can view the full data for this graph in Supplementary File S1 (sheet PC1_contribution). Thus, the greatest positive contribution is made by Regions 15, 16, 1, etc. The number of doctors changes especially quickly in Region 15. In Regions 3, 4, 6, 9, and 10, the growth rates are lower, while in Region 8 there is a trend opposite to the general trend, i.e., in recent years there has been a decrease in the number of doctors.

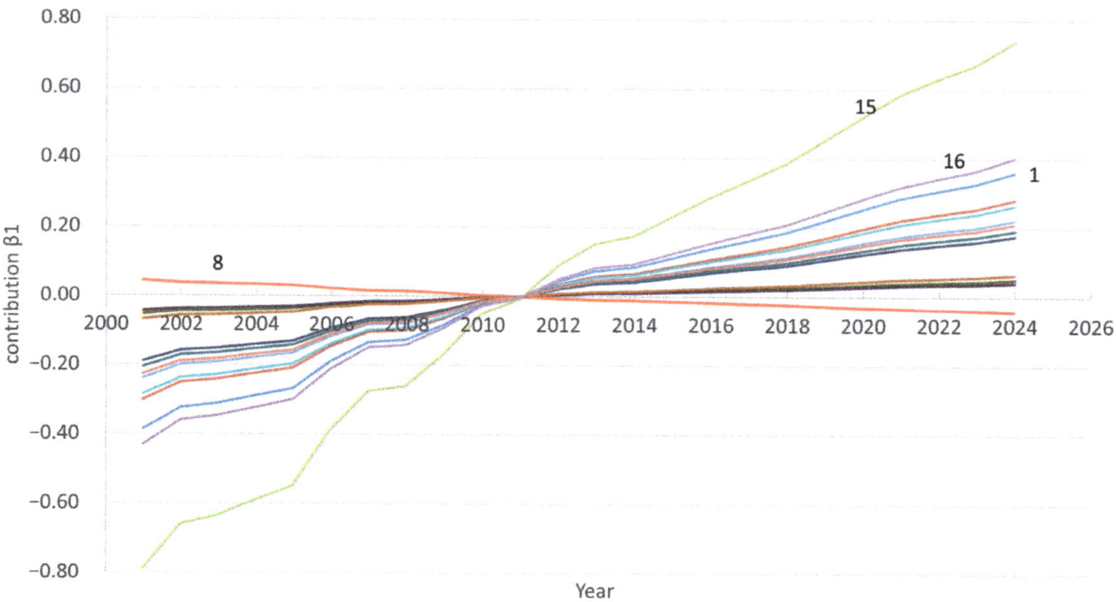

Figure 3. Contribution of the first principal component by region.

The principal component β2 explains 2% of the variations, which is significantly less than that of the first component (94.7%) but still indicates some additional variation in the data that is not explained by β1. This means that β2 describes less pronounced, but still important patterns in the number of doctors by region and year.

The β2 values show how regions influence the overall trend (Figure 2). Positive and negative values indicate a contrast between regions. Positive β2 values for Regions 7, 13, and 14 indicate that these regions have similar trends. Negative values for Regions 3, 4, 5, and 15 indicate opposite trends compared to regions with a positive β2. Regions 8, 9, 10, and 11 have weights close to zero (e.g., −0.058, 0.056, 0.009, and −0.016), indicating their weak influence on β2. These regions probably do not show significant deviations from the overall trend. k2t shows how the second component changes over time (by year). Negative k2t values are most pronounced in the period 2000–2010 (e.g., −0.172 in 2008, −0.191 in 2016). That is, in these years, Regions 3, 5, 4, and 15 had a higher number of doctors compared to regions with a positive k2t (Regions 13, 14, and 12). Positive k2t values are observed in the years 2018–2025. In these years, regions with positive weights (Regions 13, 14, and 12) could have a relatively higher number of doctors compared to regions with negative weights. If you look at the contribution of the second component by region (Supplementary File S1 (sheet PC2_contribution)), you can see "nodal points"—years when the contribution in all regions was zero, i.e., the number of doctors in these years tended to the average value. These are the years 2000, 2007, 2011, 2014, and 2018.

The third principal component β3 and the score k3t are interpreted as factors representing residual temporal fluctuations or specific regional adjustments (Figure 2). Their contribution β3*k3t captures short-term or regionalized effects, such as epidemiological events or physician migration, which complement the national trend and regional peculiarities. For instance, the negative contribution of β3 in Region 8 suggests a decline in doctor numbers, while the positive contribution in Region 5 may indicate a unique growth not explained by general trends. Since the contribution of this component to the total variance is only 1.3%, the influence of these features is insignificant.

3.2. Model Accuracy Testing

To test the accuracy of the model's forecasting, the entire time series of doctor counts in the regions was divided into two parts: training timeframe from 2000 to 2015 and testing timeframe from 2016 to 2024.

3.2.1. Goodness of Fitting on the Training Timeframe

After the model parameters were calculated on the training timeframe, the doctor counts for 2000–2015 were recalculated, and the fitting data were compared with the real data. The mean absolute percentage error (MAPE) was used as a measure of fitting accuracy. The reconstructed data, incorporating the mean doctor counts across regions and years, achieved a MAPE ranging from 1.12% to 2.73%, with an average of approximately 1.76%, indicating a strong fit to the observed data (Table 1).

Table 1. Fitting results by regions and years.

Year	MAPE	Region	MAPE
2000	1.98	1	2.49
2001	1.31	2	2.73
2002	1.56	3	1.86
2003	1.15	4	1.12
2004	1.37	5	1.63
2005	2.02	6	1.34
2006	2.58	7	2.14
2007	2.31	8	1.8
2008	1.21	9	2.14
2009	1.12	10	1.43
2010	1.6	11	1.54
2011	2.67	12	1.58
2012	1.38	13	1.95
2013	1.91	14	1.23
2014	2.09	15	1.22
2015	1.87	16	1.94
Mean	1.76		1.76

3.2.2. Forecasting Accuracy on the Testing Timeframe

We tested the model for predictive capabilities in the medium term. For this purpose, we forecasted scores k1t, k2t, and k3t for 2016–2024 using One-Step-Ahead Forecasting based on the ARIMA and LSTM methods. The reconstructed time series values for these years were compared with real data and the MAPE metric was calculated for each region and each year (Figure 4).

For the ARIMA method, the MAPE across all regions and years is 3.69%, while for the LSTM method this figure is 3.19%. This suggests that LSTM is better at forecasting the number of doctors in general.

With LSTM forecasting, the range of average MAPEs across regions was from 0.81% (Region 3) to 6.99% (Region 5). The range by year was from 2.33% (2021) to 4.18% (2020). With ARIMA forecasting, the range of average MAPEs across regions was from 1.50% (Region 7) to 9.94% (Region 15). The range by year was from 2.79% (2024) to 4.41% (2018). LSTM is more stable, since its errors vary less both across regions and across years.

LSTM has smaller peak errors (12% vs. 17.7%), making it more robust for regions with anomalous dynamics.

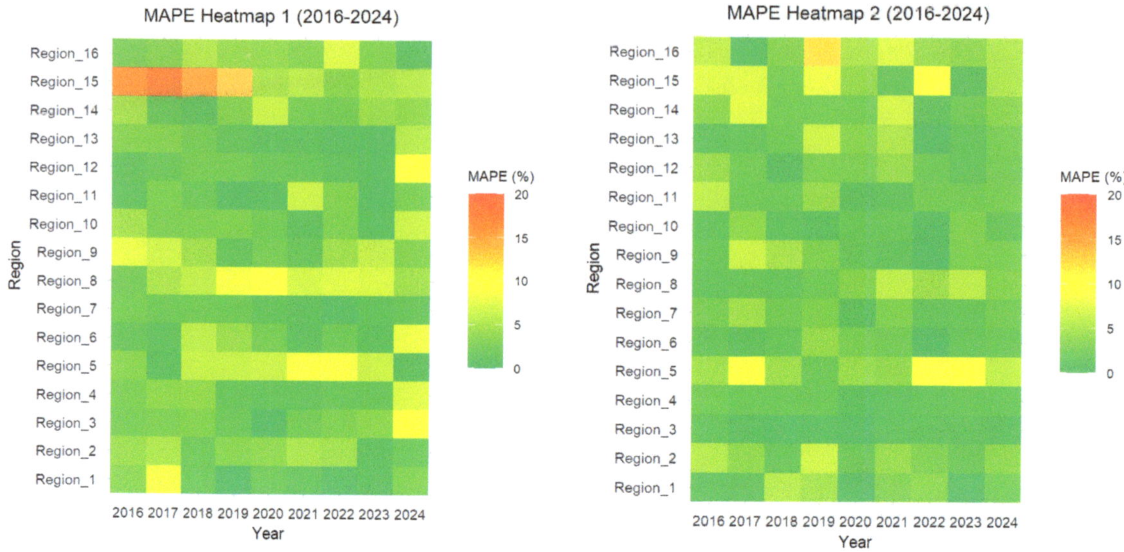

Figure 4. Model prediction accuracy of the ARIMA (Heatmap 1) and LSTM (Heatmap 2) techniques.

The advantages of LSTM were evident when analyzing data from Region 15. These regional data, covering the years 2000–2024, show a strong upward trend in the number of doctors, from 2198 doctors in 2000 to 10,540 in 2024, with an average annual growth rate of approximately 347.58 doctors per year. However, this trend is interrupted by rare but significant anomalies. In 2010–2011, the number of doctors declined from 5488 in 2000 to 5417 in 2011. This is a rare event for the region, which otherwise shows monotonic growth. After the 2011 decline, the region saw a sharp increase of 812 doctors in 2012 and another large increase of 665 doctors in 2014. These spikes are outliers compared to the average annual rate. With LSTM, the MAPE for Region 15 is 5.41%, which is significantly better than with ARIMA (9.94%). LSTM is generally preferred as it shows lower average error and more stable results.

The permutation test yielded a mean MAPE of 26.01% for permuted data, with a 95% confidence interval of [19.79%, 30.58%], reflecting a substantial increase in error when temporal patterns were disrupted. The resulting p-value of 0.000 confirmed the statistical significance of the model, suggesting that the FPCA–LSTM approach effectively captures meaningful patterns beyond random variation. These findings underscore the robustness of the hybrid methodology for time-series forecasting in healthcare resource allocation.

3.3. Forecasting Doctors Count to 2033

Based on the test results, we used the model to forecast the number of doctors for the years 2025–2033. In this case, the training timeframe included data for the years 2000–2024. Then, the scores were forecast for the period 2025–2033 by LSMT (Figure 5).

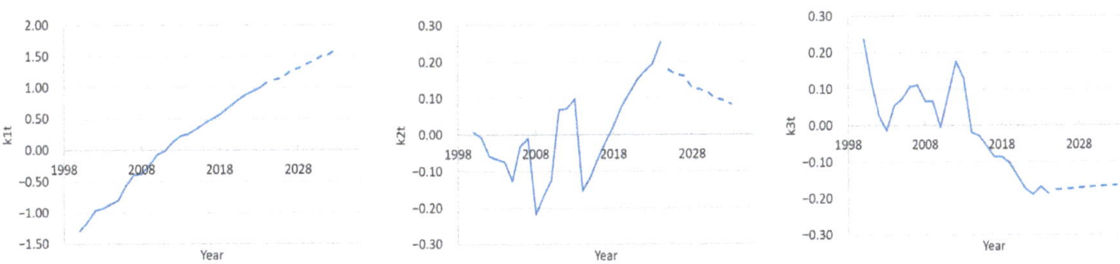

Figure 5. Principal component score forecasting by LSTM up to 2033.

The first principal component score indicates that the general trend of an increasing number of doctors in the regions will continue in the forecast period. This trend will continue to be most strongly associated with growth in Regions 15, 16, and 1 (Figure 6, contribution β1). The contribution of Region 8 will remain negative.

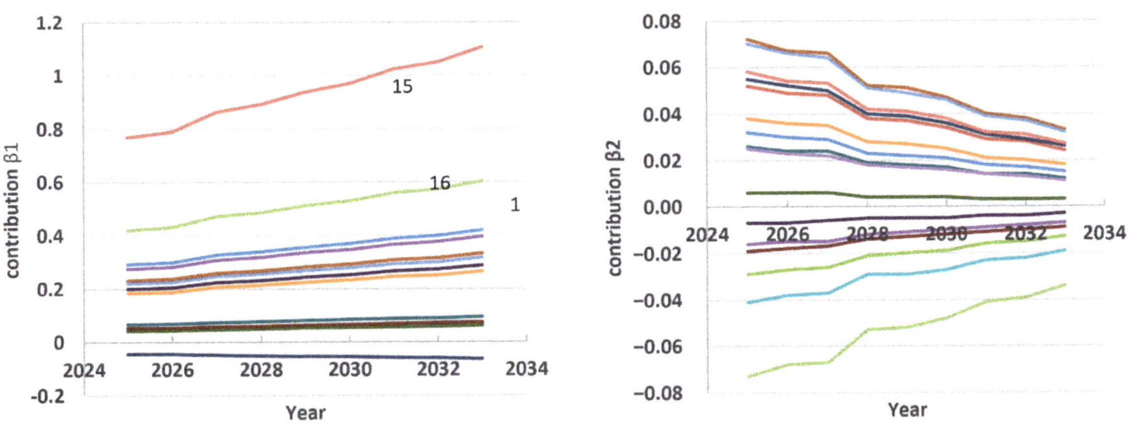

Figure 6. Contribution of the first and second principal components to the total variability.

The second principal component score, characterizing regional features, shows that in different regions the expected changes will have different dynamics. Thus, in Regions 1, 2, 6, 7, 9, 11, 12, 13, 14, and 16, in 2025–2033 the growth rate of the number of doctors will decrease, while in other regions the growth rate is expected to increase (Figure 6, contribution β2). The greatest acceleration will be observed in Region 15. In Region 8, the model predicts stagnation.

The predicted values of doctor counts for each region and each year are presented in Figure 7 and Supplementary File S1 (sheet Doctors_Forecast_2033).

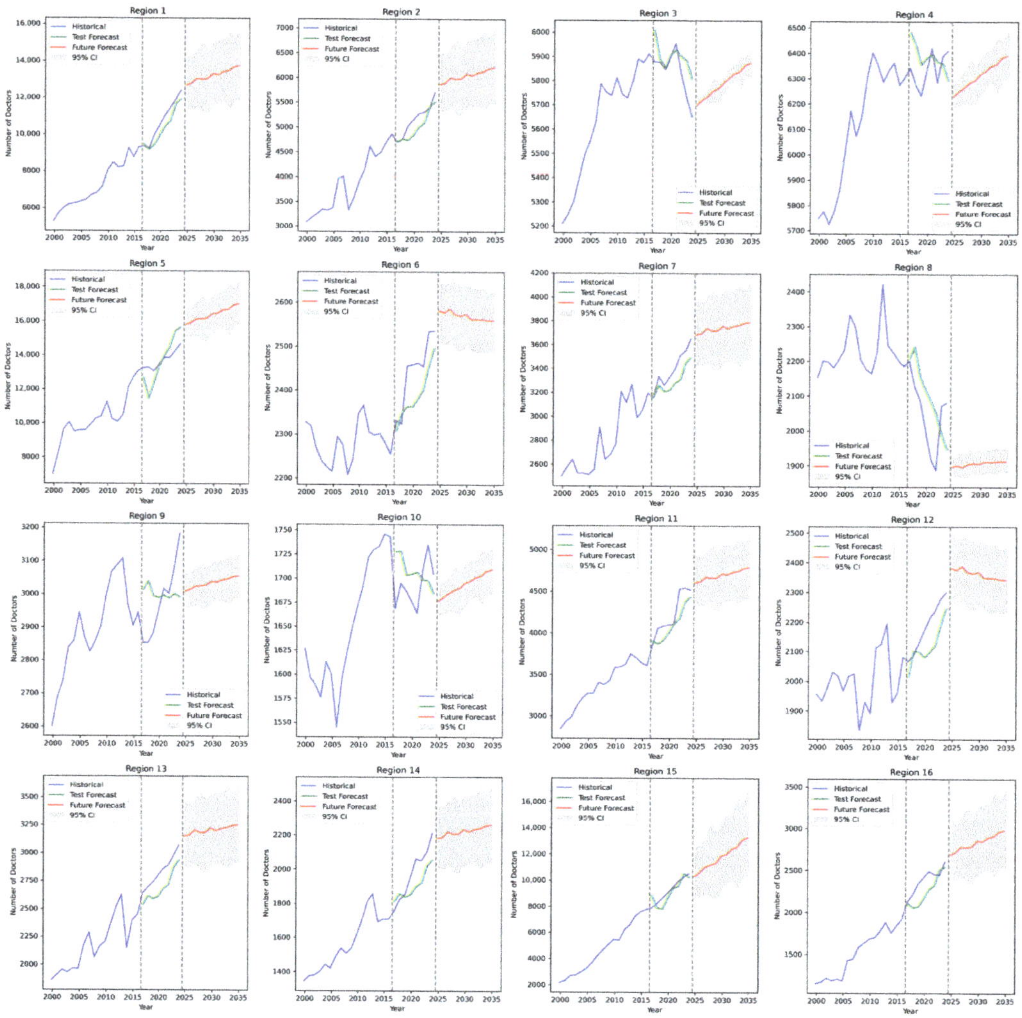

Figure 7. Prediction of regional demand for doctors.

4. Discussion

In the field of public health, FPCA studies mainly focus on the analysis of mortality, fertility, migration processes, and population size. However, the health workforce also exhibits spatial and temporal patterns. About 80% of health services in Kazakhstan are provided in the public sector. Almost half of medical students are funded by state grants. Therefore, government agencies have powerful tools to regulate the balance between the supply and demand of health resources both in the country as a whole and in individual regions. However, the problem of staff shortages and imbalances remains relevant. The growing population, the growth of chronic diseases, uneven socio-economic development of different regions, urbanization, and insufficient incentives to attract health personnel to rural areas all increase the requirements for planning and forecasting processes to meet health challenges.

Statistical and machine models (e.g., ARIMA, linear regression, neural networks) are built on historical data: they identify trends, seasonality, cycles, and correlations. The use of the FPCA method in our study allowed us to analyze medical personnel in 16 regions simultaneously while at the same time identifying national and regional trends in the dynamics of the number of doctors. We identified regions with different growth rates, showed where the most intensive growth is taking place (1, 15, 16), and identified a region in which the dynamics do not coincide with the general trend, namely, Region 8.

If the purpose of the method is forecasting, then after the stage of calculating the principal components and their coefficients, the stage of extrapolation of these scores to the forecast period begins. A wider range of univariate time series models may be used for this purpose. In this study, we used the ARIMA and LSTM methods.

While most regions were successfully modeled using ARIMA, Region 15 consistently exhibited high forecast errors. Region 15 exhibits dynamics that are out of sync with other regions. As noted, this region, the new capital of the Republic, is characterized by rapid population growth and, accordingly, increasing needs for medical personnel. The observed combination of a strong upward trend with rare anomalies (e.g., the 2011 decline) and a slowdown after 2015 made the dynamics of Region 15 less consistent with the general patterns captured by FPCA. This inconsistency led to a poor representation of Region 15 in the FPCA space, contributing to high forecast errors.

FPCA, which aims to identify general patterns across regions using a small number of principal components (in this case, three), tends to smooth out such rare anomalies. The model likely interpreted these events as noise rather than as region-specific phenomena, leading to systematic forecasting errors for Region 15. For example, during cross-validation (2016–2023), the model may not have accounted for the impact of these anomalies on the overall trend, leading to a high MAPE.

At the model testing stage, LSTM showed higher accuracy compared to ARIMA. LSTM is a type of recurrent neural network (RNN) specifically designed to work with time series. It can capture complex nonlinear dependencies in data due to its architecture with memory cells and gates (forget, input, output gates). LSTM was able to better model nonlinear dependencies inherent in some regions. In general, LSTM was more stable and robust.

Based on these results, we estimated the need for doctors by regions of Kazakhstan until 2033. It is expected that, in the medium term, the trend towards an increase in the number of doctors will continue in the Republic as a whole and in most regions. The leaders in demand will still be the new capital, the southern densely populated region and the western oil and gas region. The demand for doctors is predicted to remain unchanged in Region 8 and to decrease in Region 6.

5. Conclusions

As is the case around the world, the demand for medical specialists in Kazakhstan outpaces their supply. Young workers are flocking to large cities and industrial centers, while the imbalance between different regions is becoming more acute. Our findings may help regulators address staffing issues. Despite the importance of the results obtained, our study is not without certain limitations:

- Our calculations were based on real data of doctor counts in the regions of Kazakhstan. However, in all the analyzed years, there was a shortage of personnel in the country. Unfortunately, we do not have access to information on the number of vacancies by region in these years. Taking this information into account would allow us to obtain more accurate forecasts.
- The need for medical personnel is influenced by various socio-economic, demographic, and epidemiological factors. Taking these factors into account in FPCA is possible but

difficult, due to the uncertainty of their impact in the future. In this case, the use of scenario methods is justified.

- In our study, we predicted the total number of doctors in the regions, including general practitioners and specialists. More valuable information for regulatory authorities is the forecast of doctors by specialty. This allows for the efficient allocation of resources for training specialists.

The Ministry of Health of the Republic pays considerable attention to the problems of planning and forecasting medical personnel. Currently, methods are being introduced that take into account the socio-economic, geographical, and demographic characteristics of different regions of Kazakhstan. Our results show that the FPCA can serve as a significant tool for analyzing the situation with human resources in healthcare and can be used for an approximate assessment of future needs for medical personnel. Further development of the method with the inclusion of various external factors in the model will create a real basis for its use in the practical activities of regulatory authorities. Separate planning of medical personnel in rural and urban areas is of interest, since in sparsely populated rural areas the number of doctors cannot be determined only by the population size. It is also important to predict a possible shortage of doctors by region in order to begin training young medical specialists today. Future models should take into account the process of transferring a number of functions from a doctor to a nurse, which is gaining momentum in Kazakhstan.

Supplementary Materials: The following supporting information can be downloaded at: https://www.mdpi.com/article/10.3390/ijerph22071052/s1, File S1: input and output data.

Author Contributions: Data curation, K.A.; Formal analysis, B.O.; Methodology, B.K.; Resources, A.K.; Validation, A.A.; Writing—original draft, B.K.; Writing—review and editing, N.O. All authors have read and agreed to the published version of the manuscript.

Funding: This study received no external funding.

Institutional Review Board Statement: Not applicable.

Informed Consent Statement: Not applicable.

Data Availability Statement: The data presented in this study are available on the websites of Kazakhstan national statistics bureau https://stat.gov.kz (accessed on 1 October 2024).

Conflicts of Interest: The authors declare no conflicts of interest.

References

1. WHO. *Second Round of the National Pulse Survey on Continuity of Essential Health Services During the COVID-19 Pandemic*; World Health Organization: Geneva, Switzerland, 2021.
2. Analysis of Kazakhstan Republic Healthcare Human Resources, Astana. 2024. Available online: https://clck.ru/3Mrhbu (accessed on 1 October 2024).
3. Mukhazhanova, B.S.; Tulegenova, R.A.; Seyduanova, L.B. Approaches to improving the effectiveness of the quality of medical services. *Med. Ecol.* **2025**, *1*, 153–163. (In Russian) [CrossRef]
4. Croux, C.; RuizGazen, A. High breakdown estimators for principal components: The project-pursuit approach revisited. *J. Multivar. Anal.* **2005**, *95*, 206–226. [CrossRef]
5. Ferraty, F.; Vieu, P. *Nonparametric Functional Data Analysis*; Springer: New York, NY, USA, 2006.
6. Locantore, N.; Marron, J.S.; Simpson, D.G.; Tripoli, N.; Zhang, J.T.; Kohen, K.L. Robust principal component analysis for functional data. *Test* **1999**, *8*, 1–73. [CrossRef]
7. Kneip, A.; Utikal, K.J. Inference for density families using functional principal component analysis. *J. Am. Stat. Assoc.* **2001**, *94*, 519–533. [CrossRef]
8. Viviani, R.; Gron, G.; Spitzer, M. Functional principal component analysis of fMRI data. *Human Brain Mapp.* **2005**, *24*, 109–129. [CrossRef]
9. Hermanussen, M.; Meigen, C. Phase variation in child and adolescent growth. *Int. J. Biostat.* **2007**, *3*, 9. [CrossRef]

10. Hyndman, R.J.; Ullah, S. Robust forecasting of mortality and fertility rates: A functional data approach. *Comput. Stat. Data Anal.* **2007**, *51*, 4942–4956. [CrossRef]
11. Huang, W.; Gao, L.; Guo, W.; Cui, H.; Li, Z.; Xu, X.; Wang, G. Analysis into functional data of spectral images from bloodstains of human and two species of animal. *Forensic Sci. Technol.* **2021**, *46*, 551–558.
12. Bernardi, M.S.; Carey, M.; Ramsay, J.O.; Sangalli, L.M. Modeling spatial anisotropy via regression with partial differential regularization. *J. Multivar. Anal.* **2018**, *167*, 15–30. [CrossRef]
13. Newell, J.; McMillan, K.; Grant, S.; McCabe, G. Using functional data analysis to summarise and interpret lactate curves. *Comput. Biol. Med.* **2006**, *36*, 262–275. [CrossRef]
14. Ryan, W.; Harrison, A.; Hayes, K. Functional data analysis of knee joint kinematics in the vertical jump. *Sports Biomech.* **2006**, *5*, 121–138. [CrossRef] [PubMed]
15. Song, J.J.; Deng, W.; Lee, H.-J.; Kwon, D. Optimal classification for time-course gene expression data using functional data analysis. *Comput. Biol. Chem.* **2008**, *32*, 426–432. [CrossRef] [PubMed]
16. Dong, J.J.; Wang, L.; Gill, J.; Cao, J. Functional principal component analysis of glomerular filtration rate curves after kidney transplant. *Stat. Methods Med. Res.* **2018**, *27*, 3785–3796. [CrossRef] [PubMed]
17. Lin, Z.; Wang, J.L. Mean and Covariance Estimation for Functional Snippets. *J. Am. Stat. Assoc.* **2022**, *117*, 348–360. [CrossRef]
18. Karuppusami, R.; Antonisamy, B.; Premkumar, P.S. Functional principal component analysis for identifying the child growth pattern using longitudinal birth cohort data. *BMC Med. Res. Methodol.* **2022**, *22*, 76. [CrossRef]
19. Dey, D.; Ghosal, R.; Merikangas, K.; Zipunnikov, V. Functional Principal Component Analysis for Continuous Non-Gaussian, Truncated, and Discrete Functional Data. *Stat. Med.* **2024**, *43*, 5431–5445. [CrossRef]
20. Anderson, C.; Hafen, R.; Sofrygin, O.; Ryan, L. Members of the HBGDki community. Comparing predictive abilities of longitudinal child growth models. *Stat. Med.* **2019**, *38*, 3555–3570. [CrossRef]
21. Anderson, C.; Xiao, L.; Checkley, W. Using data from multiple studies to develop a child growth correlation matrix. *Stat. Med.* **2019**, *38*, 3540–3554. [CrossRef]
22. Han, K.; Hadjipantelis, P.Z.; Wang, J.-L.; Kramer, M.S.; Yang, S.; Martin, R.M.; Müller, H.-G.; Szczesniak, R.D. Functional principal component analysis for identifying multivariate patterns and archetypes of growth, and their association with long-term cognitive development. *PLoS ONE* **2018**, *13*, e0207073. [CrossRef]
23. Leroux, A.; Xiao, L.; Crainiceanu, C.; Checkley, W. Dynamic Prediction in Functional Concurrent Regression with an Application to Child Growth. *Stat. Med.* **2018**, *37*, 1376–1388. [CrossRef]
24. Simpkin, A.J.; Durban, M.; Lawlor, D.A.; MacDonald-Wallis, C.; May, M.T.; Metcalfe, C.; Tilling, K. Derivative estimation for longitudinal data analysis: Examining features of blood pressure measured repeatedly during pregnancy. *Stat. Med.* **2018**, *37*, 2836–2854. [CrossRef] [PubMed]
25. Dean, J.A.; Wong, K.H.; Gay, H.; Welsh, L.C.; Jones, A.-B.; Schick, U.; Oh, J.H.; Apte, A.; Newbold, K.L.; Bhide, S.A.; et al. Functional data analysis applied to modeling of severe acute Mucositis and dysphagia resulting from head and neck radiation therapy. *Int. J. Radiat. Oncol. Biol. Phys.* **2016**, *96*, 820–831. [CrossRef] [PubMed]
26. Salvatore, S.; Bramness, J.G.; Røislien, J. Exploring functional data analysis and wavelet principal component analysis on ecstasy (MDMA) wastewater data. *BMC Med. Res. Methodol.* **2016**, *16*, 81. [CrossRef] [PubMed]
27. Salvatore, S.; Frøslie, K.F.; Røislien, J.; Zuccato, E.; Castiglioni, S.; Bramness, J. A nuanced picture of illicit drug use in 17 Italian cities through functional principal component analysis of temporal wastewater data. *J. Public Health* **2016**, *24*, 165–174. [CrossRef]
28. Rostami-Tabar, B.; Hyndman, R.J. Hierarchical Time Series Forecasting in Emergency Medical Services. *J. Serv. Res.* **2024**, *28*, 278–295. [CrossRef]
29. Xie, S.; Lawniczak, A.T. Fourier Spectral Domain Functional Principal Component Analysis of EEG Signals. In *Pattern Recognition Applications and Methods (ICPRAM 2019)*; De Marsico, M., Sanniti di Baja, G., Fred, A., Eds.; Lecture Notes in Computer Science (LNIP, Volume 11996); Springer: Cham, Switzerland, 2020. [CrossRef]
30. Orozco, N.; Ortiz, S.; Ospina-Tascón, G.A. Functional Data Analysis Applications in Medicine: A Systematic Review. *WIREs Comput Stat.* **2025**, *17*, e70026. [CrossRef]
31. Sartini, J.; Zhou, X.; Selvin, L.; Zeger, S.; Crainiceanu, C.M. Fast Bayesian Functional Principal Components Analysis. *arXiv* **2024**, arXiv:2412.11340. [CrossRef]
32. Box, G.E.P.; Jenkins, G.M.; Reinse, G.C. *Time Series Analysis: Forecasting and Control*, 4th ed.; Wiley: Hoboken, NJ, USA, 2008.
33. Hochreiter, S.; Schmidhuber, J. Long Short-Term Memory. *Neural Comput.* **1997**, *9*, 1735–1780. [CrossRef]
34. Bergmeir, C.; Hyndman, R.J.; Koo, B. A note on the validity of cross-validation for evaluating autoregressive time series prediction. *Comput. Stat. Data Anal.* **2018**, *120*, 70–83. [CrossRef]

International Journal of
Environmental Research and Public Health

MDPI

Article

Equitable Healthcare Access for Type 2 Diabetes Patients Under a Low-Income Group Health Care Scheme: A Sustainable Development Goal Perspective

Sin Wei Tey [1], Kingston Rajiah [2,*], Mari Kannan Maharajan [3], Norasila Binti Zakaria [4] and Nor Haslinda Binti Ishak [5]

1 School of Postgraduate Studies, International Medical University, Kuala Lumpur 57200, Malaysia; teysinwei@gmail.com
2 School of Pharmacy and Pharmaceutical Sciences, Ulster University, Coleraine BTS2 1SA, UK
3 School of Pharmacy, University of Nottingham, Semenyih 43500, Malaysia; marikannan.maharajan@nottingham.edu.my
4 Klinik Kesihatan Ayer Molek, Melaka Tengah Health District Office, Melaka 75460, Malaysia; asilanor@gmail.com
5 Klinik Kesihatan Batu Berendam, Melaka Tengah Health District Office, Melaka 75350, Malaysia; drnorhaslinda@moh.gov.my
* Correspondence: k.rajiah@ulster.ac.uk

Abstract

Objective: The purpose of this study is to explore the factors influencing access to healthcare services among Type 2 Diabetes Mellitus (T2DM) patients enrolled in the PEKA B40 programme at a public health clinic in Melaka, Malaysia. It aims to examine how key dimensions—availability, accessibility, accommodation, and acceptance—affect patients' experiences and the utilisation of diabetes-related healthcare services. This study also seeks to identify gaps and challenges within the current healthcare delivery system, particularly for low-income populations, to inform strategies for improving equitable and sustainable access to care. Methods: This study was conducted in a public health clinic in Melaka, Malaysia. Purposive sampling was used among T2DM patients under the "Health Care Scheme for Group B40" programme in a public health clinic in Melaka, Malaysia. The study included participants with at least a 6-month history of T2DM to ensure substantial experience in accessing healthcare services. Results: Fifteen patients participated in this study. Elderly individuals, retirees, and those with average incomes demonstrated higher healthcare service utilisation. Ethnic diversity was crucial, revealing its impact on health behaviours and healthcare-seeking patterns. Primary or secondary education levels among participants highlighted the necessity for targeted health literacy efforts. Conclusions: This study highlighted notable awareness and satisfaction among patients concerning the availability, accessibility, and accommodation of services, particularly emphasising the importance of geographical proximity in healthcare services. However, challenges faced by elderly individuals in accessing social support are also highlighted. The potential of enhancing the amenities of healthcare facilities to improve patient experiences is also reflected in our results. These insights provide evidence for the effectiveness of the Malaysian healthcare system in catering to a diverse demographic and can also be helpful in refining healthcare strategies and further optimising patient-centred care in Malaysia.

Keywords: access to care; diabetes; primary care; health equity; Malaysia

1. Introduction

Access to care is pivotal in healthcare and encompasses five key dimensions: affordability, availability, accessibility, accommodation, and acceptability [1]. These dimensions ensure that healthcare services are economically feasible [2], adequately resourced with facilities, professionals, and essential medical supplies [3], geographically accessible [4], patient-centric [5] and culturally sensitive [6]. Understanding these dimensions is crucial in multiracial and multicultural societies and will be helpful in a healthcare system that is inclusive, equitable, and responsive to diverse needs.

As of 2019, approximately 3.9 million adults in Malaysia are living with diabetes, with the majority presenting with Type 2 Diabetes Mellitus (T2DM). This represents a significant public health concern, as the prevalence of diabetes among adults aged 18 and above increased from 11.2% in 2011 to 18.3% in 2019 [7]. Regarding the PEKA B40 programme, which aims to provide health services to the lower 40% income group (B40), recent data indicate that only about 10% of eligible individuals have utilised the free health screenings offered. Specifically, out of the six million Malaysians eligible under this scheme, only approximately 600,000 have availed themselves of its benefits over the past three years [8]. These statistics highlight the need for enhanced awareness and utilisation of healthcare services among T2DM patients, particularly within the B40 group, to ensure effective management and better health outcomes.

In Malaysia, despite the widespread availability of highly subsidised government healthcare facilities [9], disparities in access and inequitable health outcomes persist, particularly among socially disadvantaged groups [10], including the elderly and low-income individuals [11]. Limited access to public clinics for these groups is influenced by factors such as age, education, income and the need for care among the elderly [12]. However, detailed insights into how these factors affect the access and utilisation of healthcare services remain unexplored.

In 2019, the Malaysian government introduced the Peduli Kesihatan scheme (PeKA B40), which means "Health Care Scheme for Group B40" for the lower 40% income group to improve access to care for Non-Communicable Diseases (NCDs) [13]. The eligibility of PeKa B40 is automatic based on the set criteria, namely recipients of Sumbangan Tunai Rahmah (STR), which means "Compassion Cash Contribution", and their registered spouses who are aged 40 years and above. No separate registration is required to join PeKa B40 [14]. This scheme covers a range of benefits, including NCD screening, financial support for medical treatment, and transportation for hospital care [15], and hence, it addresses the affordability of beneficiaries. However, the dimensions of the availability, accessibility, accommodation, and acceptability of PeKa B40 beneficiaries have not been explored. Very few studies have been reported on PeKa B40 beneficiaries. Studies have stated the necessity of understanding the factors that affect the healthcare access of patients with NCDs [16,17].

Globally, the socio-economic inequalities observed in the progression of NCDs and the risk of diabetes complications are a concern [18]. In Malaysia, according to the World Health Organisation (WHO), Type 2 Diabetes Mellitus (T2DM) is one of the most common NCDs [19]. The global issue is reflected in Malaysia, as the socio-economic inequalities among the B40 group result in varied access to and utilisation of healthcare services for NCDs, especially diabetes [9–12]. Understanding the gaps in accessing and receiving appropriate healthcare is crucial for shaping policies and delivering more equitable healthcare services. Hence, this study focused on T2DM patients under the PeKA B40 programme to explore their experiences and challenges in accessing care.

2. Materials and Methods

2.1. Study Design and Sample

This study was conducted in a public health clinic in Melaka, Malaysia. Purposive sampling was used among T2DM patients under the PeKa B40 programme in Klinik Kesihatan (KK) in Melaka, Malaysia. It is a public health clinic that serves a significant population within the Melaka state and is actively engaged in the PeKa B40 programme. However, the study did not include specific data on the clinic's size or the total number of registered diabetes patients.

The study included participants with at least a 6-month history of T2DM to ensure substantial experience in accessing healthcare services. Participants were identified by confirming their eligibility using the clinic's PeKa B40 account and were approached during their visit to the pharmacy department of the clinic. The researchers aimed to achieve diversity across race, gender, and age groups. However, participant demographic information was not accessed in advance. Instead, potential participants were approached during their routine visits to the pharmacy department, and eligibility was assessed through their PeKa B40 registration status and confirmation of Type 2 Diabetes Mellitus (T2DM) history via the Pharmacy Information System. Diversity was sought progressively during the recruitment process based on observed characteristics and self-disclosed information during initial screening. While the intent was to ensure demographic variation, the study did not predefine age categories nor stratify recruitment targets by demographic quotas. Each participant who agreed to participate in the study was provided with an overview of the study, which included the study's purpose, potential risks and benefits, and the time it would take. Participation was voluntary, and participants were allowed to withdraw at any time during the interview. Written informed consent was obtained from all participants. Sampling was performed until saturation was reached. The saturation point was determined by analysing the collected data, which indicated that further collection of data may not bring any new themes. In other words, the researchers reached a point where no new themes were generated from the data collected.

2.2. Interview Guide

A semi-structured interview guide was developed by reviewing the literature on access to care [20–22]. (Refer to Supplementary Materials). Open-ended questions were used to provide interviewees with a full opportunity to convey their opinions and to obtain a greater understanding of issues. A pilot interview was conducted with two participants. The questions were rephrased based on the pilot interview. The data collected during the pilot interviews were not included in the results.

2.3. Data Collection

In-depth interviews were conducted. The interview duration was between 30 and 45 min. All interviews were audio recorded. The interview recordings were subsequently transcribed verbatim by the researcher. The accuracy of all the transcripts was checked by two researchers. The transcripts were subsequently returned to the participants for comments and corrections. The final transcripts were stored in password-protected Microsoft Office Word documents.

2.4. Data Analysis

The transcribed data were coded and analysed using thematic analysis [23], with a focus on identifying emergent themes. Initially, the data were examined for common patterns and sorted into categories based on similar trends. These categories were then coded and labelled, with notes recorded on key ideas that arose during the process. Thematic analysis was conducted following a structured approach: the researchers first familiarised themselves with the data, then generated initial codes, followed by searching for relevant themes, reviewing and refining those themes, and finally defining and naming them. The final step involved producing a comprehensive report.

2.5. Data Trustworthiness

Rigour in the study was evaluated using the criteria of credibility, dependability, transferability, and confirmability. To ensure the trustworthiness of the research, the study adhered to the Standards for Reporting Qualitative Research (SRQR) guidelines. Credibility was established using open-ended questions to elicit authentic responses from participants, allowing for a deeper understanding of their experiences. The research team achieved consensus on coding through iterative discussions, and thematic findings were validated by participants to ensure an accurate representation of their perspectives. Dependability was demonstrated by aligning the findings with the relevant literature and established theories, thereby reinforcing the consistency and reliability of the results. The research process was conducted with a high level of transparency and traceability, including detailed documentation of data collection, analysis, and key decision-making steps. This also involved maintaining logs of significant decisions, reflective notes, and the secure storage of raw data, along with records of participant feedback and peer reviews. Transferability was enhanced by providing rich, detailed descriptions of participant characteristics, the data analysis process, and original excerpts from participant dialogue, allowing readers to determine the relevance of the findings to other contexts.

3. Results

Participants' Demographic Characteristics

Participants' demographic characteristics are presented in Table 1. Fifteen in-depth interviews were conducted in total. The age of the participants ranged from 48 to 79 years, with most being older than 65 years. Nine of the participants were female. In terms of ethnicity, eight were Malay, four were Chinese, and three were Indian. In terms of education, seven received primary education and eight received secondary education. None of the participants were tertiary qualification holders. The history of T2DM among the participants ranged between 6 months and 20 years, with most of them having a diagnosis for more than 5 years. Eleven participants were either homemakers or retirees.

Table 1. Participants' demographic characteristics.

Characteristics	Participants n = 15
Age in years	48–79
Gender	
Male	6
Female	9
Ethnicity	
Malay	8
Chinese	4
Indian	3
Education level	
Primary	7
Secondary	8
Tertiary	0
Marital status	
Married/living with partner	13

Table 1. *Cont.*

Characteristics	Participants n = 15
Unmarried/living alone	2
History of Type 2 Diabetes	6 months–20 years
Employment status	
Employed	4
Homemaker/retiree	11

Table 2 lists the main themes, sub-themes and key findings.

- Main theme 1: Availability.
- Sub-theme 1.1: Utilisation of services available.

Table 2. Themes, sub-themes, and key findings.

Main Themes	Sub-Themes	Key Findings
Availability	Utilisation of service available	• Commonly known services: doctor's consultation, medication collection, blood and urine test, X-ray, and fundoscopy services. • Physiotherapy and dietitian counselling were less known to the participants.
	Ease of service utilisation	• Participants were satisfied with the medical equipment, the wide range of service coverage, and their ease of utilisation.
Accessibility	Clinic in the vicinity	• The clinic is located in the vicinity of participants' residences. • No transportation problem was reported.
	Mode of travel	• Self-drive or rely on family members. • Difficulty finding means to reach a clinic for those relied on family members.
Accommodation	Waiting time	• Aware of the need to wait. • The majority think the waiting time is acceptable; however, complaints still exist.
	After-hours and walk-in service	• No difficulty in access. • They use private clinics, hospital emergency department services, self-medicate or have not encountered the need so far.
	Frequency of follow-up	• Mixed opinions regarding the interval of follow-up.
	Facilities and amenities	• Participants are satisfied with the facilities and amenities.
Acceptance	Patients' acceptance of providers characteristics and vice versa	• No issues with acceptance, and care was delivered equally regardless of the characteristics of the providers and vice versa.
	Communication and interaction with healthcare providers	• Good interaction and communication. • Language barrier.
	Patients' perceptions of the staff	• Positive feedback on the attitude of the staff.

Participants were aware of the basic services that they routinely received for their diabetes management, such as doctor's consultations, medication collection, and blood and urine tests. X-ray and fundoscopy services were familiar to most patients, except those who had received diabetes treatment for less than a year. However, physiotherapy and dietitian counselling were less known to diabetes patients, even for those who had been on regular follow-up for a few years.

- Sub-theme 1.2: Ease of service utilisation.

Participants were satisfied with the medical equipment and services available and their ease of utilisation. A wide range of service coverage, such as X-ray and fundoscopy and co-located with dental services, was the reason for patients' satisfaction levels.

- Main theme 2: Accessibility.
- Sub-theme 2.1: Clinic in the vicinity.

Participants mentioned that the clinic is located only a short travel distance from their residence. None had transportation problems in accessing the clinic.

- Sub-theme 2.2: Mode of travel.

Some participants drove themselves to the clinic, and others relied on family members to fetch them to the clinic. None of them reported using public transport. Despite the majority of the participants having no barrier to physically reaching the clinic, a few described that they had some trouble finding people to visit the clinic. Some participants received help from others for monthly medication collection.

- Main theme 3: Accommodation.
- Sub-theme 3.1: Waiting time.

The waiting time mentioned by the participants is the time taken from registration to finish collecting medications. Participants were aware that they should wait to receive healthcare services. The waiting time in the clinic ranged from 30 min to 3 h. Most participants reported that a waiting time of 2 h was acceptable. Some participants complained about the waiting time when asked about the usefulness of services or problems encountered in utilising the services.

- Sub-theme 3.2: After-hours and walk-in service.

Participants mentioned that the clinic's opening hours from 8 am to 5 pm during weekdays were not restricting them and did not have an impact on their healthcare accessibility. None of them were concerned about after-hours accessibility to primary care service during evenings, nights, weekends, or walk-in service. When asked about the need for healthcare after-hours, most participants mentioned that they used emergency services and self-medicated. Some mentioned that they have not encountered the need so far.

- Sub-theme 3.3: Frequency of follow-up.

Regular follow-up is part of diabetes care management. The interval of time between each follow-up is determined by the doctor according to the clinical status of the patient and the treatment regimen. Generally, the time intervals for adjusting the therapeutic plan and performing laboratory tests range from two weeks for patients who require close monitoring to six months for stable patients. Most participants were satisfied with the interval given for their follow-up. However, one participant had a different opinion.

- Sub-theme 3.4: Facilities and amenities.

The examples of facilities and amenities included were the adequacy of parking lots, toilets, chairs for sitting in, and the conditions of the waiting lounge and consultation rooms. Most participants were satisfied with the facilities and amenities. Suggestions were given by some participants to increase the number of toilets and parking lots.

- Main theme 4: Acceptance.
- Sub-theme 4.1: Patients' acceptance of providers' characteristics and vice versa.

Owing to the diversity of race, culture, language, and religion in Malaysia, it is important to gain access to healthcare services. None of the participants reported issues in acceptance regarding the characteristics of the providers and vice versa. None of the participants reported any age, gender, or ethnicity preference for receiving care.

- Sub-theme 4.2: Communication and interaction with healthcare providers.

Most participants reported good interaction and communication with the healthcare providers. They agreed that they received sufficient updates about their health from the doctors, and their questions were answered clearly by the doctors. Very few participants reported a language barrier as they were not well-versed in the Malay language. Translation assistance from others, including healthcare staff, patients or family members, was gained when asked about how communications were tackled. In addition, the suggestion to establish a multiethnic healthcare team in the clinic to overcome the language barrier problem was also given by these participants.

- Sub-theme 4.3: Patients' Perceptions of the Staff.

None of the participants reported any concern about the staff. Participants commonly use the words "helpful", "friendly", and "polite" to describe the attitude of the staff.

4. Discussion

The principal findings shed light on several key aspects of healthcare delivery and patient experience within the context of diabetes management. While patients were generally aware of core services such as doctor consultations and medication collection, awareness varied for services like physiotherapy and dietitian counselling, suggesting potential areas for improvement in patient awareness. Satisfaction with available services and their ease of utilisation highlight the importance of comprehensive care provision, particularly with the inclusion of services like X-ray and fundoscopy alongside dental services. Clinic proximity was noted as favourable, although challenges in finding assistance for clinic visits or medication collection were reported, indicating potential barriers for certain patient groups. While waiting times at the clinic were generally acceptable, suggestions for improvements, such as extended hours or alternative service models, were noted. The satisfaction expressed regarding follow-up appointment frequency highlights effective collaboration between patients and providers, though personalised approaches might be warranted based on individual clinical needs. Suggestions for enhancing facilities and amenities, such as increasing toilets and parking lots, provide insights for optimising the clinic environment. The acceptance of healthcare providers' characteristics across diverse demographics reflected positively on the inclusivity of care delivery. Strategies to address language barriers, such as translation assistance, were identified as important for effective communication and accessibility. Positive perceptions of clinic staff indicated a high standard of patient-centred care.

The strength of this study is its exploration of factors influencing healthcare access for T2DM patients in the PeKA B40 programme. By integrating a range of demographic, socioeconomic, and experiential factors, this study offers valuable insights to policymakers and practitioners. The inclusion of participants from diverse demographic backgrounds enhances the generalisability of findings and offers insights into different perspectives. Qualitative data capture experiences and interactions, providing rich insights for healthcare providers and policymakers. However, despite efforts to include diverse participants, the findings may not fully generalise to all diabetes patients as it has a single-site focus.

Inequity in diabetes care is a complex challenge that requires significant effort with a special focus on social and healthcare systems. Access to healthcare services is one of the effective management strategies in the management of T2DM. The findings revealed a complex interplay between factors such as availability, accessibility, accommodation, and acceptance and how they impact T2DM patients under the PeKA B40 programme in Melaka, Malaysia. In this study, participants were over 65 years of age and predominantly homemakers or retirees. This demographic trend aligns with previous reports indicating higher healthcare utilisation among elderly individuals living independently and those with average income levels [24]. This study included participants from various ethnicities, shedding light on their health behaviours, treatment preferences, and healthcare-seeking patterns. These health-seeking patterns are related to both people's social values and culture [25]. Most participants had primary or secondary education, indicating the need for targeted health literacy initiatives. Limited educational attainment can adversely affect an individual's ability to manage diabetes effectively, adhere to treatment regimens and access healthcare services [26]. The duration of T2DM among the majority of participants exceeded five years, which points to the challenges of long-term disease management. This finding emphasises the need for ongoing support, follow-up, and education in diabetes care. The occupation status of participants, predominantly homemakers or retirees, suggests unique challenges for these groups in accessibility, aligning with global observations regarding healthcare accessibility for unemployed individuals [27]. Our study revealed participants' substantial awareness of the availability of diabetes management services, including doctor's consultations, medication collection, and blood and urine tests. This awareness is likely a result of the Malaysian government's focus on NCDs in lower-income groups [28]. However, a noteworthy observation is the limited knowledge of specialised services such as physiotherapy and dietitian counselling, irrespective of their regular follow-up for more than five years. Such gaps in awareness may arise from inadequate emphasis on holistic care or insufficient communication regarding these services. Participants expressed satisfaction with the medical equipment and services available for diabetes management, highlighting the user-friendly nature of the healthcare system. The integrated service approach used, which combines various medical services in one location, is particularly appreciated for its convenience. Geographical proximity and ease of transportation emerged as positive aspects of healthcare accessibility. The strategic location of clinics nearer to residential areas, a result of the Malaysian government's efforts to minimise urban–rural healthcare disparities [29], facilitated easy access. However, challenges in social support and medication collection highlighted the importance of community networks and direct-to-consumer prescription drug advertising (DTCA) [30]. Recognising and addressing these challenges can contribute to a more comprehensive approach to healthcare accessibility for individuals with T2DM, ensuring that both geographical and social factors are considered in optimising patient-centred care. In terms of accommodation within the healthcare setting for individuals managing T2DM, mixed perspectives were seen. Although most participants found waiting times within 2 h acceptable, complaints appeared when assessing the overall usefulness of services. The clinic's operating hours, from 8 am to 5 pm on weekdays, were generally perceived as non-restrictive, with participants expressing satisfaction with this timeframe. Interestingly, there were no concerns about after-hours primary care services or walk-in cases, with participants largely relying on emergency services and self-medication. This is mainly due to the Malaysian government's free health services at private clinics through the Madani Medical Scheme for the B40 group. The free services offered in this scheme include consultation, check-ups, medicines, procedures, and referrals at private clinics, especially at night and on weekends [31]. The frequency of follow-up, a crucial aspect of diabetes care management, received positive feedback overall, with participants expressing satisfaction with the intervals determined by doctors. The results emphasise the importance of addressing waiting times, accommodating after-hours needs, and continuously enhancing facilities and amenities to optimise the overall patient experience for those managing T2DM. In this regard, the Malaysian government was also shown to focus on primary healthcare services and community-based services to improve the delivery of healthcare services through better stakeholder engagement. Facilities and amenities received positive feedback, but suggestions for infrastructure improvements and calls for the sustainability of the healthcare system were reported. In this regard, the Malaysian government is introducing the Malaysian National Health Policy (MNHP), which aligns with global goals advocated by the WHO. Particularly, the Health White Paper (HWP) prioritises population health and aims to ensure the sustainability of the healthcare system in Malaysia [32].

The findings of this study highlight the need for policy initiatives aimed at improving healthcare service delivery for diabetes patients in Malaysia. Policymakers should prioritise initiatives that enhance the accessibility and availability of essential services, particularly for marginalised populations. Strategies to address transportation challenges and extend clinic hours could improve access to care. Additionally, policies promoting cultural competence and language diversity within healthcare settings can help address communication barriers and improve patient–provider interactions. Healthcare practitioners can utilise the insights from this study to inform their practice and enhance patient-centred care. Improving communication strategies, such as providing translation assistance or establishing multiethnic healthcare teams, can facilitate better patient–provider interactions. Practitioners should also consider the diverse needs of diabetes patients and tailor services accordingly, including personalised follow-up schedules and culturally sensitive care approaches. Addressing facilities and amenities based on patient feedback can further enhance the overall patient experience. Future research should build upon the findings of this study to further advance our understanding of healthcare service utilisation among diabetes patients in Malaysia.

Limitations

This study has several limitations that should be acknowledged. Firstly, it was conducted at a single public health clinic in Melaka, potentially limiting the generalisability of findings to other regions or healthcare settings. Detailed information about the clinic's size and the total number of T2DM patients was not reported, which restricts the contextual interpretation of the results. Secondly, while purposive sampling aimed to include participants of different racial, gender, and age backgrounds, demographic data were not accessed in advance, and recruitment was based on convenience during routine pharmacy visits. This may have introduced selection bias and limited the diversity of the sample. Thirdly, age categories were not predefined or systematically reported, which constrains the analysis of age-specific access issues. Additionally, the exclusion of newly diagnosed T2DM patients (with less than 6 months since diagnosis) may have overlooked the unique access challenges faced by this group. Finally, the reliance on self-reported data may have introduced recall or social desirability bias, particularly in participants' responses about service satisfaction and staff interactions.

5. Conclusions

This study aimed to understand the experiences and challenges of Type 2 Diabetes Mellitus patients under the PeKA B40 programme in accessing and receiving appropriate healthcare. The findings reveal several gaps and areas for improvement despite overall positive experiences. Most individuals were familiar with essential diabetes management services like doctor consultations, medication collection, and laboratory tests. However, there was limited awareness and utilisation of physiotherapy and dietitian counselling, even among long-term patients. This indicates a need for increased education and promotion of these critical services to enhance comprehensive diabetes management. Accessibility was generally satisfactory, with clinics located conveniently close to individuals' residences and most patients having reliable transportation. Yet, some individuals faced challenges in arranging visits, relying on others for transportation and medication collection, highlighting the need for better support systems for those with limited personal mobility or social support. Participants appreciated the range of services offered and found the clinic environment and medical equipment satisfactory. However, waiting times varied significantly, with some finding longer wait times unacceptable. This suggests a need for improved clinic efficiency and possibly the introduction of appointment-based systems to reduce waiting times. The clinic's operating hours were sufficient, with no significant demand for after-hours services, as participants resorted to emergency services or self-medication for urgent needs. Cultural and linguistic diversity did not significantly hinder access to care, with most participants reporting good communication with healthcare providers. However, a few faced language barriers, highlighting the importance of having a multiethnic healthcare team or translation services available.

Supplementary Materials: The following supporting information can be downloaded at https://www.mdpi.com/article/10.3390/ijerph22060817/s1. File S1: questionnaire.

Author Contributions: Conceptualisation, M.K.M. and K.R.; methodology, K.R.; software, S.W.T.; validation, M.K.M. and K.R.; formal analysis, S.W.T.; investigation, S.W.T., N.B.Z., and N.H.B.I.; resources, S.W.T., N.B.Z., and N.H.B.I.; data curation, S.W.T.; Writing—original draft preparation, S.W.T.; writing—review and editing, M.K.M. and K.R.; visualisation, M.K.M. and K.R.; supervision, M.K.M. and K.R.; project administration, S.W.T., N.B.Z., and N.H.B.I.; funding acquisition, K.R. All authors have read and agreed to the published version of the manuscript.

Funding: This research was funded by the Institute for Research, Development, and Innovation (IRDI), International Medical University, Malaysia, grant number MPP I/2021(03).

Institutional Review Board Statement: This study received ethical approval from the International Medical University Joint Committee on Research and Ethics, Malaysia (MPP I/2021(03)), 11 March 2021, and obtained permission from the National Institutes of Health, Ministry of Health Malaysia (NMRR-20-3147-57627), 22 March 2021.

Informed Consent Statement: Informed consent was obtained from all subjects involved in this study.

Data Availability Statement: The data presented in the study are stored securely at the School of Pharmacy, International Medical University. The investigators act as custodians for the data processed and generated by the study and they are also responsible for the access to any information included. Data are available upon request from the corresponding author. Due to privacy and institutional regulations, the data are not publicly accessible.

Acknowledgments: The authors thank the International Medical University and National Institutes of Health, Ministry of Health Malaysia for this research opportunity. The authors thank the Director Geneal of Health Malaysia for his permission to publish this article.

Conflicts of Interest: The authors declare no conflicts of interest.

References

1. McLaughlin, C.G.; Wyszewianski, L. Access to Care: Remembering Old Lessons. *Health Serv. Res.* **2002**, *37*, 1441–1443. [CrossRef] [PubMed]

2. Frazier, T.L.; Lopez, P.M.; Islam, N.; Wilson, A.; Earle, K.; Duliepre, N.; Zhong, L.; Bendik, S.; Drackett, E.; Manyindo, N.; et al. Addressing Financial Barriers to Health Care Among People Who are Low-Income and Insured in New York City, 2014–2017. *J. Community Health* **2023**, *48*, 353–366. [CrossRef] [PubMed]
3. Yenet, A.; Nibret, G.; Tegegne, B.A. Challenges to the Availability and Affordability of Essential Medicines in African Countries: A Scoping Review. *Clin. Outcomes Res.* **2023**, *15*, 443–458. [CrossRef] [PubMed]
4. Parvin, F.; Ali, S.A.; Hashmi, S.N.I.; Khatoon, A. Accessibility and Site Suitability for Healthcare Services Using GIS-Based Hybrid Decision-Making Approach: A Study in Murshidabad, India. *Spat. Inf. Res.* **2021**, *29*, 1–18. [CrossRef]
5. Stubbe, D.E. Practicing Cultural Competence and Cultural Humility in the Care of Diverse Patients. *FOCUS* **2020**, *18*, 49–51. [CrossRef]
6. Kuipers, S.J.; Cramm, J.M.; Nieboer, A.P. The Importance of Patient-Centered Care and Co-Creation of Care for Satisfaction with Care and Physical and Social Well-Being of Patients with Multi-Morbidity in the Primary Care Setting. *BMC Health Serv. Res.* **2019**, *19*, 13. [CrossRef]
7. Lim, L.L.; Hussein, Z.; Noor, N.M.; Raof, A.S.A.; Mustafa, N.; Bidin, M.B.L.; Ghani, R.A.; Samsuddin, S.; Yong, S.L.; Foo, S.H.; et al. Real-World Evaluation of Care for Type 2 Diabetes in Malaysia: A Cross-Sectional Analysis of the Treatment Adherence to Guideline Evaluation in Type 2 Diabetes (TARGET-T2D) Study. *PLoS ONE* **2024**, *19*, e0296298. [CrossRef]
8. Jamal, M.H.; Abdul Aziz, A.F.; Aizuddin, A.N.; Aljunid, S.M. Gatekeepers in the Health Financing Scheme: Assessment of Knowledge, Attitude, Practices, and Participation of Malaysian Private General Practitioners in the PeKa B40 Scheme. *PLoS ONE* **2023**, *18*, e0292516. [CrossRef]
9. Ku Abd Rahim, K.N.; Kamaruzaman, H.F.; Dahlui, M.; Wan Puteh, S.E. From Evidence to Policy: Economic Evaluations of Healthcare in Malaysia: A Systematic Review. *Value Health Reg. Issues* **2020**, *21*, 91–99. [CrossRef]
10. Sayuti, M.; Sukeri, S. Assessing Progress Towards Sustainable Development Goal 3.8.2 and Determinants of Catastrophic Health Expenditures in Malaysia. *PLoS ONE* **2022**, *17*, e0264422. [CrossRef]
11. Makmor, T.; Khaled, T.; Osman, A.F.; NurulHuda, M. Demographic and Socioeconomic Factors Associated with Access to Public Clinics. *J. Health Transl. Med.* **2018**, *21*. Available online: https://jummec.um.edu.my/article/view/12194 (accessed on 19 January 2024).
12. Yunus, N.M.; Manaf, N.H.A.; Omar, M.A.; Salleh, M. Determinants of Healthcare Utilisation among the Elderly in Malaysia. *Inst. Econ.* **2017**, *9*, 115–140. Available online: https://ijie.um.edu.my/index.php/ijie/article/view/4891/2749 (accessed on 19 January 2024).
13. Dr Zaliha: One Million Recipients of PeKa B40 Scheme Underwent Health Screening for NCDs Since April 2019. *Malay Mail*. 14 July 2023. Available online: https://www.malaymail.com/news/malaysia/2023/07/14/dr-zaliha-one-million-recipients-of-peka-b40-scheme-underwent-health-screening-for-ncds-since-april-2019/79807 (accessed on 19 January 2024).
14. Low Income Group Can Get Free Health Screening Through PeKa B40 Scheme, Says Khairy. *Malay Mail*. 21 February 2022. Available online: https://www.malaymail.com/news/malaysia/2022/02/21/low-income-group-can-get-free-health-screening-through-peka-b40-scheme-says/2043024 (accessed on 19 January 2024).
15. Halim, N.H.A.; Zainuddin, N.A.; Aminuddin, F.; Ahmad, F.; Hatta, S.; Saad, M.M.; Ali, R.M.; Azman, N.H.; Rahim, N.A. Navigating the Completing Cancer Treatment Incentive in Malaysia: Patient Insights and Implementation Challenges. *BMC Health Serv. Res.* **2025**, *25*, 435. [CrossRef] [PubMed]
16. Shahar, S.; Lau, H.; Puteh, S.E.W.; Amara, S.; Razak, N.A. Health, Access, and Nutritional Issues Among Low-Income Populations in Malaysia: Introductory Note. *BMC Public Health* **2019**, *19*, 552. [CrossRef]
17. Yunus, S.Z.S.A.; Puteh, S.E.W.; Ali, A.M.; Daud, F. The COVID Impact to Public Healthcare Utilization Among Urban Low-Income Subsidized Community in Klang Valley Malaysia. *Health Serv. Res. Manag. Epidemiol.* **2021**, *8*, 23333928211002407. [CrossRef]
18. Sommer, I.; Griebler, U.; Mahlknecht, P.; Thaler, K.; Bouskill, K.; Gartlehner, G.; Mendis, S. Socioeconomic Inequalities in Non-Communicable Diseases and Their Risk Factors: An Overview of Systematic Reviews. *BMC Public Health* **2015**, *15*, 914. [CrossRef]
19. WHO Malaysia. The Annual Health-Care Cost of Cardiovascular Diseases, Diabetes and Cancer in Malaysia Exceeds RM 9.65 Billion. 2022. Available online: https://www.who.int/malaysia/news/detail/09-08-2022-the-annual-health-care-cost-of-cardiovascular-diseases--diabetes-and-cancer-in-malaysia-exceeds-rm-9.65-billion (accessed on 19 January 2024).
20. Hussein, N.; Ng, C.W.; Ramli, R.; Rahim, S.S.S.A.; Mohd Arshad, M.M.; Wahab, N.A.; Abdullah, S.A. Assessing Catastrophic Health Expenditure and Impoverishment in Adult Asthma Care: A Cross-Sectional Study of Patients Attending Six Public Health Clinics in Klang District, Malaysia. *BMC Health Serv. Res.* **2024**, *24*, 327. [CrossRef]
21. Lim, M.T.; Ong, S.M.; Tong, S.F.; Bujnowska-Fedak, M.M.; Leponiemi, A.; Lionis, C.; Peritogiannis, V.; Sanfélix-Gimeno, G.; Seghieri, C.; Sęk, H.; et al. Comparison between primary care service delivery in Malaysia and other participating countries of the QUALICOPC project: A cross-sectional study. *BMJ Open* **2021**, *11*, e047126. [CrossRef]
22. WHO. *World Health Statistics 2021: Monitoring Health for the SDGs*; World Health Organization: Geneva, Switzerland, 2021. Available online: https://www.who.int/data/gho/publications/world-health-statistics (accessed on 19 January 2024).

23. Rajiah, K.; Maharajan, M.K.; Ramaya, H.; Wan Ab Rahman, W.N.A. Use of Psychotropic "Pro Re Nata" Medications by Patients Attending the Outpatient Clinic in a Hospital: A Qualitative Exploration. *Front. Med.* **2021**, *8*, 617147. [CrossRef]
24. van Doorslaer, E.; O'Donnell, O.; Rannan-Eliya, R.P.; Somanathan, A.; Adhikari, S.R.; Garg, C.C.; Harbianto, D.; Herrin, A.N.; Huq, M.N.; Ibragimova, S.; et al. Catastrophic Payments for Health Care in Asia. *Health Econ.* **2007**, *16*, 1159–1184. [CrossRef]
25. Mohd Noh, S.N.; Jawahir, S.; Tan, Y.R.; Ab Rahim, I.; Tan, E.H. The Health-Seeking Behavior among Malaysian Adults in Urban and Rural Areas Who Reported Sickness: Findings from the National Health and Morbidity Survey (NHMS) 2019. *Int. J. Environ. Res. Public Health* **2022**, *19*, 3193. [CrossRef] [PubMed]
26. Jaafar, S.; Mohd Noh, K.; Muttalib, K.A.; Othman, N.; Healy, J. *Malaysia Health System Review*; World Health Organization, Regional Office for the Western Pacific: Manila, Philippines, 2013. Available online: https://iris.who.int/bitstream/handle/10665/206911/9789290615842_eng.pdf?sequence=1 (accessed on 19 January 2024).
27. Mohd Rosnu, N.S.; Singh, D.K.A.; Mat Ludin, A.F.; Ishak, W.S.; Abd Rahman, M.H.; Shahar, S. Enablers and Barriers of Accessing Health Care Services among Older Adults in South-East Asia: A Scoping Review. *Int. J. Environ. Res. Public Health* **2022**, *19*, 7351. [CrossRef] [PubMed]
28. Isamail, N.; Said, R.; Ismail, N.W.; Haron, S.A. Non-Communicable Diseases Impact Low-Income Households in Malaysia. *Malays. J. Med. Sci.* **2024**, *31*, 124–139. [CrossRef] [PubMed]
29. Ab Hamid, J.; Juni, M.H.; Abdul Manaf, R.; Syed Ismail, S.N.; Lim, P.Y. Spatial Accessibility of Primary Care in the Dual Public-Private Health System in Rural Areas, Malaysia. *Int. J. Environ. Res. Public Health* **2023**, *20*, 3147. [CrossRef]
30. DeFrank, J.T.; Berkman, N.D.; Kahwati, L.; Cullen, K.; Aikin, K.J.; Sullivan, H.W. Direct-to-Consumer Advertising of Prescription Drugs and the Patient-Prescriber Encounter: A Systematic Review. *Health Commun.* **2020**, *35*, 739–746. [CrossRef] [PubMed]
31. The Malaysian Reserve. More People from B40 Group Benefit from MADANI Medical Scheme. *The Malaysian Reserve.* 29 August 2023. Available online: https://themalaysianreserve.com/2023/08/29/more-people-from-b40-group-benefit-from-madani-medical-scheme/ (accessed on 6 May 2025).
32. Ministry of Health Malaysia. *Health White Paper for Malaysia: Strengthening People's Health, Future-Proofing the Nation's Health System*; Ministry of Health Malaysia: Putrajaya, Malaysia, 2023. Available online: https://www.moh.gov.my/moh/resources/Penerbitan/Penerbitan%20Utama/Kertas%20Putih%20Kesihatan/Kertas_Putih_Kesihatan_(ENG)_compressed.pdf (accessed on 6 May 2025).

International Journal of
Environmental Research and Public Health

MDPI

Article

Improving Access to Radiotherapy: Exploring Structural Quality Indicators for Radiotherapy in Gauteng Province, South Africa

Portia N. Ramashia [1,*], Pauline B. Nkosi [2] and Thokozani P. Mbonane [1]

1 Department of Environmental Health, Faculty of Health Sciences, University of Johannesburg, Johannesburg 2000, South Africa; tmbonane@uj.ac.za

2 Faculty of Health Sciences, Durban University of Technology, Durban 4000, South Africa; paulinen1@dut.ac.za

* Correspondence: pramashia@uj.ac.za; Tel.: +27-11-559-6242

Abstract

Background: Radiotherapy is a critical component of effective cancer treatment, yet access remains limited in many low- and middle-income countries, including South Africa. This study explores structural quality indicators influencing radiotherapy access in Gauteng province, a region with a dual public–private healthcare system. Methods: A concurrent triangulation mixed-methods approach using a descriptive cross-sectional study was employed; for the quantitative phase, data from public and private radiotherapy facilities was analysed, and for the qualitative phase, insights were obtained from interviews with the heads of departments and members of three multidisciplinary professions in radiation oncology, namely radiation oncologists, radiation therapists, and medical physicists. Results: Findings reveal stark disparities in radiotherapy access. Gauteng province has only two major public radiotherapy facilities serving a large population, while multiple private facilities exist. The data indicate substantial differences in resource distribution, equipment accessibility, and personnel levels between public and private institutions. Bureaucratic inefficiencies, personnel shortages, and operational limitations in the public sector have surfaced as significant barriers to prompt equitable access to radiotherapy. This research shows the urgent need for focused strategies to address these systemic issues in order to improve access to radiation treatment in Gauteng province. The study's findings will inform the development of a comprehensive framework to enhance radiotherapy access and contribute to more equitable cancer care delivery in South Africa.

Keywords: radiotherapy; access; quality indicators; Gauteng province; South Africa; cancer care; healthcare system; mixed methods; resource allocation; health equity

1. Introduction

Radiotherapy is a critical component of effective cancer treatment, often playing a vital role in curative and palliative care strategies. Despite its importance, access to radiotherapy remains severely limited in many parts of the world, particularly in low- and middle-income countries [1]. The African continent, for instance, faces a significant disparity in radiotherapy access, with a considerably lower number of radiotherapy machines per capita compared to high-income regions [2,3]. This disparity contributes to poorer cancer outcomes and underscores the urgent need to improve access to radiotherapy services across Africa [4].

The availability of adequately trained and qualified personnel, including Radiation Oncologists (ROs), Radiation Therapists (RTTs), Medical Physicists (MPs), and Oncology Nurses (ONs), is crucial for workforce effectiveness [5,6]. Indicators may assess the number of staff per patient volume or per equipment unit [6]. Access to modern and well-maintained radiotherapy equipment, such as linear accelerators, brachytherapy units, treatment planning systems, and quality assurance tools, is essential, with indicators considering the age and type of equipment, maintenance records, and availability of advanced technology [4,7]. Appropriate infrastructure, including treatment rooms, simulation facilities, waiting areas, and support services, contributes to a safe and efficient environment, with indicators evaluating facility size, layout, safety features, and patient comfort. Robust information technology systems are vital for managing patient data, treatment planning, dose delivery, and quality assurance, with indicators assessing the use of electronic health records, treatment planning software, and data analysis tools. The presence of comprehensive quality management programmes ensures consistent adherence to protocols, safety standards, and continuous improvement efforts, with indicators evaluating the implementation of quality assurance procedures, incident reporting mechanisms, and staff training programmes [5].

Structural quality indicators in radiotherapy assess foundational elements that influence the delivery of high-quality care, focusing on tangible resources, organisational aspects, and infrastructure rather than processes or outcomes [6]. Key indicators include workforce availability, which evaluates the number of adequately trained personnel per patient volume or equipment unit; equipment access, which considers the age, type, and maintenance of radiotherapy tools; facilities, which assess infrastructure aspects like treatment rooms and patient comfort; information systems, which evaluate the use of technology for managing patient data and treatment planning; and quality management systems, which ensure adherence to protocols and continuous improvement through quality assurance procedures and staff training. By analysing these structural quality indicators, policymakers and healthcare providers can identify areas for improvement, allocate resources effectively, and ultimately enhance the quality and accessibility of radiotherapy services [8].

This study represents one phase of a larger research project designed to develop a comprehensive, evidence-based strategic framework for improving radiotherapy access for cancer patients in Gauteng province, South Africa. This phase examines the landscape of radiotherapy access in Gauteng province, South Africa, a region characterised by a dual public and private healthcare system, while the other phases looked at quantitative data on time intervals and patient experiences. We aim to explore the structural quality indicators of radiotherapy services and their impact on the access for cancer patients. By analysing data from both public and private radiotherapy facilities, this study provides a comprehensive assessment of the radiotherapy landscape in Gauteng province. Furthermore, we investigate the potential role of the private sector in supplementing state-provided services to improve overall access to radiotherapy for cancer patients. This research employs a concurrent triangulation mixed-methods approach, combining quantitative data analysis from radiotherapy facilities with qualitative insights from interviews conducted with key stakeholders, including radiation oncologists, radiation therapists, and medical physicists. This multifaceted approach allows for a nuanced understanding of the factors influencing radiotherapy access and quality in Gauteng province. The findings of this phase of the study will be instrumental in developing a comprehensive framework to improve access to radiotherapy by cancer patients in Gauteng province, South Africa, which is the goal of the postgraduate study that this phase is part of.

2. Materials and Methods

2.1. Study Approach and Design

This study employed a concurrent triangulation mixed-methods approach, while a descriptive cross-sectional design was used to explore the structural quality indicators of radiotherapy services in Gauteng province, South Africa, and their impact on patient access to radiotherapy. Data were collected from facilities' statistical data for the quantitative phase and interviews for the qualitative phase. The study was conducted in a month-to-month manner.

2.2. Study Setting and Population

The study employed a mixed-methods approach, combining quantitative data analysis from both public and private radiotherapy facilities with qualitative insights from interviews. While quantitative data were collected from a mix of public and private facilities, the qualitative phase focused specifically on gathering perspectives from healthcare professionals at two public radiotherapy facilities in Gauteng province. This focus allowed for a deeper exploration of the challenges and opportunities within the public sector context. For the quantitative phase, the facilities' data were acquired from heads of the radiation oncology departments (HODs) of radiotherapy departments. For the qualitative phase, the participants were HODs of the radiation oncology departments; the radiation oncologists (ROs), medical physicists (MPs), and radiation therapists (RTTs) in the public facilities.

2.3. Sampling

While the intention was to include all radiotherapy practices in Gauteng province (2 public and 20 private), logistical constraints resulted in incomplete participation. We successfully recruited 13 practices (2 public and 11 private). Six private practices were excluded due to delays in obtaining gatekeepers' permission, one practice closed during the data collection period, and another declined participation due to a busy schedule. This deviates from total population sampling, introducing the potential for bias. The practices that did not grant permission might have differed systematically from those that did. Similarly, the closure of one practice could indicate other issues not representative of the included practices, and the practice declining due to a busy schedule might have had a higher patient volume. Due to these limitations, the findings of this study should be interpreted with caution, and future research should employ more comprehensive sampling strategies to ensure greater representativeness.

2.4. Data Collection Approach

The study collected both quantitative and qualitative data to achieve the study's aim and objectives. Quantitative data were collected using a record review tool, while face-to-face interviews were used for qualitative data.

2.4.1. Quantitative Phase (Record Review)

The collected quantitative data included information on staffing, equipment, and the number of patients treated and waiting to start radiotherapy. The data collection tool was adapted from the International Atomic Energy Agency (IAEA) quality indicators tool (Table 1).

Table 1. Data collection tool.

Data Collected	Variable
C1 Average number of patients per day (January–December 2023)	Patient/Day
C2 Average number of patients per month (January–December 2023)	Patient/Month
C3 Average number of patients awaiting radiotherapy per month (January–December 2023)	Radiotherapy
D1 Number of linear accelarators	Accelerators
D2 Number of CT simulators	Simulation
D3 Number of brachytherapy units	Brachytherapy units

Table 1. *Cont.*

Data Collected	Variable
D4 Number of MRIs	MRI
D5 Number of PET scan	PET Scan
E1 Number of personnel (RO)	RO
E2 Number of personnel (MP)	MP
E3 Number of personnel (RTT)	RTT
E4 Number of personnel (ON)	ON

Abbreviations: RO = radiation oncologist; MP = medical physicist; RTT = radiation therapist; ON = oncology nurse.

2.4.2. Qualitative Phase (Interview)

Qualitative data were collected from two public radiotherapy facilities in Gauteng province through face-to-face interviews with the HODs of the radiation oncology departments and ROs, MPs, and RTTs. The intention was to also include the heads of ONs, but they were both not available. The interviews explored the challenges faced in providing radiotherapy services, including barriers related to staffing, training, and equipment. This approach provided a comprehensive understanding of the challenges and opportunities related to radiotherapy access from the perspectives of key personnel (ROs, MPs, and RTTs) involved in radiotherapy delivery.

2.5. High-Energy Units and Workload Estimation

The availability and utilisation of high-energy units (HEUs), such as linear accelerators, are critical factors in determining radiotherapy access. To assess HEU utilisation, the utilisation ratio was calculated using the following formula:

$$\text{Use of high-energy units} = \frac{Total\ number\ of\ patients\ treated\ in\ 1\ year}{Number\ of\ high\ energy\ units} \tag{1}$$

This ratio reflects the average number of patients treated per HEU annually, providing insights into equipment efficiency and potential resource strain. A higher ratio may indicate higher efficiency or, conversely, potential overutilisation and strain on resources.

To evaluate the workload of radiation therapy professionals, the following formula was used, adapted from international standards:

$$\text{Workload} = \frac{Total\ number\ of\ patients\ treated\ in\ 1\ year}{Number\ of\ workers} \tag{2}$$

This calculation compares workload distribution across different professional categories (radiation oncologists, therapists, and physicists) and between the public and private sectors. By comparing calculated workloads to established benchmarks or guidelines, the staffing levels were assessed to determine whether they were adequate to meet patient demand and maintain quality care. This analysis also informed the broader investigation into resource allocation and its impact on radiotherapy access in Gauteng province.

2.6. Data Analysis

2.6.1. Quantitative Phase Analysis

Data were entered into Microsoft Excel and then analysed using IBM SPSS Version 29 software. Frequencies and descriptive statistics were used to analyse and calculate key quality indicators of radiotherapy, including the staff-to-equipment-to-patient ratio and the average number of patients waiting to start treatment. Categorical variables were summarised with counts and percentages for the ratios; median, minimum, and maximum values were used. The statistics were run for the entire population and then were split by facility type (public or private).

2.6.2. Qualitative Phase Analysis

The qualitative interviews were transcribed and analysed using a thematic analysis approach to explore the key challenges and barriers to radiotherapy access as perceived by the HODs and key stakeholder professionals in radiotherapy departments.

2.7. Ethical Considerations

The relevant institutional ethics review board approved the study, and all participants provided informed consent before they participated in the study.

3. Results

This study provides a comprehensive assessment of structural quality indicators in radiotherapy services in Gauteng province. This section integrates these findings to provide a nuanced perspective on the factors influencing access to and quality of radiotherapy services. Employing a concurrent triangulation mixed-methods approach, the results reveal notable disparities in radiotherapy access between public and private facilities. Key themes that emerged from this integrated analysis include limited radiotherapy capacity impacting waiting times and treatment efficacy, disparities between the public and private sectors affecting technology availability and resource allocation, and systemic issues such as bureaucratic inefficiencies and communication breakdowns. These findings highlight the need for comprehensive strategies that address both structural and systemic barriers to ensure equitable access to quality radiotherapy for all patients in Gauteng. The following sections will present the quantitative data that highlight these disparities, followed by qualitative insights from interviews with the heads of the radiation oncology departments in the public facilities, which provide context and explain the underlying factors contributing to these challenges.

3.1. Quantitative Phase Results

This quantitative analysis aims to provide a comprehensive view of the radiotherapy landscape in Gauteng province, South Africa, by examining key characteristics of both public and private radiotherapy facilities. The results reveal notable differences in patient volume, equipment availability, and staffing levels between the two sectors. As shown in Table 2, the two public radiotherapy facilities in this study had a substantially higher average number of patients per day (mean = 102.50) compared to the private facilities (mean = 31.18) [1,4,9,10]. This noticeable disparity in patient load between the public and private facilities suggests a potential strain on resources and service provision within the public radiotherapy sector.

Significant variations were also observed in the availability of critical radiotherapy equipment. While all facilities reported having at least one CT simulator, the analysis of the data revealed that brachytherapy units, essential for internal radiation therapy, were present in both public facilities but only available in a limited capacity within the private sector. Similarly, access to MRI machines, which facilitate advanced treatment planning and tumour visualisation, was more prevalent in public facilities than private facilities [1]. This limited capacity is further exacerbated by systemic challenges such as bureaucratic delays in procuring new equipment, as reported in interviews, and insufficient investment in infrastructure, leading to longer waiting times and potentially compromising treatment efficacy.

Table 2. Descriptive analysis of public (N = 2) and private (N = 11) radiotherapy facilities.

Variables	Public Facilities					Private Facilities				
	Mean	Mode	SD [1]	Min [2]	Max [3]	Mean	Mode	SD	Min	Max
Patient/Day	102.50	100 [a]	3.54	100	105	31.18	12	12.86	12	52
Patient/Month	179.50	179 [a]	0.71	179	180	45.91	15	31.56	15	125
Radiotherapy	115.00	56 [a]	83.44	56	174	3.73	0	9.32	0	30
Accelerators	4.50	4 [a]	0.71	4	5	1.27	1	0.47	1	2
Simulation	1.00	1	0.01	1	1	1.00	1	0.01	1	1
Brachytherapy units	1.00	1	0.01	1	1	0.27	0	0.47	0	1
MRI	0.50	0 [a]	0.71	0	1	0.27	0	0.47	0	1
PET Scan	0.50	0 [a]	0.71	0	1	0.09	0	0.30	0	1
RO	3.00	2 [a]	1.44	2	4	4.18	3	2.18	1	9
MP	6.50	6 [a]	0.71	6	7	1.45	1	0.52	1	2
RTT	22.00	21 [a]	1.41	21	23	6.27	3 [a]	2.61	3	11
ON	15.50	15 [a]	0.71	15	16	0.18	0	0.41	0	1

[1] SD—Standard deviation.; [2] Min—Minimum. [3] Max—Maximum. [a] Multiple modes exist. Abbreviations: RO = radiation oncologist; MP = medical physicist; RTT = radiation therapist; ON = oncology nurse.

This difference highlights the importance of considering not just the total number of machines but also their availability relative to the population they serve. To further illustrate this point, our analysis revealed that public radiotherapy facilities had a higher average number of linear accelerators compared to private centres. Specifically, there were 4.5 linear accelerators in the public sector and 1.27 in the private sector in average per facility. However, to account for differences in patient populations served, we calculated the number of linear accelerators per 1000 patients. This normalised metric showed that the public sector had 2.09 linear accelerators per 1000 patients, while the private sector had 2.31 linear accelerators per 1000 patients. This difference in linear accelerator availability, as highlighted by the normalised metric, is reflected in the HEU utilisation ratios presented in Table 3 and the normalised linear accelerator availability in public and private sectors provided in Table 4. These disparities are perpetuated by policy gaps and governance issues that result in unequal funding allocations in public hospitals, as indicated by qualitative data.

$$Linear\ Accelerator\ per\ patients = \frac{number\ of\ linear\ accelerators}{total\ patients} \times 1000 \quad (3)$$

The workload of radiation oncologists, therapists, and medical physicists in both public and private facilities was analysed to examine the impact of patient volume on resource allocation and utilisation. As shown in Table 5, the workload is calculated as the average number of patients treated per year for each radiation oncologist, therapist, and medical physicist. Public facilities exhibit a considerably higher average workload for radiation oncologists (540–1048 patients/year) compared to private facilities (60–201 patients/year). This disparity is particularly striking when considering the recommended workload ranges of 250–300 patients per year for radiation oncologists. The radiation therapists in workload public and private facilities ranged between 93 and 103 patients/year and 55–115 patients/year, respectively; these ranges are within the recommended range of 100–150 patients per year. However, although the ranges are within the recommended range, it is important to note that these workload figures may be higher than currently represented due to variations in the scope of responsibilities for radiation therapists across the different centre types. For instance, therapists in public facilities are often required to work on a broader range of equipment, including brachytherapy units, which are less common in private facilities. These findings underline the significant strain placed on healthcare professionals within the public sector due to the higher patient volume.

Table 3. High energy unit (linear accelerator) utilisation in public and private radiotherapy centres.

Centre ID	Centre Type (Public/Private)	Total Patients Treated/Year (Average)	Number of HEUs	HEU Utilisation Ratio (Patients/HEU) [1]
1	Private	600	1	600
2	Private	540	2	270
3	Private	504	1	504
4	Private	744	2	372
5	Private	804	1	804
6	Private	276	1	276
7	Public	2160	4 (3) [2]	540 (720)
8	Private	432	1	432
9	Private	180	1	180
10	Private	300	1	300
11	Private	180	1	180
12	Private	1500	2	750
13	Public	2148	5 (3) [2]	430 (716)

[1] Reference range (patients/HEU) 200–500; [2] number of HEUs in use.

Table 4. Normalised linear accelerator availability in public and private sectors (linear accelerators per 1000 patients).

Sector	Number of Linear Accelerators	Patients Treated	Linear Accelerators per 1000 Patients
A [1]	14	6060	2.31
B [1]	9 (6) [2]	4308	2.09 (1.39)

[1] Sector A = private; B = public; [2] LINACs in use.

Table 5. Workload ratio for public and private radiotherapy facilities.

	Centre Type (Public/ Private)	Average Patients Treated/Year	Number of Radiation Oncologists	Number of Radiation Therapists	Number of Medical Physicists	Radiation Oncologist Workload (Patients/ Year) [1]	Radiation Therapist Workload (Patients/ Year) [2]	Medical Physicist Workload (Patients/ Year) [3]
1	Private	600	3	4	1	200	150	600
2	Private	540	3	7	2	180	77	270
3	Private	504	7	9	2	72	56	252
4	Private	744	5	11	2	149	68	372
5	Private	804	4	7	2	201	115	402
6	Private	276	4	5	1	69	55	276
7	Public	2160	4	21	7	540	103	309
8	Private	432	4	6	1	108	72	432
9	Private	180	1	3	1	180	60	180
10	Private	300	3	5	1	100	60	300
11	Private	180	3	3	1	60	60	180
12	Private	1500	9	9	2	167	167	750
13	Public	2148	2	23	6	1048	93	358

[1] Recommended: 250–300. [2] Recommended: 100–150 [3] Recommended: 300–400.

3.2. Qualitative Phase Findings

The interviews with the heads of the radiotherapy departments from the two public facilities echo the quantitative results. The thematic analysis of the qualitative data highlights specific barriers related to limited radiotherapy facilities, government bureaucracy and tendering challenges, staff shortages and remuneration disparities, and operational challenges. These systemic issues further exacerbate the challenges faced by public radiotherapy facilities and hinder their ability to provide timely and effective care, resulting in longer waiting times for treatment in the public sector, potentially leading to disease progression and poorer outcomes and widening the health equity gap between different socioeconomic groups in the province.

3.2.1. Limited Radiotherapy Facilities

Limited facilities have been expressed as a considerable challenge and limitation to radiotherapy. The radiation oncology healthcare professionals mentioned that there are limited treatment facilities for cancer patients, with only two facilities in Gauteng province accommodating many patients. The limited facilities then result in delays in receiving radiation therapy within the recommended timeframe. As the quantitative data indicate, the higher patient load per machine in the public sector likely contributes to these delays. The delay is further compounded by the fact that the existing facilities also serve patients from other provinces without radiotherapy centres. As is seen in the following excerpt:

> *"The major issue here in Gauteng province is the population that we have. We have many patients diagnosed with cancer, and we only have two facilities, for therefore our patients are not going to be getting radiation within the recommended period"*
>
> (CMJAH Healthcare Professional 1).
>
> *"Okay, so Gauteng province has only two major academic facilities which provide healthcare to the majority of the population in South Africa. So, 85% of the patients do not have access to medical services and rely on the public health system"*
>
> (SBAH Healthcare Professional 3).

This lack of resources is not merely a matter of funding, it is also tied to systemic issues such as bureaucratic inefficiencies and a lack of coordinated planning, further straining the capacity of the department to provide timely and effective care.

3.2.2. Government Bureaucracy and Tendering Challenges

Inefficient bureaucratic processes and tendering issues create significant obstacles for public radiotherapy facilities. Tender and procurement processes were expressed as another challenge, which often impacted the timeline for equipment used in treating cancer patients. The payment process in the procurement cycle can be a significant challenge due to delays and bureaucratic red tape, causing frustration and inefficiencies. There are challenges with equipment repairs and payment of invoices. The payment process is seen as overly complicated due to multiple levels of interference and tender rules. The process involves requesting quotes, creating purchase orders, and receiving services or goods from suppliers. However, delays often occur when submitting documents for purchase order numbers or navigating complex procurement procedures. These challenges contribute to extended timelines for acquiring equipment or services, impacting operational efficiency. For instance, malfunctioning machines cause delays at a radiotherapy facility. These challenges cause prolonged waiting times due to machines being down and limited in number. As seen in the following quotes:

> *"...there's an issue in planning, we need a solution around how planning needs to work, we need to sort of solve the issue regarding staffing and getting that, you know ... So it*

wasn't difficult things. Unfortunately, it's a bureaucracy that is very slow moving to try and get any of those things done. So it was very simple to diagnose what the issue was, but then to actually get people actioning any of this is a very long process"

(CMJAH Healthcare Professional 2).

"So, even getting the two compact Linacs onto the tender, which I started when I started here in 2021, only ended at the beginning of this year. The Brachytherapy was even longer, that was a five-year tendering process. That started before I even arrived here and only finished at the beginning of this year"

(CMJAH Healthcare Professional 2).

"Even though the tendering system, the idea was to empower those ones who want to initiate their businesses. The bureaucracy that comes with all these things do need to be looked at. But... The tenders are awarded to people who are not...I do not know whether I should say competent. Or who do not have products they can supply. They become third party."

(SBAH Healthcare Professional 1).

"So, the delay arises when you submit the required documents to say we are requesting that we get a PO for the service provider to be able to come and attend to the problem arising. So that, to me, has been an issue ..."

(SBAH Healthcare Professional 1).

"So, I think, yeah, I think in terms of equipment as well. I think procurement processes are extremely laborious and painful as well. When I started, I was involved as a chairperson of the steering committee for the acquisition of Brachytherapy for the province. We started the process in October 2019. It was only completed this year, at the beginning of the year, in 2024, and that is because the whole process is just so complex"

(SBAH Healthcare Professional 3).

3.2.3. Staff Shortages and Remuneration Disparities

Staff shortages, driven by remuneration disparities and challenging working conditions, emerged as a critical barrier to providing timely and effective radiotherapy care. These shortages are supported by quantitative data indicating that radiation oncologists in public facilities handle a considerably higher average workload (540–1048 patients/year) compared to their counterparts in private facilities (60–201 patients/year), exacerbating the strain caused by inadequate compensation and challenging working conditions. Healthcare professionals expressed that specialists were underpaid compared to other provinces, mainly due to an occupational-specific dispensation (OSD) introduced by the Department of Health, specifically in the Gauteng province. Therefore, participants expressed a need for healthcare professionals working in specialised areas to be paid accordingly. As seen in the following quote:

"... the remuneration of the staff in Gauteng province, not CMJAH alone, is different from other provinces. Therapists here are still paid as diagnostic radiographers. I do not know why things are done that way because there is this; I do not know whether it is a policy or what that says equal pay for equal jobs, which Gauteng province health is not practising. So, if these therapists are working in a speciality, they should be paid as specialists"

(CMJAH Healthcare Professional 1).

The remuneration issues then result in specialists seeking employment opportunities in the private sector or other provinces, as stated by two other professionals:

"... because this is what has happened here, where the biggest challenge was with the therapist, and they were leaving because of this payment issue, right, but in truth, staffing issues are just a problem throughout the specialities"

(SBAH Healthcare Professional 3).

"So, all these potential workers that wanted to stay with us go back to the private sector, and I think we are going to run into problems because eventually, this private sector is going to be totally overly, they are going to be full"

(SBAH Healthcare Professional 2).

The staff shortages do not only apply to radiation therapists. There is not enough incentive for all qualified specialists in the government sector. The challenging work environment and lack of financial rewards are discouraging for staff who have dedicated years to their studies and careers. The current criteria for radiation therapists do not align with the qualifications of recent graduates, leaving them without entry-level job opportunities. Some provinces have adjusted their rules, but Gauteng Province Health has not. Despite promises to address the issue, it has not been resolved, leading to a situation where qualified individuals cannot secure positions due to outdated regulations. This payment issue has led to staff leaving, affecting all specialities in the facility. Challenges with remuneration and working conditions have led to an imbalance in relation to available healthcare professionals who are available to treat patients. The remuneration and working conditions are part of the reason for the long waiting list. Healthcare professionals leaving the public sectors in Gauteng province and seeking opportunities in other provinces result in challenges with limited staff members, which then impacts the delivery of service. Some participants have expressed that, ultimately, there is a need for more specialists in South Africa since there are only a few available. The following quotes from healthcare professionals support this:

"... It can be easily resolved. We have tried numerous times with the Department of Health. There has been a memo sent out by Western Cape and KZN ... You know, they have amended their rules, even though DPSA has not amended theirs, and said that they can recruit people who do not have the OSD match requirements, even though they have a four-year degree. However, Gauteng Health refuses to do that. My personal opinion, I think it is maybe because of trade unions and because it might spill over into other disciplines where similar problems exist"

(SBAH Healthcare Professional 3).

"The second thing, I think, is that we do have a staffing issue. So if you are to compare us to the IAEA requirements for staffing, and that is also outdated, you know, and has not been updated, I think we are way, way under par. ... there is one full-time consultant, and then there are two doctors who come in to do one-day sessions. One of them might be leaving, so that is one thing. Then, two registrars are qualifying and will soon have to register as specialists. Nevertheless, the biggest thing is that they do not have any incentive to stay because the public sector does not pay lucrative salaries".

(SBAH Healthcare Professional 2).

"And so if you had to compare what they could earn in the private sector basically, they could earn one month's salary by just treating five patients, excluding overheads and stuff like that. So I think it is not inviting for them because, you know, the environment is frustrating because there are so many challenges. And then they basically, it is not financially lucrative, and they have studied a long time to get there"

(SBAH Healthcare Professional 2).

"As we speak, we do not have therapists that can operate all the linear accelerators. So, in my view, if we had enough staff to operate the equipment, we were going to be able to make a difference in these patients that are waiting for treatment"

(CMJAH Healthcare Professional 1).

"... but the biggest challenge currently is the lack of staff to be able to treat all those radiation patients. So, we have five fully functioning linear accelerators currently, but not enough staff to operate all the machines. Up until the beginning of July, we only worked three of our linear, linear accelerators, and then we have like three fully qualified with a comm serve, helping out sometimes after the school holidays."

(SBAH Healthcare Professional 2).

Addressing the human resource issue is crucial. Staff shortages are causing delays in patient treatment and limiting operational effectiveness. Staffing inadequacies also hinder the ability to conduct research and develop local policies. It was emphasised that having skilled individuals is as essential as having equipment.

3.2.4. Operational Challenges

Healthcare professionals highlighted challenges in the workflow and communication within their radiation oncology department. They mentioned the need for improved multidisciplinary teamwork, more structured protocols, better communication between staff and management, and involving all stakeholders in decision-making. They also emphasised the importance of collaborative planning involving therapists, doctors, and medical physicists to streamline processes and ensure efficient patient care. The following quotes support this:

"The other thing is communicating needs from your end user, I mean us now, and the executive or, you know, that communication sometimes is lost, like, for instance, I will make an example. Say the head of oncology, who is the head of the department, goes and sits with whoever is there, and they say, this is what is needed. However, the problem really is that in oncology, unfortunately, it is a multidisciplinary team, so the communication among professionals from all disciplines should be something that is really addressed"

(CMJAH Healthcare Professional 3).

"And the other one, as I am thinking, would be teamwork if the planners, not planners alone, planners, doctors and medical physics. If we can work together as a team and do these patients together, it will speed up the process. Furthermore, you know, when we work together as a team, even if communication improves, then we will enjoy our work as currently, the way I see things, there are lines drawn between the therapist, the doctor and the medical physicist. More especially between therapists and medical physicists, you will find that when a plan has some challenges, or maybe the medical physics is putting something on a plane, the medical physicist will bring the file back to the therapist instead of communicating directly with the consultant involved in order to resolve that issue, which then delays the treatment of a patient. So, I strongly feel that we need to improve in that as well"

(CMJAH Healthcare Professional 1).

"It feels like we are all working in silos, and that is not good for patients"

(CMJAH Healthcare Professional 3).

"I think there will always be a little strain between the radiographers and physicists because, I cannot say it, but it always seems like physics think they are more clever than radiographers, but it is not really the case. Also, because of the strain, we are constantly

putting out fires because of poor communication between the teams ... As a team, it is a collaboration we all bring to the table to get this patient's plan planned"

(SBAH Healthcare Professional 2).

Collaborative work was considered necessary even between radiography facilities in the province, as participants deemed it necessary for effective patient treatment. One healthcare professional believed that collaborative work could mean learning from each other. As seen in the following quote:

"Even though, when we went to Steve Biko during the fire, there were things that our doctors would say no to. Furthermore, Steve Biko's doctors were doing things like Steve Biko; they would give one single shot of 8Gy, and the patient goes, and here our doctors felt no, no, no with 8Gy single shot is too much for the patient. We want to give it bits by bits. So, such things. If then, that will make both centres consultants get together and they come up with one plan"

(CMJAH Healthcare Professional 1).

Efficiency in the referral process can help reduce delays and streamline patient care, as discussed in the following quote:

"They face the same the same issues. But what I would say is things that they can control, like when they refer patients, try to refer the patients, quickly to us, and then the other thing is, when they refer patients to us, to send everything that the patient needs, needs to come with biopsy, scans. Because what happens sometimes is that when the patients come without that, the patients will stay the entire day here, see, wait to see the doctor. The doctor will then write a letter back to their referring doctor and say, "Please, can you send the whatever, you know, CT scan of this patient, or whatever" right? Or, please, can you do a CT scan of this patient? It's, you know, and it's frustrating for the patients as well, going up. So, I think if those things that the doctors could just be a bit better"

(CMJAH Healthcare Professional 2).

Healthcare professionals discussed the challenges in planning and treating participants in the medical system, proposing a centralised hub with satellite facilities for oncology and diagnostics. They suggested creating a system to streamline communication and information sharing between facilities to avoid the duplication of services and improve efficiency. Participants also discussed the importance of proper information transfer between healthcare providers for effective patient care.

"I think, because it sounds like a Steve Biko, they do not have a long waiting period like us. Maybe if we can have a pool where we're all going to take from it to treat these patients, it might help. So a pool, we just have, we have a centralised planning system, so to say, this is the patient that has just been diagnosed, ... then we all take from that pool to plan the patient, and it goes to the machine. Because I understand Steve Biko has some patients that are waiting to be put on the machine, and with us, we do not have such patients. Instead, we are having a challenge in terms of planning"

(CMJAH Healthcare Professional 1).

"... However, what I would say is things that they can control, like when they refer patients, try to refer the patients quickly to us, and then the other thing is, when they refer patients to us, to send everything that the patient needs, needs to come with biopsy, scans. What happens sometimes is that when the patients come without that, the patients will stay the entire day here, waiting to see the doctor. The doctor will then write a letter back to their referring doctor and say, "Please, can you send the whatever ... you know...,

a CT scan of this patient, it is frustrating for the patients as well, going up and down. So, I think if those things are addressed, the doctors could be a bit better"

(CMJAH Healthcare Professional 2).

4. Discussion

This study examined radiotherapy access in Gauteng province, South Africa, revealing significant disparities between the public and private sectors. The quantitative analysis of high-energy unit utilisation demonstrated higher workloads and a potential strain on resources in public facilities compared to private facilities. Furthermore, workload distribution analysis revealed substantial variations among radiotherapy professionals, with some exceeding recommended standards while others fell short. Qualitative findings corroborated these results, highlighting key barriers to timely and effective radiotherapy services, including limited facilities, bureaucratic tendering processes for equipment acquisition, staff shortages with remuneration disparities, and operational challenges such as equipment breakdowns and inadequate maintenance. These systemic issues exacerbate the challenges faced by public radiotherapy facilities, contributing to longer waiting times [4,11]. Addressing these systemic issues will require a comprehensive, multifaceted approach involving policy reforms, targeted investments, and collaborative efforts between the public and private sectors.

Another key challenge is the stark imbalance in the distribution of facilities between the public and private sectors. There are only two public radiotherapy facilities compared to 20 private facilities serving a population of 15.83 million [12,13]. These results translate to a population-to-facility ratio of 7.9 million people per centre in the public sector. This disparity is further compounded by variations in radiotherapy capacity within each sector. Public facilities, on average, operate with four linear accelerators and one brachytherapy unit staffed with 22 radiotherapists.

In contrast, private facilities, on average, have 1.27 linear accelerators and 0.27 brachytherapy units, with 2.27 radiotherapists. These figures underscore the significant high patient load and potential resource strain in public facilities. Benchmarking these ratios against international standards, such as the IAEA recommendation of one megavoltage machine per 250,000–400,000 population, reveals a substantial shortfall in radiotherapy capacity within Gauteng province, particularly in the public sector [1]. This scarcity of resources contributes directly to extended waiting times and potentially compromises the quality of care delivered.

The limited radiotherapy facilities observed in Gauteng province echo a global trend, particularly pronounced in LMICs, where access to radiotherapy remains a significant challenge [14–16]. The findings of this study indicate a potential shortage of radiotherapy resources in Gauteng province. For context, it is important to consider the number of linear accelerators available relative to the patient population. In Gauteng province, approximately 4308 patients receive radiotherapy treatment annually. With a total of 9 linear accelerators (of which 6 are currently in use), this translates to 2.09 linear accelerators per 1000 patients when considering all machines and 1.39 linear accelerators per 1000 patients when considering only those in operation. This falls slightly short of the recommendation of 2.2 linear accelerators per 1000 patients, highlighting a need to maintain the current infrastructure to meet the demands of the population. The number of machines needed can be calculated based on how many fractions can be delivered per machine per year divided by the number of fractions per patient [1]. While public and private facilities may serve different patient populations, the resource imbalance clearly indicates a need for strategic investment and resource allocation to ensure equitable access to timely and effective radiotherapy services across the province.

A critical constraint on radiotherapy service delivery in Gauteng province is the severe shortage of qualified personnel, particularly within the public sector. This scarcity spans across key roles, including radiation oncologists, medical physicists, and radiation therapists. Interview data revealed a significant disparity in remuneration between the public and private sectors for these positions. Healthcare professionals in the public sector frequently cited lower salaries and less favourable working conditions compared to their private sector counterparts, leading to an exodus of skilled personnel to private institutions or other provinces. This trend has resulted in increased workload and burnout among remaining staff in the public sector, ultimately impacting the quality of patient care. The brain drain further exacerbates the strain on the already limited public radiotherapy services, resulting in increased workloads for remaining staff, potential compromises in patient care, and extended waiting times for treatment. In addressing the critical workforce shortage, it is essential to implement strategies that will attract and retain qualified professionals in public facilities; competitive salaries and benefits packages are necessary. Furthermore, to mitigate the impact of these workforce shortages and improve the efficiency of radiotherapy service delivery, exploring the use of artificial intelligence (AI) technologies might be beneficial. AI can automate tasks such as contouring or treatment planning and optimise treatment plans and workflows [17,18].

While the shortage of qualified personnel poses a significant challenge, these human resource issues are often exacerbated by bureaucratic hurdles and inefficiencies in the procurement and maintenance of essential radiotherapy equipment. As Ambe notes in a study on the role of public procurement to socioeconomic development, "*public procurement activities suffer from neglect, a lack of direction, poor co-ordination, a lack of open competition and transparency, differing levels of corruption, and most importantly, not having a cadre of trained and qualified procurement specialists who can conduct and manage procurement in a professional, timely and cost-effective manner*" [19].

These bureaucratic processes, including lengthy tendering procedures and complex administrative requirements, further complicate the already strained radiotherapy service in Gauteng province. Streamlining procurement practices and increasing transparency could help address these challenges and improve access to life-saving treatment in the region. While streamlining procurement practices is crucial, the impact of these bureaucratic challenges extends beyond acquisition to the operational realities within radiotherapy facilities [20,21]. The lack of timely maintenance and repairs, often a direct result of these inefficiencies, creates significant operational hurdles that further impede service delivery.

Moreover, beyond staffing and procurement challenges, healthcare professionals expressed significant concerns about operational issues stemming from poor communication, lack of teamwork, and collaboration within the radiation oncology multidisciplinary departments. One interviewee noted that there are siloed approaches within these departments, with insufficient coordination between key personnel like ROs, RTTs, and MPs, often leading to suboptimal treatment planning and delivery. This observation aligns with findings, highlighting the prevalence of communication breakdowns between these professional groups and their negative impact on patient care and echoing the concerns raised in a study by Selby et al. regarding the fragmentation of care in multidisciplinary oncology settings [5,22]. Another interviewee's comment, "*We are constantly putting out fires because of communication breakdowns*", highlights the urgency of addressing these issues. As Buchman et al. suggest, fostering a culture of interdisciplinary collaboration through regular multidisciplinary team meetings and targeted training programmes can significantly improve communication, teamwork, and, ultimately, patient outcomes in radiation oncology service delivery [23]. These challenges are not unique to Gauteng. Studies show that disparities in access to radiotherapy services persist, especially in low- and middle-income countries.

Proposed solutions include task-shifting, which may improve radiotherapy access and reduce waiting times in the region.

This study contributes to the growing body of evidence [14,24–26] demonstrating the negative impact of limited radiotherapy capacity on cancer outcomes in LMICs. The long waiting times experienced by patients in Gauteng province due to insufficient facilities may lead to disease progression and reduced treatment efficacy, ultimately exacerbating existing health disparities. The potential consequences of limited radiotherapy access to patient outcomes are highlighted. Exploring alternative service delivery models, such as task-shifting, may offer potential strategies to improve radiotherapy access and reduce waiting times in Gauteng province. These strategies will include the framework that will be developed following this phase of the postgraduate research study aimed at improving access to radiotherapy and must consider the unique contextual factors, including economic and health system constraints, that shape radiotherapy service delivery in the region.

This study employed a convenience sampling method, which, while practical, introduces potential limitations regarding the generalizability of the findings. As detailed in the methodology section, delays in obtaining gatekeepers' permission resulted in the exclusion of six private practices. This exclusion could potentially bias the sample, particularly if these practices share common characteristics that differ from the included practices. For example, if the excluded practices were predominantly high-volume centres, our findings might underestimate the actual utilisation of HEUs in the private sector. Additionally, one practice closed during the data collection period, further limiting the sample size and potentially affecting the representativeness of the private sector. Finally, one practice declined participation due to a busy schedule. While understandable, this non-response could introduce selection bias, as busier practices might have different resource allocation strategies or staffing patterns compared to less busy practices. These limitations should be considered when interpreting the study's findings and generalising them to the broader radiotherapy landscape in Gauteng province. Future research with a larger, more representative sample is needed to confirm these findings and explore the nuances of HEU utilisation and workload across diverse practice settings.

5. Conclusions

In conclusion, addressing the challenges in Gauteng's radiotherapy services, including bureaucratic inefficiencies, human resource shortages, and operational constraints, necessitates a comprehensive, multifaceted approach encompassing policy reforms, targeted investments, and robust public–private collaboration. This research underscores the urgent need for such interventions to improve access and equity in radiotherapy for cancer patients in Gauteng province.

To build upon these findings, the next phase of this research will focus on developing an actionable strategic framework. This framework will integrate quantitative data on time intervals, qualitative insights into patient experiences, and structural quality indicators to provide a practical roadmap for improving radiotherapy services. By synthesising results from all phases, this framework aims to guide decision-making and resource allocation, ensuring that interventions are evidence-based and patient-centred.

Ultimately, this research seeks to contribute to a more equitable and efficient cancer care system, not only in Gauteng but also in similar LMICs facing comparable challenges. By translating research into actionable strategies, we can strive to ensure that all patients have timely access to the life-saving benefits of radiotherapy, regardless of their socioeconomic status or geographic location.

Author Contributions: Conceptualisation, P.N.R., T.P.M. and P.B.N.; methodology, P.N.R.; data curation, P.N.R.; writing—original draft preparation, P.N.R.; writing—review and editing, P.N.R., T.P.M. and P.B.N. All authors have read and agreed to the published version of the manuscript.

Funding: The principal researcher (P.N.R) received a research grant in support of the PhD studies from the National Research Foundation of South Africa (NFSG23031582533).

Institutional Review Board Statement: This study was conducted according to the guidelines of the UJ. This article is part of the first author's PhD study at the University of Johannesburg (UJ); the proposal complied with the Faculty of the Health Sciences standards at the UJ (HDC-01-154-2023) and was registered in the National Health Research Database (NHRD), ref no.: GP_202311_078). The Faculty of Health Sciences Research Ethics Committee (REC) at the University of Johannesburg granted ethical clearance (REC-2509-2023, 28 November 2023) for the study.

Informed Consent Statement: Informed consent was obtained from all subjects involved in the study.

Data Availability Statement: All data in this study are provided in the main manuscript.

Acknowledgments: The authors would like to acknowledge J. de Klerk, biostatistician from the UJ Statistical Consultation Service (STATKON), for the support in developing the data collection tool and analysis of the data and K. Moilwa of Oracle Research Consulting for the qualitative data transcriptions and coding.

Conflicts of Interest: The authors declare no conflicts of interest. The funders had no role in the design of the study; in the collection, analyses, or interpretation of data; in the writing of the manuscript; or in the decision to publish the results.

References

1. Zubizarreta, E.H.; Fidarova, E.; Healy, B.; Rosenblatt, E. Need for radiotherapy in low and middle income countries—The silent crisis continues. *Clin. Oncol.* **2015**, *27*, 107–114. [CrossRef] [PubMed]
2. Vanderpuye, V.; Hammad, N.; Martei, Y.; Hopman, W.M.; Fundytus, A.; Sullivan, R.; Seruga, B.; Lopes, G.; Sengar, M.; Brundage, M.D.; et al. Cancer care workforce in Africa: Perspectives from a global survey. *Infect. Agents Cancer* **2019**, *14*, 11. [CrossRef] [PubMed]
3. Akinwande, A.M.; Ugwuanyi, D.C.; Chiegwu, H.U.; Idigo, F.; Ogolodom, M.P.; Anakwenze, C.P.; Abi, R.; Odukoya, O. Radiotherapy services in low resource settings: The situation in Nigeria. *SAGE Open Med.* **2023**, *11*, 20503121231153758. [CrossRef] [PubMed]
4. Ndlovu, N. Radiotherapy treatment in cancer control and its important role in Africa. *Ecancermedicalscience* **2019**, *13*, 942. [CrossRef]
5. Sternick, E.S. Development of a comprehensive radiation oncology quality and safety program. *Front. Oncol.* **2014**, *4*, 30. [CrossRef]
6. Salma, N.S.; Raveendran, V.; Ranjith, C.P.; Anjana, P.T.; Gupta, T.; Laskar, S. Structural Quality Indicators in Radiation Oncology: Insights and Implications. *Clin. Oncol.* **2024**, *38*, 103624. [CrossRef]
7. Mdletshe, N. Perceptions of Radiotherapy Employees on Radiotherapy Costing in KZN Health Provincial Hospitals. Doctoral Dissertation, University of Kwazulu-Natal, Durban, South Africa, 2017.
8. Foroudi, F.; Kron, T. Importance of quality in radiation oncology. *J. Med. Imaging Radiat. Oncol.* **2017**, *61*, 660–661. [CrossRef]
9. Bhatia, R.; Balogun, O.D.; Simonds, H.; Vanderpuye, V.; Shah, M.M.; Yamoah, K.; Dominello, M.M.; Hanna, N.; Grover, S. Radiation therapy current practice capacity and needs assessment in Africa. *Int. J. Radiat. Oncol. Biol. Phys.* **2019**, *105*, E453. [CrossRef]
10. Stecklein, S.R.; Taniguchi, C.M.; Melancon, A.D.; Lombe, D.; Lishimpi, K.; Banda, L.; Mwaba, C.; Pupwe, G.; Mwale, M.; Munkupa, H.; et al. Radiation sciences education in Africa: An assessment of current training practices and evaluation of a high-yield course in radiation biology and radiation physics. *JCO Glob. Oncol.* **2020**, *6*, 1631–1638.
11. Lievens, Y.; Borras, J.M.; Grau, C. Provision and use of radiotherapy in Europe. *Mol. Oncol.* **2020**, *14*, 1461–1469. [CrossRef]
12. OPINION: Stark Realities Facing Cancer Patients at Charlotte Maxeke Hospital, Spotlight. Available online: www.spotlightnsp.co.za (accessed on 9 August 2023).
13. Available online: https://bmr.co.za/2024/08/20/mid-2024-population-projections-for-south-africa (accessed on 11 November 2024).

14. Grover, S.; Xu, M.J.; Yeager, A.; Rosman, L.; Groen, R.S.; Chackungal, S.; Rodin, D.; Mangaali, M.; Nurkic, S.; Fernandes, A.; et al. A systematic review of radiotherapy capacity in low-and middle-income countries. *Front. Oncol.* **2015**, *4*, 380. [CrossRef] [PubMed]
15. Yap, M.L.; Zubizarreta, E.; Bray, F.; Ferlay, J.; Barton, M. Global access to radiotherapy services: Have we made progress during the past decade? *J. Glob. Oncol.* **2016**, *2*, 207–215. [CrossRef]
16. Bishr, M.K.; Zaghloul, M.S. Radiation therapy availability in Africa and Latin America: Two models of low and middle income countries. *Int. J. Radiat. Oncol. Biol. Phys.* **2018**, *102*, 490–498. [CrossRef]
17. Korreman, S.; Eriksen, J.G.; Grau, C. The changing role of radiation oncology professionals in a world of AI–just jobs lost–or a solution to the under-provision of radiotherapy? *Clin. Transl. Radiat. Oncol.* **2021**, *26*, 104–107. [CrossRef]
18. Krishnamurthy, R.; Mummudi, N.; Goda, J.S.; Chopra, S.; Heijmen, B.; Swamidas, J. Using Artificial Intelligence for Optimization of the Processes and Resource Utilization in Radiotherapy. *JCO Glob. Oncol.* **2022**, *8*, e2100393. [CrossRef] [PubMed]
19. Ambe, I.M. The role of public procurement to socioeconomic development. *Int. J. Procure. Manag.* **2019**, *12*, 652–668.
20. Balogun, O.; Rodin, D.; Ngwa, W.; Grover, S.; Longo, J. Challenges and prospects for providing radiation oncology services in Africa. *Semin. Radiat. Oncol.* **2017**, *27*, 184–188. [CrossRef] [PubMed]
21. Maitre, P.; Krishnatry, R.; Chopra, S.; Gondhowiardjo, S.; Likonda, B.M.; Hussain, Q.M.; Zubizarreta, E.H.; Agarwal, J.P. Modern radiotherapy technology: Obstacles and opportunities to access in low-and middle-income countries. *JCO Glob. Oncol.* **2022**, *8*, e2100376. [CrossRef]
22. Selby, P.; Popescu, R.; Lawler, M.; Butcher, H.; Costa, A. The value and future developments of multidisciplinary team cancer care. *Am. Soc. Clin. Oncol. Educ. Book* **2019**, *39*, 332–340. [CrossRef]
23. Buchman, S.; Evans, J.M.; Mackinnon, M.; Gradin, S.; Wright, F.C. Bridging silos: Delivering integrated care to patients with cancer in Ontario, Canada. *Psycho-Oncology* **2018**, *27*, 2673–2676. [CrossRef]
24. Datta, N.R.; Samiei, M.; Bodis, S. Radiation therapy infrastructure and human resources in low-and middle-income countries: Present status and projections for 2020. *Int. J. Radiat. Oncol. Biol. Phys.* **2014**, *89*, 448–457. [PubMed]
25. Zietman, A. Bringing radiation therapy to underserved nations: An increasingly global responsibility in an ever-shrinking world. *Int. J. Radiat. Oncol. Biol. Phys.* **2014**, *89*, 440–442. [PubMed]
26. Efstathiou, J.A.; Heunis, M.; Karumekayi, T.; Makufa, R.; Bvochora-Nsingo, M.; Gierga, D.P.; Suneja, G.; Grover, S.; Kasese, J.; Mmalane, M.; et al. Establishing and delivering quality radiation therapy in resource-constrained settings: The story of Botswana. *J. Clin. Oncol.* **2016**, *34*, 27–35. [CrossRef] [PubMed]

International Journal of
Environmental Research and Public Health

MDPI

Article

Social Determinants and Health Equity Activities: Are They Connected with the Adaptation of AI and Telehealth Services in the U.S. Hospitals?

Pearl A. Pinera [1], Pearl C. Kim [1], Fye A. Pinera [1] and Jay J. Shen [1,2,*]

[1] Department of Healthcare Administration and Policy, School of Public Health, University of Nevada, Las Vegas, NV 89119, USA; pinerp1@unlv.nevada.edu (P.A.P.); pearl.kim@unlv.edu (P.C.K.); pinera@unlv.nevada.edu (F.A.P.)
[2] Center for Health Disparities Research, School of Public Health, University of Nevada, Las Vegas, NV 89119, USA
* Correspondence: jay.shen@unlv.edu

Abstract

In recent decades, technological shifts within the healthcare sector have significantly transformed healthcare management and utilization, introducing unprecedented possibilities that elevate quality of life. Organizational factors are recognized as key drivers in technology adoption, but involvement of hospitals in community-oriented activities and promotion of health equity are underexplored. This study investigated the impact of community social determinant activities and health equity activities on the adoption of AI and telehealth services within U.S. hospitals. The data were collected from the 2021 American Hospital Association (AHA) annual survey and were analyzed using multiple logistic and linear regression models to examine activities related to addressing population health, particularly social determinants and health equity, and their impacts on the adoption of AI and telehealth among U.S. hospitals. The results indicate a significant positive association between the community social determinant indicator and health equity indicator in adopting AI and telehealth services. Organizational factors were also major drivers of AI and telehealth adoption. The active incorporation of hospital strategies that address social determinants and promote health equity leads to the integration of advanced technologies and improves hospital conditions, enabling more adaptability to the changing healthcare landscape, which enhances healthcare services and accessibility.

Keywords: artificial intelligence; telehealth; social determinants; health equity; hospital

1. Introduction

The widespread acceptance of technology in the healthcare sector over the past decades has led to a paradigm shift in healthcare management and utilization, contributing to enhanced patient outcomes across a broader continuum of care. The implementation of technologies such as artificial intelligence (AI) is promptly gaining traction in many medical disciplines, functioning as clinical support systems for many healthcare providers [1]. Simultaneously, the integration of telehealth has introduced significant progress in the delivery of virtual care services, further elevating healthcare processes and overall accessibility [2]. Growing health technology adoption in healthcare highlights public concerns with the received quality of care and safety risks within U.S. hospitals [3]. These have driven healthcare organizations to embrace advanced innovative solutions that prioritize patient safety and elevate care delivery.

The development of AI in 1956 significantly boomed to support human input in various settings [4] and healthcare has been no exception. AI is a designed computer system that executes human intelligence across numerous healthcare operations and has shown incredible results in different healthcare areas including service management, logistic processes, predictive medicine, diagnostic treatment and prognosis evaluation, clinical decision-making, and medical research [5]. The utilization of AI services in many healthcare operations has improved patient safety and the received quality of care, especially with rising healthcare-associated infections, adverse drug events, and diagnostic errors [6]. Additionally, with the increasing U.S. healthcare costs, integration of AI has been seen as a potential asset to reduce healthcare spending by billions of dollars in the next few years [7]. As a result, hospitals embrace the adoption of AI to streamline healthcare processes, including mitigating healthcare expenses.

Similarly, the utilization of telehealth technologies has flaunted remarkable outcomes in healthcare, particularly during the onset of the COVID-19 pandemic [8]. While U.S. hospital admissions rose with COVID-19 patients, together with complications from cardiac events and other common health conditions [9], telehealth and remote monitoring have become significant tools for managing patient care from a distance. During this period, the majority of telehealth adoption was associated with the need to provide continuity of care for paused inpatient services and an absence of hospital spaces amid the mandatory "stay-at-home" protocols [8,10]. Regardless of the decline in telehealth utilization at the end of 2021 [11], telehealth services continue to reach many healthcare practices including managing chronic geriatrics, mental health, and other specialized areas of care [12–14]. Despite these innovative solutions, certain hospitals still lag in the adoption of telehealth and AI, creating barriers to healthcare service delivery and exacerbating existing health disparities [15,16]. These disparities underline the need for greater technology adoption within hospitals, ensuring equitable access to care and enhancing health outcomes among broader patient demographics.

Institutional theory argues that legitimacy in environments is crucial for organizations to exist and grow [17]. Organizations often respond to changes in their surrounding environments (e.g., geographic area, local policy, population and community, and market competition) for maintaining and strengthening their legitimacy. Therefore, changes being made, such as technology adoption among hospitals, are influenced by environmental and community factors. Telehealth utilization among U.S. hospitals is significantly affected by several state-level policies related to service reimbursements, including market dynamics and technology capacity [18]. Similarly, AI adoption among hospitals is shaped by factors such as market share, hospital characteristics, and performance outputs [19]. Adding the restrictions and barriers based on hospitals' cultural stances and overall healthcare structure, technology implementation becomes more challenging. In particular, U.S. hospitals exhibit multifaceted organizational cultures, instead of one major cultural type, with these hospitals embodying strong multidimensional cultures, using higher quality measurements, and giving patient-centered care [20]. Additionally, the complexity of diverse networks of the U.S. healthcare system raises concerns ranging from delivery and access to the overall healthcare framework. This has led to creating disparities in the overall provision of healthcare, affecting mostly less-resourced and underserved populations.

Moreover, in response to the need for broader patient demographics in communities, many hospitals, to gain and strengthen their legitimacy, are actively involved in population health by implementing strategies that address upstream social determinants of health and the core causes of health inequity/disparities [21,22]. These approaches provide a foundation for navigating the complexities of healthcare delivery and improving health outcomes [23]. Despite the importance of these initiatives to address population health, their impact on the adoption of technologies such as AI and telehealth services remains under-examined. This underscores the importance of further investigation into how these hospital activities related to social determinants and health equity may impact or hinder the adoption of technologies in healthcare settings. According to institutional theory, we hypothesized that, for maintaining and strengthening legitimacy, hospitals that are able to do well in one area, such as addressing community social determinants needs, will also be likely to do well in other areas such as AI and technology adaptation, because they often have the mindset, resources, and experiences to do so.

Nevertheless, although numerous studies have investigated the significance of AI and telehealth technologies, there is a literature gap in exploring the relationship between social determinants efforts on the adoption of AI and other technologies in hospitals. This has led to a growing lack of acknowledgement of the importance of hospitals' involvement in activities aimed at narrowing disparities and underlying social factors across various areas. Additionally, with the current status of the U.S. healthcare system framework that continues to stir conflicts related to equitable access and delivery of care, the integration of new technologies across larger diverse demographics has become more challenging. Therefore, examining the significance of social determinant indicator- and health equity indicator-related hospital activities is currently needed to improve hospitals' strategies focusing on addressing population health to assess greater technological adoption across all healthcare areas. The aims of this study were to (a) examine the association between social determinants and health equity activities with regard to the adoption of AI and telehealth services; (b) evaluate the association of these activities with the utilization of AI, telehealth, and the overall volume of virtual services; and (c) identify organizational factors that might relate to these technologies' adoption in U.S. hospitals.

2. Materials and Methods

2.1. Data Source

This study chose various types of hospitals across the United States, considering ownership, market characteristics, bed size, geographic locations, and hospital groups. The aspects of hospital community social determinant indicator and health equity indicator were stated as the independent variables (manipulated variable), while the AI and telehealth services were articulated as the dependent variables (observed variable). Data for this study were obtained using the 2021 American Hospital Association (AHA) annual survey, which represents various types of hospitals, healthcare networks, patients, and communities [24]. The AHA annual survey is a valuable resource for identifying AI services, telehealth, remote patient monitoring, and behavioral or social determinants of health services [25]. The year 2021 was chosen for the period of this study as it was the only year that information on AI-related activities was available, and it also provided the latest data on health equity activities and other initiatives demonstrating equity efforts within U.S. hospitals. The final sample size included 4061 hospitals.

2.2. Dependent Variables

Five dependent variables were selected to illustrate whether hospitals adopted AI or telehealth and to assess the extent of use of technologies, such as AI, telehealth, and virtual services in hospital operations. The use of AI and telehealth were treated as dichotomous variables to demonstrate a hospital's status regarding the adoption of these technological tools. The dependent variable of using AI was sourced using the AHA questionnaire, which asked whether a hospital uses AI or machine learning in any of the activities (predicting staffing needs, predicting patient demand, staff scheduling, automating routine tasks, and optimizing administrative and clinical workflows). The dependent variable of using telehealth was sourced using the AHA questionnaire, which asked hospitals to check whether it offers any different types of telehealth services (e.g., consultation and office visits, eICU, stroke care, psychiatric and addiction treatment, remote patient monitoring, other virtual care). These two variables referred to the condition of hospitals integrating AI or telehealth into their services and practices. Other dependent variables included the number of AI activities, the number of telehealth services, and the overall number of virtual services which were cited as continuous variables. The number of AI activities highlights the total records of AI appearance with regard to hospital operations. On the other hand, the number of telehealth services refers to the overall number of remote services delivered via digital health platforms. Finally, the overall number of virtual services incorporates all of the services offered virtually, including AI and telehealth.

2.3. Independent Variables

Independent variables were selected to indicate hospitals' activities related to social determinants and health equity. To measure hospitals' involvement in addressing social determinants of health and promoting health equity, we assessed two key indicators: the social determinant indicator and the health equity indicator. All independent variables were obtained using the 2021 AHA annual survey, which records all necessary comprehensive information of U.S. hospitals' activities.

The two independent variables were composite indicator of social determinant activities and composite indicator of health equity activities, based on Section F of the AHA annual survey. According to the AHA survey questionnaire design, the first independent variable, the community social determinant composite indicator focused on addressing social determinants that are non-medical factors that influence the health of individuals. AHA has recognized different social determinants of health that implicate healthcare access, including economic stability, neighborhood and built environments, education, social and community context, biology, and health behavior [26]. This social determinant indicator variable exhibited 28 community social determinant-related programs/activities (e.g., housing, food security, transportation, interpersonal violence, employment, education) reported by U.S. hospitals in the AHA 2021 annual survey, ranging from 0 to 28, illustrating the various community social determinant activities that hospitals are involved in. The second independent variable, the health equity composite indicator, focused on accountability and commitment of hospitals in assessing the hospital's strategies towards health equity goals such as addressing health disparities, equitable access to care, diverse representation, and culturally appropriate patient care. This health equity indicator encompassed 24 health equity actions/activities (e.g., having a health equity strategic plan, implementing and meeting health equity goals, and using DEI (diversity, equity, and inclusion) in decision-making), ranging from 0 to 24, highlighting the extent of hospital engagement in activities that promote equitable access to care and diversity. These activities primarily focused on managing health disparities and inequalities, aiming to achieve equitable health outcomes.

2.4. Statistical Analysis

Multiple logistic regression was used for analyzing the two dichotomous dependent variables and multiple linear regression was used for analyzing the three continuous dependent variables. Covariates being considered in the multivariable models included the hospital's bed size (6–49 beds, 50–199 beds, 200–399 beds, and 400 beds or more), ownership (public, investor-owned, and non-for-profit private), type (specialty hospital, children's hospital, mental health hospital, long-term care hospital, acute short-term hospital, and rural and non-rural hospital), and local market competition (competitive market, mild-concentrated market, and concentrated market). In response to the right tail distributions of both the number of AI services and the number of telehealth services, sensitivity analysis was conducted by taking the log of the two continuous dependent variables, respectively, and rerunning the regression models, which yielded similar results in terms of statistical significance of the independent variables.

3. Results

Table 1 illustrates the trends and characteristics of AI and telehealth adoption in U.S. hospitals including social determinants and health equity activities from 2021. AI adoption was observed at about 24.62%, with an average of 0.68 AI services and a standard deviation (SD) of 1.41. On the other hand, telehealth adoption was significantly higher at about 84.54%, with an average of 3.06 telehealth services and an SD of 2.71. The average number of all virtual services was 65,553, with an SD of 304,790. In terms of hospital activities, the mean number of social determinant activities was about 13.26, with an SD of 8.59 while health equity was about 8.66, with an SD of 8.01. Furthermore, 36.81% of hospitals had a bed size of 50–199 beds and approximately 80.06% of hospitals were short-term acute general hospitals. Additionally, the majority of hospitals were not-for-profit (60.72%, with (39.94%) identified as teaching hospitals, located mainly in rural areas (37.36%), and structured as concentrated markets (64.57%)).

Table 1. Characteristics of AI and telehealth adoption in U.S. hospitals, 2021 (n = 4061).

Variables	Percent
Response Variable	
Use of AI	24.62%
Number of AI services, mean (SD)	0.68 (1.41)
Use of telehealth	84.54%
Number of telehealth services, mean (SD)	3.06 (2.71)
All virtual services, mean, (SD), (n = 2893)	65,553 (304,790)
Main Independent Variable	
Community social determinant score, mean (SD)	13.26 (8.59)
Health equity score, mean (SD)	8.66 (8.01)
Hospital Characteristics	
Hospital Size	
6–49 beds	35.16%
50–199 beds	36.81%
200–399 beds	17.36%
400–500 and more beds	10.66%
Hospital Type	
Mental health hospital	6.55%
Children's hospital	2.27%
Specialty hospital	7.57%
Long-term care hospital	3.55%
Short-term acute general hospital	80.06%
Hospital Ownership Type	
Investor-owned	18.96%
Not-for-profit	60.72%
Public	20.32%
Teaching hospital	39.94%
Rural hospital	37.36%
Hospital Market Type	
Competitive market	19.16%
Mild concentrated market	16.28%
Concentrated market	64.57%

Source: American Hospital Association, 2021; Note: AI = artificial intelligence; SD = standard deviation.

Table 2 shows the associations between social determinants and health equity activities of hospitals and their adoption of AI and telehealth. A one-point increase in the community social determinant indicator was associated with a 7.0% increase in the odds of adopting AI (odds ratio [OR] = 1.070, 95% confidence interval [CI] = [1.054, 1.086]) and a 7.7% increase in the odds of adopting telehealth services (OR = 1.077, CI = [1.060, 1.093]). Similarly, a one-point increase in the health equity indicator was associated with an 8.5% increase in the odds of adopting AI (OR = 1.085, CI = [1.070, 1.1001]) and a 4.6% increase in the odds of adopting telehealth services (OR = 1.046, CI = [1.026, 1.067]). In addition, this study showed that small hospitals were less likely to adopt AI. Public and investor-owned hospitals were less likely to adopt both AI and telehealth compared to their non-for-profit counterparts. Rural hospitals had a higher likelihood of adopting telehealth and hospitals within competitive markets tended to adopt AI compared to their counterparts in concentrated markets (Table 2). The results related to organizational factors are also shown in Table 2.

Table 2. Organizational factors and adoption of AI and telehealth in U.S. hospitals (n = 4061).

	AI			Telehealth		
Variables	OR	95% CI	p-Value	OR	95% CI	p-Value
Main Independent Variables						
Community Social Determinants	1.07	[1.05, 1.09]	<0.0001	1.08	[1.06, 1.09]	<0.0001
Health Equity	1.09	[1.07, 1.10]	<0.0001	1.05	[1.03, 1.07]	<0.0001
Hospital Characteristics						
Hospital Size						
≥ 400 beds (reference)						
6–49 beds	0.59	[0.44, 0.79]	0.0368	0.22	[0.12, 0.41]	<0.0001
50–199 beds	0.59	[0.45, 0.78]	0.0144	0.35	[0.20, 0.64]	0.1214
200–399 beds	0.70	[0.53, 0.93]	0.9596	0.38	[0.20, 0.70]	0.4483
Hospital Group						
General hospital (reference)						
Mental health hospital	0.60	[0.36, 0.98]	0.1276	0.53	[0.39, 0.72]	0.6532
Children's hospital	0.92	[0.54, 1.57]	0.6587	0.70	[0.38, 1.30]	0.1782
Specialty hospital	0.91	[0.60, 1.37]	0.5944	0.36	[0.26, 0.48]	0.0085
Long-term care hospital	0.78	[0.41, 1.46]	0.8116	0.23	[0.16, 0.35]	<0.0001
Hospital Ownership						
Not-for-profit (reference)						
Investor-owned	0.40	[0.30, 0.52]	0.0010	0.45	[0.34, 0.58]	0.0288
Public	0.43	[0.31, 0.60]	0.0281	0.34	[0.26, 0.44]	<0.0001
Rural Hospital	1.01	[0.83, 1.22]	0.9580	2.52	[1.95, 3.25]	<0.0001
Market Competition						
Concentrated (reference)						
Competitive	1.64	[1.30, 2.06]	0.0046	0.90	[0.69, 1.16]	0.5874
Mild concentrated	1.41	[1.11, 1.79]	0.4046	0.93	[0.70, 1.23]	0.8832

Source: American Hospital Association, 2021; Note: OR = odds ratio; CI = 95% confidence interval; AI = artificial intelligence.

Table 3 demonstrates the associations between hospitals' community social determinants and health equity activities and their impacts on the numbers of AI and telehealth services, as well as the volume of all virtual services. A 10-point increase in the community social determinant activity indicator was associated with an increase of 0.22 in the new type of AI services and 0.52 in the new type of telehealth services, respectively. Similarly, a 10-point increase in the health equity activity indicator was associated with an increase of 0.49 in the new type of AI services and 0.75 in the new type of telehealth services, respectively. Moreover, an increase of one point in the community social determinant activity indicator was associated with an increase of 749 virtual service volume, whereas an increase of one point in the health equity activity indicator was associated with an increase of 3125 for all virtual service volume. The results related to organizational factors are also displayed in Table 3.

Table 3. Equity-focused hospital community activities associated with utilization of AI and telehealth and volume of all virtual services in U.S. hospitals, 2021.

Variables	Coefficient	SE	*p*-Value
Number of AI Services (n = 4061)			
Main Independent Variables			
Community Social Determinants	0.022	0.003	<0.0001
Health Equity	0.049	0.003	<0.0001
Hospital Characteristics			
Hospital Size	0.117	0.028	<0.0001
Hospital Group			
Short-term acute general hospital (reference)			
Mental hospital	−0.208	0.095	0.0293
Children's hospital	0.006	0.147	0.9684
Special hospital	−0.157	0.086	0.0689
Long-term hospital	−0.119	0.115	0.3020
Teaching Hospital	−0.138	0.052	0.0083
Hospital Location			
Non-rural hospital (reference)			
Rural hospital	0.038	0.046	0.4013
Hospital Ownership			
Non-for-profit (reference)			
Investor-owned	−0.198	0.064	0.0019
Public	−0.305	0.056	<0.0001
Market Competition			
Concentrated (reference)			
Competitive	0.184	0.055	0.0008
Mild concentrated	0.118	0.058	0.0421
Number of Telehealth Services (n = 4061)			
Main Independent Variables			
Community Social Determinants	0.052	0.005	<0.0001
Health Equity	0.075	0.006	<0.0001
Hospital Characteristics			
Hospital Size	0.490	0.046	<0.0001
Hospital Group			
Mental hospital	−0.386	0.159	0.0151
Children's hospital	−0.636	0.245	0.0095
Special hospital	−0.384	0.143	0.0073
Long-term hospital	−0.485	0.192	0.0115
Teaching Hospital	0.368	0.087	<0.0001
Rural Hospital	0.736	0.076	<0.0001
Hospital Ownership			
Investor-owned	−1.231	0.106	<0.0001
Public	−0.784	0.094	<0.0001
Market Competition			
Competitive	0.131	0.091	0.1506
Mild concentrated	0.439	0.097	<0.0001
Number of All Virtual Services (n = 2893)			
Main Independent Variables			
Community Social Determinants	749	929	0.4202
Health Equity	3125	895	0.0005
Hospital Characteristics			

Table 3. *Cont.*

Variables	Coefficient	SE	*p*-Value
Hospital Size	59,885	7646	<0.0001
Hospital Group			
Mental hospital	2859	27,686	0.9177
Children's hospital	47,630	39,996	0.2338
Special hospital	9361	24,132	0.6981
Long-term hospital	2067	34,056	0.9516
Teaching Hospital	16,121	14,594	0.2694
Rural Hospital	10,095	12,448	0.4175
Hospital Ownership			
Investor-owned	−34,373	18,473	0.0629
Public	−13,454	15,341	0.3805
Market Competition			
Competitive	386	14,941	0.9794
Mild concentrated	−5065	16,212	0.7548

Source: American Hospital Association, 2021; Note: AI = artificial intelligence; SE = standard error.

4. Discussion

The adoption trends of AI and telehealth among U.S. hospitals draw attention to the significance of hospital strategies to address social determinants and health inequalities. As hospitals engage in these population health-related activities, technology adoption increases, matching hospitals' focus to recognize initiatives that are centered on social determinants of health and health equity, meeting population needs and demands. Our findings demonstrate that hospital indicator-related activities addressing social determinants and health equity are consistently and positively associated with the adoption and use of AI and telehealth services.

Several key factors may help to interpret this association. Primarily, hospitals' strategic alignment with priorities centered on community initiatives and achieving equitable care served as a major driver. U.S. hospitals that respond to community health needs, as evaluated through community health assessments, improve population health and modify their healthcare services in response to community concerns [27]. For example, utilizing healthcare services for vulnerable individuals that are unique to their healthcare needs may influence hospitals to adopt technology-driven and innovative solutions to cater to a broader patient demographic. Relatedly, Carroll-Scott, A, 2017 [14] demonstrates that hospitals' inclusion of health equity in their assessment of community health needs reflects the growing trend of population health strategies that elevate healthcare costs and enhance patient outcomes. Additionally, hospitals committed to breaking barriers through community-oriented activities contribute to improved quality care by effectively tailoring services to the needs of specific populations [28]. The rapidly changing social environment, including the increasing availability of technology, may also influence the strategies of hospitals to become more adaptive and embrace new technologies to provide preeminent healthcare services and treatment. Emerging state health policies, particularly those related to reimbursement methods, may also account for driving the adoption of telehealth and AI within hospitals [19,29]. Other possible underlying factors may include comprehensive administrative support, a well-trained healthcare workforce, and adequate hospital financial resources.

Another significant finding of our study is the positive association between hospital activities related to social determinant indicators and health equity indicators and the increased number of AI and telehealth services, as well as the volume of virtual services. In other words, the extent and abilities of providing these services may be related to hospitals' strategic goals, particularly those focused on addressing social needs and health disparities through social determinants and health equity activities. Research highlights the significance of hospital boards' involvement in strategic decision-making, contributing to hospitals being able to navigate the complex and evolving external healthcare environment [30]. Such involvement ensures that hospitals' strategies are aligned with external forces and opportunities, hence enhancing the ability to respond in the rapidly changing healthcare landscape. For instance, the changing patient demographics have driven the need to improve quality healthcare and access for growing minority populations in the U.S., both racially and ethnically [31]. Shifts in disease patterns and their impacts on the population have also imposed changes in terms of healthcare delivery, technology, and health policy. Notably, the COVID-19 pandemic has created a massive impact on ramping up healthcare innovation approaches, facilitating the adoption of new collaboration methods, dynamic care strategies, and public approval of innovative solutions [32]. As healthcare continues to evolve, there is a growing focus on hospital policies that implement community engagement addressing upstream social determinants such as income, housing, insurance, and education. Hospitals' strategies addressing non-medical factors play a huge part in improving community health outcomes [33]. Furthermore, integrating initiatives that address disparities has been shown to increase health equity, elevating the provision of equitable healthcare and accessibility. These efforts may drive hospitals to allocate specific services and develop healthcare approaches that align with population needs and preferences in advancing innovative solutions.

In addition, several organizational factors were found to be associated with the adoption of AI and telehealth in hospitals. In regard to hospital bed size, larger hospitals tend to be more likely to adopt AI and telehealth, which is consistent with the existing literature [18,19]. This is likely due to their capabilities to acquire greater technological resources and integrate innovative solutions more quickly, allowing them to adapt seamlessly to emerging healthcare trends. Hospital type was also associated with the use of AI and telehealth. Short-term acute general hospitals, in particular, tend to be more likely to adopt technologies compared to other hospitals. This may be due to the higher patient volume and the demand of various advanced care interventions, which promote the adoption of new technologies. In terms of hospital ownership, not-for-profit private hospitals are more reluctant to offer AI and telehealth services. This is likely due to their mission-driven focus and commitment to serving the community with quality patient-centered care [34]. Not-for-profit private hospitals are more likely to adopt various forms of AI than their counterparts with for-profit non-private hospitals because doing so enhances their capacity to deliver quality patient care that reflects their mission and goals [35]. Not-for-profit hospitals being tax-exempt solidifies their status and benefits them by including access concepts to their mission statement and quality services, whereas for-profit non-private hospitals exclude cost-effectiveness into their mission which strives to prioritize revenue and investors' returns [36], which might hinder AI adoption. Therefore, for-profit ownership is more likely to be in a less non-adoption category when it comes to AI. Similarly, not-for-profit private hospitals are also more likely to implement telehealth services than their for-profit counterparts, which is consistent with the existing literature [37]. Additionally, not-for-profit private hospitals expand operations to reach a broader patient demographic, allowing individuals wider access to more holistic healthcare services. Rural hospitals are also more motivated to offer telehealth services to provide complex medical care and to enable remote specialist consultations for distant patients who face barriers to accessing healthcare [37]. Particularly, telehealth allocates rural hospitals with a value-driven approach to care for patients in remote areas. In contrast, they may not be able to adopt AI quickly due to their limited resources and market demand. Finally, competition may stir market dynamics that force hospitals to adopt recent AI technologies. In more competitive markets, hospitals are urged to adopt the latest technologies to retain their market advantage. Competitive hospitals commonly implement AI to enhance clinical outcomes, increase revenue streams, and maintain their competitive position [38]. Furthermore, competitive tensions drive hospitals to acquire technologies that attract and retain more patients and better address the unique needs of a broader patient demographic.

As hospitals move forward to address population health and reduce disparities, strategies focused on targeting community social needs in combination with health equity activities may need to be incorporated into hospitals' strategic goals. The findings of this study are relevant for significant policy implications regarding healthcare management and the adoption of emerging technologies such as AI and telehealth in U.S hospitals. For instance, the allocation of financial support and resources to hospitals that engage in these population-focused activities can encourage healthcare organizations and other health institutions to incentivize greater technology adoption to address the barriers faced by marginalized patients. Additionally, policies that support value-based payment systems, such as the merit-based incentive payment system, can provide financial incentives for hospitals that prioritize improved care processes and patient engagement in care. Therefore, policy makers should recognize the importance of hospitals' involvement in activities related to addressing the social determinants of health and promoting health equity in driving technology adoption. Hospitals that adopt technologies to enhance care for broader patient demographics could encourage greater reimbursement rates, allowing hospitals continued focus on activities that address the population [28]. These engagements can collectively promote the adoption of technology on a larger scale.

5. Study Limitations

The limitations of this study underscore the importance of further research in several areas. First, this study utilizes cross-sectional data from 2021, restricting the generalization of hospital's related activities that address population health and the adoption of AI and telehealth in other years. Although associations were observed based on the reliance on a cross-sectional study, it may be insufficient to fully determine the order of events that occurred over time, and a longitudinal study would be needed to track these changes in events. Second, this study only relies on data from the AHA 2021 survey, which could overlook other significant key factors impacting AI and telehealth adoption. As the data were only retrieved from a single year, some hospitals might not have reported all activities related to the social determinants of health/health equity and technology implementations, leading to an incomplete understanding of hospitals' engagement in both areas. Third, some hospitals have limited capabilities to implement AI services, creating barriers to respond to AI-related questions, resulting in missing data and complicating the measure of AI services within hospitals. Fourth, the number of AI services offered by hospitals was restricted to just five related measures, which hindered comprehensive assessment of the AI services available within hospitals. More extensive information on AI services may need to be obtained to better evaluate hospitals' activities related to addressing population health. Another limitation of this study is the absence of a focus on commercial insurance within the U.S. system, which results in a lack of understanding of social equity in terms of patient delivery. Future research is merited to investigate the role of commercial insurance in addressing the healthcare needs of the underserved population. Finally, although this study highlights the importance of hospitals' activities related to addressing social determinants and health equity, it does not comply with other organizational factors, particularly external forces that might drive technological adoption. Future research should take into account a broader scope of technological drivers.

6. Conclusions

In conclusion, this study presents evidence that hospitals that actively engage in activities that address social determinants and promote health equity are positively associated with the adoption and utilization of AI and telehealth services. Increased technology adoption within these hospitals informs the significance of strategies addressing non-clinical factors that affect health and an advancement in equitable inclusive patient care, striving to improve overall healthcare delivery. By engaging in community activities that address the social determinants of health and health equity, hospitals can enhance their capabilities to improve care delivery and access and reduce disparities regarding barriers stopping individuals from attaining the highest levels of care. This motivates hospitals to prioritize improved care processes and patient engagement through a broader continuum of care. Therefore, hospitals can enhance their capacity to adopt emerging technologies and be more adaptive as a healthcare organization. The findings also support the need to address specific healthcare challenges, such as rural healthcare access, that often hinder underserved populations from obtaining timely medical attention and the broader impact of technology adoption within hospitals. Within the structure of the U.S. healthcare system, technology implementation is significant in many areas and addressing population health and reducing disparities are two of the many aspects that mean that effective widespread technology adoption is crucial among healthcare organizations.

Author Contributions: Conceptualization, J.J.S. and P.C.K.; methodology, J.J.S.; software, J.J.S.; validation, P.A.P., P.C.K. and J.J.S.; formal analysis, J.J.S.; investigation, P.A.P. and F.A.P.; resources, J.J.S.; data curation, J.J.S.; writing—original draft preparation, P.A.P. and F.A.P.; writing—review and editing, P.A.P., P.C.K. and J.J.S.; visualization, P.C.K.; supervision, J.J.S.; project administration, J.J.S. All authors have read and agreed to the published version of the manuscript.

Funding: This research received no external funding.

Institutional Review Board Statement: Not applicable, a non-human subject research.

Informed Consent Statement: Not applicable, a non-human subject research.

Data Availability Statement: Data is unavailable due to the data purchasing agreement with the American Hospital Association.

Conflicts of Interest: The authors declare no conflict of interest.

References

1. Yu, K.-H.; Beam, A.L.; Kohane, I.S. Artificial intelligence in healthcare. *Nat. Biomed. Eng.* **2018**, *2*, 719–731. [CrossRef] [PubMed]
2. Sharma, A.; Pruthi, M.; Sageena, G. Adoption of telehealth technologies: An approach to improving the healthcare system. *Transl. Med. Commun.* **2022**, *7*, 20. [CrossRef] [PubMed]
3. Bleich, S. Medical errors: Five years after the IOM report. *Issue Brief (Commonw Fund)* **2005**, *830*, 1–15.
4. Moor, J. The Dartmouth College Artificial Intelligence Conference: The Next Fifty Years. *AI Mag.* **2006**, *27*, 87–91. [CrossRef]
5. Mukherjee, J.; Sharma, R.; Dutta, P.; Bhunia, B. Artificial intelligence in healthcare: A mastery. *Biotechnol. Genet. Eng. Rev.* **2023**, *40*, 1659–1708. [CrossRef] [PubMed]
6. Bates, D.W.; Levine, D.; Syrowatka, A.; Kuznetsova, M.; Craig, K.J.T.; Rui, A.; Jackson, G.P.; Rhee, K. The potential of artificial intelligence to improve patient safety: A scoping review. *NPJ Digit. Med.* **2021**, *4*, 54. [CrossRef] [PubMed]
7. Bohr, A.; Memarzadeh, K. The rise of artificial intelligence in healthcare applications. In *Artificial Intelligence in Healthcare*; Academic Press: Cambridge, MA, USA, 2020; pp. 25–60. [CrossRef]
8. Kim, P.C.; Tan, L.F.; Kreston, J.; Shariatmadari, H.; Keyoung, E.S.; Shen, J.J.; Wang, B.L. Socioeconomic factors associated with use of telehealth services in outpatient care settings during the COVID-19. *BMC Health Serv. Res.* **2024**, *24*, 446. [CrossRef] [PubMed]
9. Ramphul, K.; Singh Dhaliwal, J.; Sombans, S.; Passi, J.K.; Aggarwal, S.; Kumar, N.; Sakthivel, H.; Ahmed, R.; Verma, R. Trends in admissions for COVID-19 in the United States between April 2020 and December 2021 and cardiovascular events. *Arch. Med. Sciences. Atheroscler. Dis.* **2024**, *9*, e60–e65. [CrossRef]

10. Wosik, J.; Fudim, M.; Cameron, B.; Gellad, Z.F.; Cho, A.; Phinney, D.; Curtis, S.; Roman, M.; Poon, E.G.; Ferranti, J.; et al. Telehealth transformation: COVID-19 and the rise of virtual care. *J. Am. Med. Inform. Assoc. JAMIA* **2020**, *27*, 957–962. [CrossRef] [PubMed]
11. Andino, J.J.; Eyrich, N.W.; Boxer, R.J. Overview of telehealth in the United States since the COVID-19 public health emergency: A narrative review. *mHealth* **2023**, *9*, 26. [CrossRef] [PubMed]
12. Doraiswamy, S.; Jithesh, A.; Mamtani, R.; Abraham, A.; Cheema, S. Telehealth Use in Geriatrics Care during the COVID-19 Pandemic-A Scoping Review and Evidence Synthesis. *Int. J. Environ. Res. Public Health* **2021**, *18*, 1755. [CrossRef] [PubMed]
13. Leonard, C.; Liu, W.; Holstein, A.; Alliance, S.; Nunnery, M.; Rohs, C.; Sloan, M.; Winchester, D.E. Informing Use of Telehealth for Managing Chronic Conditions: Mixed-Methods Evaluation of Telehealth Use to Manage Heart Failure During COVID-19. *J. Am. Heart Assoc.* **2023**, *12*, e027362. [CrossRef] [PubMed]
14. Mesa, A.; Grasdal, M.; Leong, S.; Dean, N.A.; Marwaha, A.; Lee, A.; Berger, M.J.; Bundon, A.; Krassioukov, A.V. Effect of the COVID-19 pandemic on individuals with spinal cord injury: Mental health and use of telehealth. *PM & R* **2022**, *14*, 1439–1445. [CrossRef]
15. Green, B.L.; Murphy, A.; Robinson, E. Accelerating health disparities research with artificial intelligence. *Front. Digit. Health* **2024**, *6*, 1330160. [CrossRef] [PubMed]
16. Saeed, S.A.; Masters, R.M. Disparities in Health Care and the Digital Divide. *Curr. Psychiatry Rep.* **2021**, *23*, 61. [CrossRef] [PubMed]
17. DiMaggio, P.J.; Powell, W.W. The Iron Cage Revisited: Institutional Isomorphism and Collective Rationality in Organizational Fields. *Am. Sociol. Rev.* **1983**, *2*, 147–160. [CrossRef]
18. Adler-Milstein, J.; Kvedar, J.; Bates, D.W. Telehealth Among US Hospitals: Several Factors, Including State Reimbursement And Licensure Policies, Influence Adoption. *Health Aff.* **2014**, *33*, 207–215. [CrossRef] [PubMed]
19. Pham, P.; Zhang, H.; Gao, W.; Zhu, X. Determinants and performance outcomes of artificial intelligence adoption: Evidence from U.S. Hospitals. *J. Bus. Res.* **2024**, *172*, 114402. [CrossRef]
20. Lee, J.Y.; McFadden, K.L.; Lee, M.K.; Gowen, C.R. U.S. hospital culture profiles for better performance in patient safety, patient satisfaction, Six Sigma, and lean implementation. *Int. J. Prod. Econ.* **2021**, *234*, 108047. [CrossRef]
21. Begun, J.W.; Potthoff, S. Moving Upstream in U.S. Hospital Care Toward Investments in Population Health. *J. Healthc. Manag.* **2017**, *62*, 343–353. [CrossRef] [PubMed]
22. Carroll-Scott, A.; Henson, R.M.; Kolker, J.; Purtle, J. The Role Of Nonprofit Hospitals In Identifying And Addressing Health Inequities In Cities. *Health Aff.* **2017**, *36*, 1102–1109. [CrossRef] [PubMed]
23. Lemont, B.; Puro, N.; Franz, B.; Cronin, C.E. Efforts by critical access hospitals to increase health equity through greater engagement with social determinants of health. *J. Rural. Health* **2023**, *39*, 728–736. [CrossRef] [PubMed]
24. American Hospital Association. *About the AHA*; American Hospital Association: Chicago, IL, USA; Available online: https://www.aha.org/ (accessed on 8 August 2024).
25. American Hospital Association. AHA Annual Survey Database. AHA Data. Available online: https://www.ahadata.com/aha-annual-survey-database (accessed on 8 August 2024).
26. American Hospital Association. Social Determinants of Health. Available online: https://www.aha.org/system/files/2018-04/value-initiative-icd-10-code-social-determinants-of-health.pdf (accessed on 8 August 2024).
27. Cramer, G.R.; Singh, S.R.; Flaherty, S.; Young, G.J. The Progress of US Hospitals in Addressing Community Health Needs. *Am. J. Public Health* **2017**, *107*, 255–261. [CrossRef] [PubMed]
28. Kang, R.; Hasnain-Wynia, R. Hospital commitment to community orientation and its association with quality of care and patient experience. *J. Healthc. Manag.* **2013**, *58*, 277–288. [CrossRef] [PubMed]
29. Venkatesh, K.P.; Raza, M.M.; Diao, J.A.; Kvedar, J.C. Leveraging reimbursement strategies to guide value-based adoption and utilization of medical AI. *NPJ Digit. Med.* **2022**, *5*, 112. [CrossRef]
30. Ford-Eickhoff, K.; Plowman, D.A.; McDaniel, R.R. Hospital boards and hospital strategic focus: The impact of board involvement in strategic decision making. *Health Care Manag. Rev.* **2011**, *36*, 145–154. [CrossRef] [PubMed]
31. Natale-Pereira, A.; Enard, K.R.; Nevarez, L.; Jones, L.A. The role of patient navigators in eliminating health disparities. *Cancer* **2011**, *117* (Suppl. S15), 3541–3550. [CrossRef] [PubMed]
32. Guarcello, C.; Raupp, E. Pandemic and Innovation in Healthcare: The End-To-End Innovation Adoption Model. *BAR Braz. Adm. Rev.* **2021**, *18*, e210009. [CrossRef]
33. Crossley, M.; Tyler, E.T.; Herbst, J.L. Tax-Exempt Hospitals and Community Health under the Affordable Care Act: Identifying and Addressing Unmet Legal Needs as Social Determinants of Health. *Public Health Rep.* **2016**, *131*, 195–199. [CrossRef]
34. Asagbra, O.E. Factors Associated with the Adoption of Health Information Technologies to Increase Patient Engagement in US Hospitals. *J. Organ. Psychol.* **2019**, *19*, 24–38. [CrossRef]
35. Bin Abdul Baten, R. How are US hospitals adopting artificial intelligence? Early evidence from 2022. *Health Aff. Sch.* **2024**, *2*, qxae123. [CrossRef] [PubMed]

36. Bolon, D.S. Comparing Mission Statement Content in For-Profit and Not-For-Profit Hospitals: Does Mission Really Matter? *Hosp. Top.* **2005**, *83*, 2–9. [CrossRef]
37. Gaziel-Yablowitz, M.; Bates, D.W.; Levine, D.M. Telehealth in US hospitals: State-level reimbursement policies no longer influence adoption rates. *Int. J. Med. Inform. (Shannon Irel.)* **2021**, *153*, 104540. [CrossRef]
38. Ali Mohamad, T.; Bastone, A.; Bernhard, F.; Schiavone, F. How artificial intelligence impacts the competitive position of healthcare organizations. *J. Organ. Change Manag.* **2023**, *36*, 49–70. [CrossRef]

International Journal of
Environmental Research and Public Health

MDPI

Article

Exploring Managers' Insights on Integrating Mental Health into Tuberculosis and HIV Care in the Free State Province, South Africa

Christo Heunis * and Gladys Kigozi-Male

Centre for Health Systems Research & Development, University of the Free State, P.O. Box 339, Bloemfontein 9301, South Africa; kigozign@ufs.ac.za
* Correspondence: heunisj@ufs.ac.za

Abstract: The integration of mental health (MH) services into tuberculosis (TB) and HIV care remains a significant challenge in South Africa's Free State province. This study seeks to understand the perspectives of public health programme managers on the barriers to such integration and to identify potential strategies to overcome these challenges. Data were collected between February and October 2021 using qualitative methods including four individual semi-structured interviews and two focus group discussions with a total of 15 managers responsible for the MH, primary healthcare, TB, and HIV programmes. Thematic data analysis was guided by an adapted version of the World Health Organization's "building blocks" framework encompassing "service delivery", "workforce", "health information", "essential medicines", "financing", and "leadership/governance". Additionally, the analysis underscored the crucial role of "people", acknowledging their significant contributions as both caregivers and recipients of care. Managers highlighted significant concerns regarding the insufficient integration of MH services, identifying structural barriers such as inadequate MH management structures and staff training, as well as social barriers, notably stigma and a lack of family treatment adherence support. Conversely, they recognised strong management structures, integrated screening, and social interventions, including family involvement, as key facilitators of successful MH integration. The findings emphasise the need for a whole-system approach that addresses all building blocks while prioritising the role of "people" in overcoming challenges with integrating MH services into TB and HIV care.

Keywords: managers' insights; mental health integration; TB; HIV; building blocks; barriers; facilitators

1. Introduction

A prevalent issue confronting healthcare systems in numerous low- and middle-income countries (LMICs) is the significant disparity between the demand for mental health (MH) services and the availability of such treatments [1,2]. A primary objective of the World Health Organization's (WHO) Comprehensive Mental Health Action Plan 2013–2030 is to provide integrated and responsive MH care services in community-based settings [3]. Integrated primary healthcare (PHC) is a complex and multifaceted concept [4]. The World Health Report 2005 [5] (p. 108) stated that the goal of integration is "to tackle the need for complementarity of different independent services and administrative structures, so as to achieve common goals". The report outlined integration at three levels: at the patient level as "case management"; at the service delivery point where "multiple interventions are provided through one delivery channel"; and at the systems level by "bringing together the management and support functions of different sub-programmes, and ensuring complementarity between different levels of care" [5] (p. 109). Thus, integration influences programme financing, planning, and delivery, ultimately impacting the achievement of health goals. Integrated care aims to elevate the quality of care, resulting in better health outcomes and greater patient satisfaction throughout their treatment journey, with the added potential for cost savings. However, despite these worthy aspirations, putting integrated care into practice is fraught with complex challenges.

Health managers often face significant obstacles, such as poor information sharing, a lack of time and personnel to spur programmes, and confusion over who is responsible for patient care [6–8]. These issues make it difficult to seamlessly integrate care across various programmes, levels of care, and organisations. While achieving functional integration of health services is considered an attainable goal [9], it is contingent upon several critical intersecting capabilities within the health system. These include ensuring fully operational frontline health services, adequately trained and motivated healthcare personnel, access to appropriate technology, and the decentralisation of authority and decision-making processes to lower cadres of frontline managers and staff [9]. Decentralisation facilitates the adaptation of integration processes to suit local contexts.

The transition to democracy in post-apartheid South Africa requires more attention to MH [10]. However, the field of MH care continues to generate significant public health concerns [11]. The Mental Health Care Act No. 17 of 2002 [12] was founded on the basic tenets set out by the WHO in 1996 to guide MH care law [13]. By setting a deinstitutionalisation agenda on par with countries like Brazil [14], the Act requires users to be treated as close to their place of domicile and in the least restrictive manner possible. By implication, a "human rights-driven ethos in patient care" era had arrived in South Africa [15] (p. 69). The integration of MH care services into PHC services requires fundamental change in the health system, from "one of human rights violations and poor health outcomes associated with care delivered through psychiatric institutions" to "one which respects human rights and promotes good health outcomes and recovery through the delivery of [MH] care in the [PHC] system" (p. 5) [16]. The 2022 World Mental Health Report stated that "[MH] is a lot more than the absence of illness: it is an intrinsic part of our individual and collective health and well-being... Ultimately, there is no health without [MH]" [17] (p. vi).

South Africa has a growing burden of non-communicable diseases (NCDs) where deaths due to major NCDs such as cardiovascular diseases, cancer, diabetes, and chronic lower respiratory diseases increased by 58.7% over 20 years, from 103,428 in 1997 to 164,205 in 2018 [18]. Kenge (2022) thus questioned whether the hospital-based model of prevention and control of MH disorders is suitable [19] (p. 19). The prevention and control of NCDs—including MH disorders—might better be integrated into other existing health services, notably PHC services as the foundation of universal health care.

The National Mental Health Policy Framework and Strategic Plan (MHPF&SP) 2013–2020 [20] was implemented by the National Department of Health to generate momentum towards the transformation and integration of MH care. MH services are meant to be offered as a key component of the PHC Package. The MHPF&SP 2013–2020 guided provinces in promoting MH, preventing mental illness, and providing treatment and rehabilitation for diverse MH disorders. It directed that MH care services should be decentralised and integrated into existing programmes through task sharing at the PHC level, with a view to increasing prevention, screening, self-management, care, treatment, and rehabilitation. Specialist district MH care and community-based teams had to be established to provide psychological services with appropriate accreditation and staffing in line with the PHC Re-engineering Strategy [21]. Selected key staff in every PHC facility had to be trained to provide basic MH care services under routine supervision and mentoring, with referral as appropriate.

However, the recently introduced National Mental Health Policy Framework and Strategic Plan (MHPF&SP) 2023–2030 [22] recognises significant under-investment in MH care across South Africa. This has led to substantial disparities in the accessibility of services and resources for MH care, perpetuating the historical legacy of colonial and apartheid-era MH systems that heavily relied on psychiatric hospitals. While progress has been made with the integration of MH into general healthcare in some provinces, nationally, major shortfalls in human resources characterise MH care at the PHC level [23]. While most provinces endorse the importance of integrating MH into PHC and some PHC nurse training initiatives have been undertaken, there is urgent need to strengthen the MH training of general health staff.

It is also a concern that there are presently only five indicators for MH included in the District Health Information System, viz. "[MH] caseload", "PHC mental disorders treatment rate-new", "[MH] separation rate", "[MH] involuntary admission rate", and the recently added "child and adolescent attempted suicide rate". A qualitative study investigating the use of newly developed, contextually appropriate MH indicators in PHC facilities revealed that their implementation was generally perceived as feasible across three South Asian and three Sub-Saharan African countries, including South Africa (e.g., service utilisation by disorder [psychosis, bipolar disorder, depression, alcohol use disorder, epilepsy, suicide attempts], follow-up, and referral) [24]. This feasibility was attributed largely to the simplicity of the forms and the ongoing support provided during the design and implementation stages.

Further regarding the new MHPF&SP 2023–2030, while the deinstitutionalisation of MH care has made some progress in South Africa, the process has been devoid of concomitant development of PHC and community-based MH care services. This has led to a high number of people living with MH disorders facing housing insecurity, being in prison, and being constantly faced by "revolving door patterns of care" [25] (p. 403). MH services for children and adolescents are severely lacking. Substance use disorders treatment services are also in short supply with weak coordination between sectors.

In 2016, an inquest into the deaths of 144 MH care users and the disappearance of 44 others, who had been treated at Life Esidimeni hospitals in Gauteng province, revealed that approximately 1500 MH care users were haphazardly discharged or transferred to inadequate facilities without proper documentation [26]. This led to the abrupt discontinuation of their treatment. This sad event underscored the severe lack of continuity in MH care in South Africa, with many individuals effectively "lost" within the system. Coupled with the absence of a national clinical programme guideline for MH, this represents a significant challenge to the country's healthcare system [27].

A growing body of evidence highlights the challenges in MH policy implementation in South Africa [11,28,29]. MH is often perceived as being less prioritised, inadequately resourced, and insufficiently supported compared to other critical public health programmes, such as HIV and maternal and child health [29]. This deficiency in policy implementation exacerbates existing inequalities and inequities in public health. The overarching goal of deinstitutionalisation cannot be humanely achieved without the development and implementation of effective models for delivering MH services at the PHC level [10,30].

Although research in this area is expanding within developing countries, significant gaps remain in the literature, particularly concerning LMICs that face a combined affliction from both TB and NCDs, threatening population health and further straining already stressed health systems [31]. Individuals with poor MH often exhibit higher rates of TB and HIV compared to those without MH issues. Conversely, individuals with TB or HIV are more prone to MH problems [32], which can result in decreased treatment adherence and increased mortality rates [33]. This bidirectional relationship, particularly with depression, has been extensively documented in both TB and HIV contexts. Given the significant overlap in vulnerable populations, any strategy aimed at eradicating TB and HIV must comprehensively address the MH and psychosocial needs of affected individuals and those at risk. It is therefore clear that effective management of mental illness, TB, and HIV requires an integrated and coordinated approach, including mental and behavioural healthcare services.

Studies have highlighted the significance of understanding the factors that impact healthcare implementation from the perspective of managers [34,35]. In South Africa, the delineation of management roles, with provincial-level managers overseeing and district managers ensuring frontline service delivery, underscores the crucial role of "leadership/governance" in enhancing the effectiveness of the district-based PHC system and achieving shared objectives. The current study examines public health programme managers' insights into the challenges of integrating MH services into TB and HIV care in South Africa's Free State province. The research questions specifically sought to identify the barriers and facilitators perceived by these managers that influence the integration of MH into TB and HIV care, and to propose solutions to overcome these challenges. As far as could be established, this is the first qualitative study focusing on programme managers' views on the integration of MH into PHC services in South Africa.

In line with previous research related to public health systems being strengthened in the Free State [36,37], this analysis was guided by the WHO's health systems strengthening framework. This framework emphasises six key "building blocks" crucial to a functioning health system: "service delivery", "health information", "workforce", "essential medicines", "financing", and "leadership/governance" [38,39]. As all the building blocks are regarded as fundamental, the framework offers no weighting of the importance of the individual building blocks.

However, uncertainty persists regarding the optimal use of the building blocks framework to address fragmentation and inefficiencies in public health systems in LMICs. Mounier-Jack et al. [40] recommend that researchers adapt the framework to suit specific contexts. Collectively, the building blocks constitute the structural elements of the health system. However, de Savigny and Adam [41] (p. 32) suggest that the "missing ingredient" in the building blocks framework may be the role of "people", not only as mediators and beneficiaries but also as active agents driving the system. A qualitative study applying the building blocks framework to assess health systems strengthening in Zambia highlighted the central role of people across all building blocks [42]. While the WHO building blocks framework primarily addresses structural and systemic aspects of health systems, it does acknowledge and integrate the critical role of "people", both as healthcare providers and as recipients of health services. Highlighting the role of people facilitates the adaptation of health services to better meet their specific needs, thereby enhancing their societal relevance. This approach aligns with the foundational principles of PHC, such as equity, social justice, participatory decision-making, and intersectoral collaboration.

In South Africa, conditions such as HIV [43], TB [44], as well as MH disorders [45] are highly stigmatised, profoundly influencing the daily experiences of both healthcare providers and clinic service users. To address the people-related barriers—such as stigmatisation and inadequate family support for treatment adherence—frequently highlighted by managers in the current study and to incorporate the corresponding facilitators, a decision was made to add a seventh component, "people", to the building block analytical framework.

2. Materials and Methods

2.1. Design

The study utilised an exploratory qualitative design, including individual semi-structured interviews (SSIs) and focus group discussions (FGDs) with health programme managers operating at both the provincial and district levels within the Free State province's public healthcare system. As stated, the study design was guided by the WHO's health systems strengthening framework which highlights six "building blocks" of the health system: "service delivery", "health information", "workforce", "essential medicines", "financing", and "leadership/governance" [38,39].

2.2. Setting

With a population of 2,964,412 in 2022 [46], the Free State is one of South Africa's nine provinces. The province accounted for 4,038,494 PHC headcounts in the 2021/22 period, representing 4.8% of the national PHC headcount of 84,511,186 [47] (pp. 196–199). However, according to the Health Systems Trust, the province reported lower PHC utilisation rates compared to national averages, with 1.8 visits per year in 2019/20 versus 2.0 visits nationally, and 1.6 visits per year in 2021/22 versus 1.7 visits nationally. Furthermore, the PHC professional nurse clinical workload in the Free State was higher in 2021/22, with 23.4 clients per nurse per day, exceeding the national rate of 21.9.

Regarding TB, the Free State reported 5569 cases of drug-susceptible TB out of a total of 121,883 cases in South Africa in 2021 [47] (pp. 144–146), accounting for 4.6% of the national total. The province's TB programme's performance fell below national averages across several key indicators: TB treatment initiation rate for clients aged five years and older in 2021/22 (90.6% vs. 93.4% nationally), drug-susceptible TB client loss to follow-up rate in 2021 (14.3% vs. 13.0% nationally), drug-susceptible TB death rate in 2021 (13.4% vs. 8.3% nationally), drug-susceptible TB treatment success rate in 2021 (71.3% vs. 77.9% nationally), multi-drug resistant TB client death rate in 2020 (26.6% vs. 17.5% nationally), multi-drug resistant TB treatment success rate in 2020 (56.1% vs. 60.8% nationally), TB symptom screening rate for clients aged five years and older in 2021/22 (89.3% vs. 95.8% nationally), and extremely drug-resistant TB client loss to follow-up rate in 2020 (25.0% vs. 17.8% nationally).

Concerning HIV, the Free State accounted for 415,029 out of 7,975,940 people living with HIV in South Africa in 2022, representing 5.2% of the national total [47] (pp. 153–161). According to the Health Systems Trust, the HIV prevalence rate in the overall population in 2022 was 14.7% in the Free State, which was higher than the national prevalence of 13.5%. Nevertheless, the Free State's HIV programme demonstrates robust performance relative to the national programme across several key metrics. These include antiretroviral treatment coverage in 2020 (80.9% vs. 75.0% nationally), clients remaining on antiretroviral treatment in 2022 (75.7% vs. 67.7% nationally), HIV viral load suppression in 2020 (70.6% vs. 64.0% nationally), and antenatal clients initiated on antiretroviral treatment in 2021/22 (97.7% vs. 95.0% nationally). However, the HIV testing coverage rate in the Free State in 2022 was notably lower at 75.5% compared to the national rate of 82.9%, suggesting lower provider screening for HIV—including HIV screening among patients with MH disorders—and initiation of testing.

In the realm of MH care, the Free State has reported a strikingly higher MH separation rate of 20.1%, representing the proportion of clients admitted to hospitals for MH-related conditions, in contrast to the national rate of 3.8% [47] (p. 127). Previous studies in this province have exposed a fragmented MH network that remains largely hospital-centric, with authority and influence concentrated in a single specialist psychiatric hospital [48]. As previously discussed, the MH information system in the province is markedly underdeveloped. This shortcoming has led to the exclusion of MH indicators from health programmes at the PHC level, including those targeting TB and HIV. This omission, in itself, highlights a significant lack of prioritisation of MH care management and services within the province.

2.3. Participant Sampling, Recruitment

A non-probability purposive sampling approach was used to select 15 MH, PHC, TB, and HIV programme managers across the provincial and district levels of the health system. The sample sizes were chosen to achieve data saturation rather than the generalisability of findings. The Head of Department of the Free State Department of Health granted us permission to access the participants, who were recruited with assistance from their line managers. A study authorisation letter was presented to the line managers, who were then asked to distribute the letter and invite eligible managers to participate in the study. The line managers informed the managers about the voluntary nature of participation and requested to share their contact information with the research team. Subsequently, appointments for the SSIs and FGDs were scheduled with the participants to ensure minimal disruption to their work routines and duties.

2.4. Data Collection

Semi-structured guides featuring open-ended questions were crafted to elicit comprehensive and nuanced responses from participants, thereby enabling a thorough exploration of their perspectives. The questions included: "What, in your view, are the major barriers to integrating MH into TB and HIV care" and "What, in your view, are the major facilitators of integration of MH into TB and HIV care?"

Data were collected between February and October 2021. Experienced fieldworkers conducted the SSIs, while the first and second authors led the FGDs. All interviews and discussions, lasting about one and two hours, respectively, were audio-recorded with participants' informed consent.

Initially, the plan was to conduct all data collection in person. However, the COVID-19 pandemic and the resulting protective measures, such as travel restrictions and social distancing [49], required a shift in approach. A hybrid methodology was adopted, combining both in person and virtual interactions. The pandemic also led to many health managers being reassigned to COVID-19 response roles, complicating fieldwork coordination. As a result, activities were staggered to comply with COVID-19 guidelines and accommodate participants' availability. Virtual interviews and conferencing became a common practice for qualitative data collection during the pandemic [49,50]. While both the FGDs in the current study were conducted in person, upholding guidelines for social distancing and personal protection, two of the SSIs took place remotely. Throughout the process, strict ethical standards were upheld to ensure the protection of participants' rights and privacy, regardless of the data collection method used [50].

2.5. Data Analysis

The discussions and interviews were audio-recorded and transcribed, and thematic analysis was performed by two independent coders following the methodology established by Braun and Clarke [51]. The study utilised the WHO health systems strengthening building blocks framework as its analytical lens [38–42], applying the individual blocks as predefined themes. Through careful coding, subthemes were identified and categorised into barriers and facilitators to integrating MH into TB and HIV care. To ensure the trustworthiness of the findings, data integrity principles were rigorously upheld, including triangulating data from both interviews and FGDs. Furthermore, a third coder reviewed the subthemes iteratively and engaged in discussions with the primary coders to achieve consensus.

2.6. Ethics Statement

This study received ethical clearance from the Health Sciences Research Ethics Committee at the University of the Free State (UFS-HSD2019/1574/2611-0003). Written informed consent was obtained from participants in data collection and handling aligned with the Declaration of Helsinki [52].

3. Results

This section presents the insights of provincial and district public health programme managers on the integration of MH into TB and HIV healthcare services within the Free State province. A total of 15 managers responsible for the MH, PHC, TB, and HIV programmes participated in the study: four in the individual SSIs and eleven in two FGDs, respectively, involving five TB programme and six HIV programme managers. Demographically, eight of the FGD participants were female and six were aged between 51 and 60 years. Five of the respondents had over 15 years of experience in their positions, with one respondent not specifying their experience. Additionally, seven participants held a bachelor's degree. As depicted in Table 1, the identified subthemes underscored both the barriers impeding and the facilitators promoting the integration of these services across the WHO building blocks, with the inclusion of "people", as perceived by the respondents.

Table 1. Subthemes highlighting managers' perceptions of barriers to and facilitators of integration of MH into TB and HIV care.

Building Block	Barrier	Facilitator
Service delivery	• Lack of MH support for diseases other than HIV • Limited role of NGOs and CBOs • Communication gaps between initiating and receiving facilities during down referral	• Decentralise and deinstitutionalise MH care • Establish a proper MH management structure • Establish support groups for TB-HIV-MH patients
Workforce	• Deficits in staff MH training • Staff not prioritising MH • Lack of district MH specialist teams	• Improve staff MH training and retraining • Re-establish district MH specialist teams
Health information	• Unawareness/non-use of TB-HIV-MH screening tool	• Integrate screening for TB, HIV, and MH • Formalise inclusion of MH data elements into TB-HIV-MH screening
Essential medicines	• Lack of nutritional support for patients on treatment	• Utilise CHWs to distribute medicine to patients' homes
Financing	• Insufficient resources and lack of dedicated funding for MH	• Utilise NGOs and CBOs more effectively
Leadership/ governance	• Limited MH management structure and lack of subdistrict MH managers	• Adopt a multisectoral approach to improve training of MH care providers
People	• Stigmatisation • Lack of family treatment adherence support • Patients refraining from taking responsibility for their own health	• Increase family involvement • Partner with traditional and religious leaders

Abbreviations: CBO, community-based organisation; CHW, community health worker; MH, mental health; NGO, non-governmental organisation; TB, tuberculosis.

3.1. Service Delivery

3.1.1. Service Delivery Barriers

The first barrier perceived to hinder the integration of MH into TB and HIV services under the pre-defined "service delivery" theme was lack of MH support for diseases other than HIV, explained as:

> *"For our HIV patients we do have the buddy system where we encourage them to have someone to talk to... But when we look at other diseases that are also deadly as HIV, we really don't give that support"* (HIV FGD participant 6).

The second perceived barrier under "service delivery" was the limited role of non-governmental organisations (NGOs) and community-based organisations (CBOs), articulated as:

> *"[NGOs and CBOs] are crucial in terms of taking long term care and making sure that the patients adhere to treatment and go for follow up visits to [PHC] or to the specialist... and I know in our province we don't have enough"* (HIV FGD participant 4).

The third perceived barrier related to the "service delivery" building block was the communication gaps between initiating and receiving facilities during down referral. A participant observed:

> *"When you discharge a [MH] patient from a psychiatric complex; they just discharge the patient, but they don't report to the clinic to say, 'today we discharged so and so. You must have a follow-up at your clinic on these dates.' If that back referral is not done actively we will miss them. The problem is that they sometimes give the discharge letter to the patients in their hands, but they do not go back to the clinic... The down referral sometimes breaks the system and that causes the defaulters"* (SSI participant 2).

In summary, the service delivery barriers observed by the managers included a lack of MH support for non-HIV diseases, insufficient involvement of NGOs and CBOs in patient care, and communication gaps during patient discharge that lead to missed follow-ups and treatment defaults.

3.1.2. Service Delivery Facilitators

The first facilitator perceived to advance the integration MH into TB and HIV services related to the "service delivery" building block was to decentralise/deinstitutionalise MH care. A participant remarked:

> *"The institutions that are decentralising [multi-drug resistant TB] patients need to be supported because as patients are decentralised from the institution they should also have some plan in terms of how are they going to be supported in terms of [MH]"* (HIV FGD participant 6).

The second perceived facilitator related to "service delivery" was to establish a proper MH management structure. This was emphasised by a participant who stated:

> *"Currently the [MH] directorate consists of two people. And it is really struggling in terms of resources. It used to have a complete structure from provincial level, district level and subdistrict and obviously it goes together with the budget so that we can have specific activities aiming to address specific areas of concern"* (HIV FGD participant 4).

The third perceived facilitator under "service delivery" was to establish support groups for TB-HIV-MH patients. This was elaborated as follows by a participant:

> *"I think we should not undermine the impact of a support group. In our adherence guidelines which is cutting across all, it is not only for HIV/TB, but also for [MH] and other chronics, there is what we call enhanced counselling. Where people need some extra support and there is also the support group issue where you can put people in a group to relate to each other and get some extra support. We found that over the years it is a really good idea"* (HIV FGD participant 7).

To summarise, the managers believed that advancing the integration of MH into TB and HIV services required decentralising MH care, establishing a robust MH management structure, and creating support groups for patients.

3.2. *Workforce*

3.2.1. Workforce Barriers

The first barrier perceived to hinder the integration of MH into TB and HIV care, related to the "workforce" building block, was deficits in staff MH training. This was articulated as follows by participants:

> *"Most colleagues feel that [MH] is a specialised disease which is not applicable at their level, especially in the [PHC] setting. So, it is going to take some time to get people to understand that there are certain things in [MH] which can be treated at the level of [PHC]"* (TB FGD participant 4).

> *"I believe that the integration level is very minimal mainly due to lack of skills within our PHC setting. The majority of nurses are not clued up with [MH]. And we know there are limited clinicians who are specialists in that area of [MH]. Hence, the integration level is very slow"* (HIV FGD participant 3).

The second perceived barrier related to the "workforce" building block was staff not prioritising MH, reflected on as:

> *"You know, it is only a few who understand the priority; that [MH] should be prioritised. But I can say most of them don't see it that way"* (SSI participant 1).

The third perceived barrier under "workforce" was lack of MH specialist teams, shared as:

"We are supposed to have more specialist teams but due to financial implications we could not appoint them yet" (SSI participant 2).

Briefly, the major workforce-related barrier was the lack of MH training among staff. Reportedly, many healthcare workers viewed MH as a specialised field not relevant to their roles in PHC, leading to a slow integration process. They needed time to understand that some MH issues can be managed at the PHC level. Another important barrier was the lack of prioritisation of MH. The managers observed that only a few healthcare workers recognised its importance, while most did not see it as a priority. Additionally, financial constraints were seen to have prevented the appointment of necessary MH specialist teams, further hindering integration efforts.

3.2.2. Workforce Facilitators

The main facilitator perceived to advance the integration of MH into TB and HIV care related to the "workforce" building block was to improve staff MH training and retraining. Participants motivated this as follows:

"They should be skilled [in] how to care for [MH] care users, how to manage the down referrals and the importance of our [MH] care users to adhere to treatment [...] I think skilling of our professionals at [PHC] level will really be helpful" (SSI participant 1).

"Lately I have realised that instead of doing more campaigns for communities, we need to re-train our health professionals because I think there is lack of skill regarding the provision of the service. That is our biggest need, retraining" (SSI participant 2).

The key facilitator for integrating MH into TB and HIV care perceived by the managers was to enhance staff training and retraining. Participants emphasised the need for healthcare professionals to be skilled in managing MH care users, handling referrals, and ensuring treatment adherence. They highlighted that retraining health professionals was more crucial than community campaigns due to a significant skill gap in service provision.

3.3. *Health Information*

3.3.1. Health Information Barriers

Regarding the "health information" building block, the primary barrier perceived to impede the integration of MH into TB and HIV care was unawareness/non-use of the TB-HIV-MH screening tool. This was articulated by a participant as follows:

"We should start to insist that most of the screening tools must be used. It could have been that they have only been concentrating on TB and HIV and neglecting the MH screening tool. So, it should be insisted and given more impetus to be able to get a better outcome" (TB FGD participant 4).

In summary, the main perceived health information-related barrier to integrating MH into TB and HIV care was the lack of awareness and use of the TB–HIV–MH screening tool. Participants emphasised the need to prioritise and consistently use this tool to improve outcomes.

3.3.2. Health Information Facilitators

The corresponding principal facilitator identified by respondents for advancing the integration of MH into TB and HIV care was to integrate screening for TB, HIV and MH and to formalise the inclusion of MH data elements into TB-HIV-MH screening. This was elaborated by participants as follows:

"I think integration of the screening tool at the entry level of each PHC facility should be introduced because some facilities are not aware of that H form that is integrated with all the diseases to screen" (TB FGD participant 5).

"[CHWs] have already been trained on [MH]. They do it already. But you see... again, it was not a formal data element. You must have a formal data element to get it done consistently" (SSI participant 2).

The main health-information-related facilitator for integrating MH into TB and HIV care perceived by the managers was the need for consistent combined screening for TB, HIV, and MH at PHC facilities using the available tool that many healthcare workers do not seem to be aware of. Additionally, formalising the inclusion of MH data elements in these screenings was seen to be crucial for consistency. Participants highlighted the need for awareness and formal processes to ensure effective integration and consistent care.

3.4. Essential Medicines

3.4.1. Essential Medicines Barriers

Regarding the "essential medicines" building block, while the managers did not express specific concerns about the availability of and access to medications for MH, TB, and HIV, they did highlight challenges related to treatment support. Specifically, they voiced concerns about the lack of nutritional support to patients on treatment. As one participant remarked:

> *"As they are on treatment, they are complaining of hunger because they are not working. So, I think food parcels are the better solution for them"* (TB FGD participant 1).

In summary, while managers did not report issues with the availability of essential medicines for MH, TB, and HIV, they did express concerns about the lack of nutritional support for patients undergoing treatment. They suggested providing food parcels to address patients' complaints of hunger.

3.4.2. Essential Medicines Facilitators

The principal facilitator identified for the "essential medicines" building block was to utilise CHWs to distribute medication to patients' homes. As one participant advised:

> *"If they did not come for their treatment the [CHWs] go to them to give them their treatment and advise them that they should take their treatment regularly. It is an ongoing service that they do in the community"* (TB FGD participant 3).

To put it briefly, the main strategy perceived by the managers to ensure access to essential medicines was using CHWs to deliver medications directly to patients' homes.

3.5. Financing

3.5.1. Financing Barriers

The primary barrier perceived to hinder the integration of MH into TB and HIV services, related to the "financing" building block, was insufficient resources and a lack of dedicated funding for MH. This issue was conveyed as follows:

> *"Normally when they talk about the budget, they prioritise HIV and TB"* (SSI participant 3).

The main financial barrier to integrating MH into TB and HIV services perceived by the managers was the lack of resources and dedicated funding for MH. This was often because budgets prioritise HIV and TB over MH.

3.5.2. Financing Facilitators

The main facilitator perceived to advance the integration of MH into TB and HIV care under the "financing" building block was to utilise NGOs and CBOs more effectively. This was articulated as follows:

> *"I think we must have more funding available for NGOs to render specific services. For example, we must license NGOs to accommodate [MH] care users... but we don't find them to become compliant. There are thirteen criteria, norms and standards that they must meet before we can license them. [But] how can you enforce an NGO or a service provider to become compliant, but you don't fund them?"* (SSI participant 3).

As perceived by the managers, in order to better integrate MH into TB and HIV care, it is crucial to utilise NGOs and CBOs more effectively. This requires increasing funding for these organisations so they can meet compliance standards and provide necessary services. Without sufficient funding, NGOs and CBOs struggle to be compliant and support MH care users.

3.6. Leadership/Governance

3.6.1. Leadership/Governance Barriers

The primary barrier perceived to hinder the integration of MH–PHC–TB–HIV services, related to the "leadership/governance" building block, was the limited MH management structure and lack of subdistrict MH managers. This was elucidated as follows:

> *"The structure of the [MH] directorate at the provincial level is very slim and it is not approved as yet"* (HIV FGD participant 1).

The main perceived obstacle to integrating MH into TB and HIV services was the weak leadership and governance structure. Specifically, the managers remarked on the limited MH management framework and a lack of MH managers at the subdistrict level. This issue was highlighted by the fact that the MH directorate at the provincial level was understaffed and not yet officially approved.

3.6.2. Leadership/Governance Facilitators

The primary facilitator identified for advancing the integration of MH–PHC–TB–HIV services within the "leadership/governance" building block was to adopt a multisectoral approach to improve MH care provider training. This was conveyed as follows:

> *"Capacitation should not be left on the shoulders of the [Department of Health]. This should be a multidisciplinary approach from all government, private, universities, etc."* (HIV FGD participant 6).

The key facilitator perceived by the managers for integrating MH–PHC–TB–HIV services under the "leadership/governance" framework was to adopt a multisectoral approach to enhance MH care provider training involving collaboration across government, private sectors, and universities, rather than relying solely on the Department of Health.

3.7. People

3.7.1. People Barriers

The first barrier perceived to hinder the integration MH–PHC–TB–HIV services related to the added component, "people" was stigmatisation, explained as:

> *"I think within our communities [MH patients] are perceived as outcasts. Even their immediate family members also perceive them as outcasts because they lack understanding of what this person is going through; what is happening to this person"* (HIV FGD participant 3).

The second perceived barrier related to the added component was lack of family treatment adherence support, elaborated as:

> *"[Sighs], it is a very difficult thing. Families and caretakers are dealing with [MH] patients every day. But I don't think they give support to the user that they must get. A simple example, if they can ensure that [MH] care patients or users maintain their treatment they will not end up in defaulting. The moment they default treatment they end up in hospital systems"* (SSI participant 2).

The third perceived barrier related to "people" was patients refraining from taking responsibility for their own health, clarified as:

> *"What about your own commitment and your own responsibility to take your treatment? And that is not only for TB but for any patient. If you don't take your treatment it*

is not the professional nurse's, social worker's responsibility. You must take your own responsibility..." (SSI participant 2).

In summary, stigmatisation was perceived to represent a significant barrier, as MH patients are often viewed as outcasts by their communities and even their families, who lack understanding of their conditions. Another perceived factor was the lack of family support for treatment adherence. Families and caretakers often struggle to help MH patients maintain their treatment, leading to treatment default and hospitalisation. Additionally, patients frequently fail to take responsibility for their own health. This issue is compounded by fears related to other conditions, such as TB, which can result in neglect of MH treatment.

3.7.2. People Facilitators

The main facilitator perceived to advance the integration MH–PHC–TB–HIV services related to the added component, was to increase family involvement, voiced as:

"*We also encourage, for instance if it's an elderly or a mentally challenged person, the family to be part of the medical consultations or whatever that will be discussed. Because if we are talking to a mentally challenged patient the message won't be clear*" (HIV FGD participant 5).

Another perceived facilitator related to the "people" building block was to partner with traditional and religious leaders, as depicted by a participant:

"*There is another element that we are forgetting. The traditional health people and the religious people. Your pastors and the inyangas in the community. Most of our people receive advices from religious or traditional help. And we need to capacitate them in terms of not only treatment adherence but also the mental support. We cannot run away from that because our communities do consult them*" (HIV FGD participant 4).

To summarise, the primary "people"-related facilitator for integrating MH–PHC–TB–HIV services according to the managers was to increase family involvement in medical consultations, especially for elderly patients or patients with intellectual disabilities, to ensure clear communication. Additionally, partnering with traditional and religious leaders was seen as crucial for supporting treatment adherence and MH within the community.

4. Discussion

This study examines the barriers and facilitators influencing the integration of MH into TB and HIV care as perceived by the Free State public health programme managers within the framework of the health system building blocks. The argument ultimately posits that a whole-system approach—encompassing all six building block elements, with an added emphasis on the "people" component—is crucial for the successful integration of MH services into these healthcare domains.

4.1. Service Delivery

4.1.1. Service Delivery Barriers

Lack of MH support for diseases other than HIV: A significant barrier to the integration of MH care, as perceived by managers in the current study, was the disparity in support provided to patients with MH conditions compared to those with HIV. While mechanisms like the "buddy system" for HIV patients were well-established, similar support structures for other serious conditions, including MH disorders, were conspicuously lacking. This imbalance undermined the provision of comprehensive care for patients with multimorbidities, underscoring the pressing need for a more equitable and integrated support system. The perceived barrier, "lack of MH support for diseases other than HIV", identified by Free State managers is consistent with the directives of South Africa's Mental Health Care Act of 2012 [12]. The Act designates PHC as the primary entry point for MH services and prioritises the integration of MH care into general health services. The MHPF&SP 2023–2030 [22] further underscores the urgent need to strengthen this integration.

Limited involvement of NGOs and CBOs: The primary and community-based MH care systems in South Africa are both underfunded and under-resourced [53]. The Free State managers pointed out that the limited involvement of NGOs and CBOs represented a major challenge in integrating MH into TB and HIV services. These organisations were perceived to be vital for providing long-term MH care and ensuring that patients adhere to their treatment plans. The perceived barrier was consistent with the principles outlined in the MHPF&SP 2013–2020 [20] (pp. 19–20), which stresses the necessity of intersectoral collaboration, including partnerships with NGOs, to address the social determinants of health.

Communication gaps during down referral: Effective communication between initiating and receiving healthcare facilities is essential for seamless patient management, particularly during the down-referral process. The National Referral Policy [54] (p. 16) stipulates that both the referring facility and the receiving facility must document all outgoing and incoming referrals in a designated referral register. The communication gap observed by the Free State programme managers, where discharges from psychiatric facilities reportedly often occurred without proper notification to follow-up clinics, likely significantly contributed to patient non-adherence and systemic failures. This issue highlighted the critical need for integrated protocols and systematic approaches to ensure that patients were consistently tracked and supported post discharge.

4.1.2. Service Delivery Facilitators

Deinstitutionalising and decentralising MH care and supporting CBOs: The managers in the current study identified deinstitutionalising and decentralising MH care, along with enhancing the role of CBOs, as pivotal components in the broader strategy to integrate MH care into PHC. This perspective aligns with the MHPF&SP 2023–2030, which advocates for the gradual downsizing and replacement of long-term custodial specialist MH facilities with a comprehensive network of community-based residential and day care centres. However, the policy stipulates that deinstitutionalisation should only proceed once these essential community-based facilities are fully established, a requirement reportedly unmet in the Free State province. In 2009, Petersen et al. [55] noted that, akin to other LMICs, South Africa's efforts to achieve deinstitutionalisation and comprehensive, integrated MH care was hindered by the lack of MH resources within the PHC Package and the inefficient utilisation of existing resources.

Establishing a proper MH management structure: The Free State managers' recommendation to establish a robust MH management structure as a critical facilitator for integrated care aligns with the MHPF&SP 2013–2020 directive [20] (p. 31) to strengthen the capacity of district health management teams in planning, implementing, supervising, monitoring, and evaluating MH programmes at both district and community levels. Previous research in the Western Cape province has highlighted the pivotal role of district facility managers in developing and executing district MH information systems and policies, which are essential for improving health service outcomes at the district level [56].

Establish support groups for TB–HIV–MH patients: The Free State managers' recognition of the importance of the role of social support, particularly through self-help groups, as a facilitator of MH improvement is strongly supported by research. For instance, a study in Myanmar found that participation in self-help groups served as a protective factor against depressive symptoms among people living with HIV [57]. Similarly, research in Zimbabwe on vulnerable young mothers revealed that engagement in self-help groups enhanced MH by strengthening peer support and fostering hope for the future [58]. In the United Kingdom, a study on men's experiences with peer support groups for managing mental distress found that these groups provided a secure environment—a "safe space"—where men could challenge traditional masculine norms by exchanging personalised MH support and adopting specific roles within the group [59].

4.2. Workforce

4.2.1. Workforce Barriers

Staff MH training deficits: The issue of inadequate MH training among PHC nurses, as highlighted by the Free State managers, aligns with findings of a study to assess MH literacy of PHC workers in South Africa and Zambia showing moderate MH literacy, which may hinder their ability to adequately recognise MH conditions, but with a wide range from low to high MH literacy [60]. The findings in the Free State also resonate with a recent international literature review that identified significant MH knowledge gaps and learning needs among PHC nurses [61]. This review underscored the necessity for PHC nurses to actively identify their MH learning needs and engage in targeted education to adequately prepare them for meeting the increasing demands for MH services.

Staff not prioritising MH: Not considering MH as one of the priorities within district health services has also been reported in a study on district managers' perspectives of MH information processing and utilisation at the PHC level in the Western Cape [56]. This oversight reflects a broader issue within the health system where MH is often marginalised despite its critical impact on other public health challenges. Staff must be attuned to the fact that beyond stigma and social isolation, mental illness persists as a "silent driver of the global TB epidemic" [62].

Lack of MH specialist teams: As reported by the managers, the Free State province, which consists of five districts, had only one district MH specialist team. This is despite the MHPF&SP 2013–2020 [20] (p. 23) directive that district specialist MH teams should be established to support non-specialist PHC staff and community-based workers. The new MHPF&SP 2023–2030 [22] (p. 36) emphasises that district MH specialist teams are responsible for building capacity among users—patients and their families—to provide appropriate self-help and peer-led services, such as support groups facilitated by NGOs.

4.2.2. Workforce Facilitators

Improving staff MH training and retraining: The approach suggested by the Free State managers aligns with the MHPF&SP 2023–2030 [22] (p. 28), which mandates that all health staff receive basic MH training, including anti-stigma education, along with regular supervision and mentoring. Provincial Departments of Health are tasked with expanding the MH workforce, and a task-shifting approach is emphasised, where trained non-specialist workers provide evidence-based psychosocial interventions under the guidance of specialists [22] (p. 28).

Re-establishing district MH specialist teams: This perceived facilitator of the Free State managers resonates with the MHPF&SP 2023–2030 [22] (p. 24) emphasis on the importance of district MH specialist teams. These teams are tasked with developing and implementing district MH plans, utilising all available resources within the district, and incorporating tools and lessons from South African innovations in district MH plans.

4.3. Health Information

4.3.1. Health Information Barriers

Non-awareness/use of TB–HIV–MH screening tool: This perceived barrier corroborates the findings of a study on the views of facility managers on the use of MH information for planning services in the Western Cape province showing that MH information processing systems were fragmented and inadequate for decision-making [56]. According to this study, a lack of knowledge in information processing and utilisation, as well as poor information infrastructure and networking were associated with poor understanding about MH, not considering MH as one of the priorities within the district health services, and a lack of higher officials' interest in the development of the MH programme.

Surprisingly, the Free State managers did not seem to be aware of two recognised screening guidelines: firstly, the 2023 Adult Primary Care guideline [63]—a prescribed guideline in South Africa in PHC settings for the screening, assessment, and management of diseases, and secondly, the Mental Health Gap Action Programme (MHGaP), recommended by the WHO for use by healthcare professionals [1].

4.3.2. Health Information Facilitators

Integrating screening for TB, HIV, and MH: This proposed facilitator aligned with the MHPF&SP 2013–2020 [20] (p. 29) call for routine screening and treatment of physical illnesses during all consultations for individuals with mental illness. The new MHPF&SP 2023–2030 [22] (p. 24) again emphasises that MH interventions will be included in the core package of district health services. This should involve a task-sharing approach where trained non-specialist workers deliver evidence-based psychosocial interventions, including routine screening for mental illness during pregnancy and for other identified high-risk groups, along with a stepped approach to management and referral.

4.4. Essential Medicines

4.4.1. Essential Medicines Barriers

Lack of nutritional support for patients on treatment: This perceived barrier resonates with a study in the USA showing that medically appropriate food support may improve MH for people living with HIV [64]. As shown in a review of studies in Africa that included co-infected adults and children, nutritional support is also important to minimise the harmful effects of food insecurity in HIV-TB populations [65]. This underscores the importance of integrating nutritional support into healthcare strategies to enhance MH outcomes and address the broader impacts of food insecurity on individuals with HIV–TB co-infection.

4.4.2. Essential Medicines Facilitators

Utilising CHWs to take medicine to patients' homes if they do not collect it from the clinic: This suggested facilitator is supported by a study in the Western Cape province that showed that home delivery of medication by CHWs was feasible at scale and affordable [66]. The integration of CHWs into home delivery of medication demonstrates significant potential to enhance medication adherence and access.

4.5. Financing

4.5.1. Financing Barriers

Insufficient resources and a lack of dedicated funding for MH: According to the Free State managers, insufficient resources and inadequate dedicated funding for MH presented substantial challenges. These perceptions are consistent with the MHPF&SP 2013–2020 observation that inadequate MH financing significantly impedes progress [20] (p. 13). Research carried out across six sub-Saharan African countries, including South Africa, and South Asian nations, highlights critical obstacles to sustainable MH financing, including inadequate funding levels, pervasive inequalities in access, and entrenched poverty [67].

4.5.2. Financing Facilitators

Utilising NGOs and CBOs effectively: As suggested by the Free State managers, effective use of NGOs and CBOs is crucial in the delivery of decentralised MH services. Despite government subsidies allocated to approximately 2000 MH NGOs in South Africa, the lack of coordination between government departments and these NGOs has resulted in fragmented care delivery [68].

4.6. Leadership/Governance

4.6.1. Leadership/Governance Barriers

Limited MH management structure and lack of subdistrict MH managers: In South Africa's district health management context, which is continuously shaped by major healthcare reforms from the National Department of Health, many managers lack the competencies required for effective leadership [69]. Research has shown that healthcare managers within districts are often selected from health professional backgrounds. While this provides valuable contextual insight, they frequently lack formal management training, thereby limiting their managerial effectiveness. A 2015 study on health system governance aimed at supporting integrated MH care in South Africa highlighted significant deficiencies in managerial and planning capacities at both provincial and district levels, particularly regarding the development and implementation of integrated MH care plans [70].

4.6.2. Leadership/Governance Facilitators

Adopt a multisectoral approach to improve MH care provider training: Respondents in the current study emphasised the need for a multisectoral approach to training MH care providers at the PHC level. They argued that responsibility for this training should extend beyond the Department of Health to include universities and the private sector. Given the increasing demands of MH care, there is a critical need to fundamentally revise undergraduate nursing education to better prepare students for MH care delivery, particularly within the TB and HIV programmes. However, the South African Nursing Council has significantly reduced the content and clinical hours in undergraduate nursing curricula, focusing narrowly on foundational theory and basic interpersonal skills. As a result, newly qualified nurses are inadequately prepared to provide effective MH care.

4.7. People

4.7.1. People Barriers

Stigmatisation: Respondents in the current study reported that MH patients are often viewed as "outcasts", a perception consistent with findings by Mathias et al. (2024) [68], which reveal that in Ghana, India, and South Africa, mental illness is frequently interpreted through religious and traditional frameworks, attributing it to moral failings, taboo violations, or malevolent forces such as sorcery. These interpretations reinforce conservative moral codes and perpetuate stigma. The pervasive stigma surrounding mental illness often discourages individuals from seeking care due to fear of judgement and discrimination. This reluctance significantly contributes to the underutilisation of MH services, presenting major obstacles to the effective integration of these services into TB and HIV care settings.

Lack of family treatment adherence support: From the perspective of the Free State programme managers, the lack of family support for treatment adherence emerged as a significant barrier to integrating MH services with TB and HIV care. Inadequate family support can severely impact the management of MH disorders, TB, and HIV. Research consistently underscores the critical role of family involvement in improving treatment outcomes. For example, a study in China found that TB patients who received regular supervision and spiritual encouragement from family members demonstrated higher adherence to treatment protocols [71]. Similarly, research in Uganda showed that strong family cohesion was strongly associated with greater self-efficacy in adhering to antiretroviral treatment [72]. Furthermore, a multi-ethnic Asian cohort study observed that significant psychological distress early in HIV care was a predictor of future non-adherence to antiretroviral treatment, emphasising the need for early detection and intervention for psychological distress in people living with HIV [73]. The study advocated for integrating MH interventions with adherence strategies to improve HIV treatment outcomes.

Patients refraining from taking responsibility for their own health: The Free State managers observed that TB patients with MH disorders often refuse both MH and TB treatments, underscoring a significant barrier to integrating MH services into TB care. This issue reflects broader concerns about the expectation that individuals should be solely accountable for their adverse health outcomes. Levy (2019) [74] challenged this notion by arguing that it forms an inadequate foundation for policy. The capacity to make responsible health choices is often inequitably distributed, influenced by social and economic disparities. Therefore, it is flawed to place sole responsibility on individuals for making poor health choices. Instead, accountability should rest with those who influence the distribution of resources and shape broader circumstances, as they indirectly contribute to adverse health outcomes and also possess the means to address these underlying inequities.

Moreover, the low level of MH literacy among the South African population [75] exacerbates this issue. Without an adequate understanding of MH, individuals are less likely to recognise symptoms, seek help, or adhere to treatment plans. This lack of literacy further undermines the expectation that patients should take full responsibility for their health outcomes. Improving MH literacy is essential to empower individuals to make informed health decisions and to support the integration of MH services into TB and HIV care effectively [76]. Wiedermann et al. (2023) [77] presented well-founded recommendations to bolster MH support within educational systems, especially during crises like the COVID-19 pandemic. These authors champion a proactive and comprehensive approach to MH, suggesting the integration of MH education into the core curriculum to help students develop coping mechanisms and emotional intelligence. Additionally, they emphasised the necessity of training educators to recognise and address MH issues, and advocate for interdisciplinary collaboration among various stakeholders.

4.7.2. People Facilitators

Increasing family involvement: The managers in the current study identified increasing family involvement as a crucial facilitator for the integration of MH services, recognising the significant role families play in providing emotional and practical support. This involvement creates a nurturing environment that enhances treatment adherence and overall well-being. Evidence from an Ethiopian study supports this view, showing that TB/HIV co-infected patients had a lower quality of life across all domains compared to patients with HIV but without active TB. The study found that strong family support was significantly associated with improvements in most quality-of-life domains [78].

Partnering with traditional and religious leaders: Recent findings from diverse settings—including Ghana, India, the occupied Palestinian territories, and South Africa—highlight that essential MH resources extend beyond formal healthcare systems to include religious groups, and faith-based organisations [68]. The Free State programme managers believed that partnering with traditional and religious leaders is crucial for the effective integration of MH services into TB and HIV programmes. In Sub-Saharan Africa, there is a widespread belief that traditional healers have special skills to diagnose and treat both physical and emotional ailments stemming from social misconduct, spirits, spells, and sorcery—domains where allopathic doctors are often seen as inadequate [79]. In South Africa, traditional healers are also often seen to be more accessible than biomedical providers and play a vital role in addressing emotional and spiritual well-being.

Recognising the paucity of allopathic MH care providers in South Africa's public sector (for example, only 0.4 psychiatrists and 0.3 psychologists per 100,000 people at the time), Audet et al. (2017) [79] commended innovative solutions, such as task sharing models being proposed in the government's MHPF&SP 2013–2020 [20]. These authors however emphasised that despite these innovative policies, challenges persisted in implementing allopathic–traditional MH care integration. Van Rooyen et al.'s (2015) [80] (p. 4) research highlighted that the negative attitudes of allopathic health practitioners towards traditional healers emanated from "unscientific methods" used by the traditional health practitioners in treating MH patients, the "interference" of traditional healers with the efficacy of hospital MH treatment, and "delays" by traditional healers in referring MH patients to hospital.

Campbell-Hall et al. (2010) [81] emphasised the importance of creating collaborative models that integrate traditional and Western MH care systems in South Africa. These authors explored the perceptions of service users and providers in a rural sub-district of KwaZulu–Natal province and proposed the following steps to foster a functional relationship between these two systems. Firstly, adopting a collaborative approach that respects the domains of both traditional and Western practices, finding mutually reinforcing intersections. Secondly, Western practitioners should adopt a "meaning-centred" approach, which involves understanding the user's perspective and negotiating treatment plans that may include traditional methods. Thirdly, addressing the need for alternative arrangements to bring together different MH service providers, suggesting the establishment of a multisectoral MH advisory group to facilitate integration at district and sub-district levels. Such groups should include representatives from traditional practitioners to ensure participatory processes.

4.8. Limitations

While qualitative studies, including FGDs and SSIs with public health programme managers, offer valuable insights, they are not without limitations. A notable limitation is the restricted generalisability of findings to other contexts or provinces. Qualitative research, relying on the subjective perspectives and experiences of participants, is susceptible to bias from both participants and researchers. The quality of data can vary based on factors such as participants' willingness to share, the skill of the facilitator or interviewer, and group dynamics. In FGDs, dominant voices may overshadow others, leading to a partial or skewed understanding of the issues. Furthermore, the interpretive nature of qualitative research poses challenges for reproducibility and validation, as various researchers may differently interpret findings.

According to de Savigny and Adam [41], a health system cannot function effectively if its components are considered in isolation. Instead, it is the complex relationships and dynamic interactions among these components—how each one influences and is influenced by the others—that create an integrated and functional system. To fully understand a health system, one must examine both the configuration and interplay of its components, and how these interactions collectively enable the system to achieve its intended goals. The current exploratory study falls short of this comprehensive perspective as it primarily identifies key perceived barriers and facilitators to integrating MH services into TB and HIV services. However, it lays the groundwork for future research that could more deeply investigate the cross-cutting effects of these barriers and explore strategies to address them. Future qualitative research could, for example, examine how managerial perspectives influence the implementation of integrated MH–TB–HIV interventions, such as by promoting awareness and encouraging the routine use of integrated TB–HIV–MH screening tools.

5. Conclusions

This study highlights significant gaps in the integration of MH services with TB and HIV care in South Africa's Free State province. Programme managers identified substantial structural barriers, such as inadequate MH management frameworks, and social obstacles, including stigma and insufficient family support for treatment adherence. Despite these challenges, the study emphasises the crucial role of robust management structures and integrated screening processes as key facilitators for successful integration.

The Free State's underperformance in MH care, evidenced by a notably high rate of MH separation, underscores the urgent need for a comprehensive, system-wide strategy. Such a strategy must address both structural and social barriers that hinder MH integration. In the province's public health sector, where the integration of MH services with TB and HIV care remains inadequate, a fragmented approach is unlikely to yield significant improvements. The province's suboptimal TB outcomes and insufficient HIV testing coverage indicate deeper systemic interdependencies that require a cohesive, coordinated response.

A whole-system approach is imperative, conceptualising the healthcare system as an interconnected network where changes in one area inevitably affect others. By addressing all six building blocks of the health system and emphasising the central role of "people"—both as healthcare providers and recipients—this approach offers a more comprehensive and effective strategy for tackling the root causes of integration challenges.

Author Contributions: Conceptualisation, G.K.-M.; methodology, G.K.-M. and C.H.; validation, G.K.-M. and C.H.; formal analysis, C.H. and G.K.-M.; data curation, C.H.; writing—original draft preparation, C.H.; writing—review and editing, C.H. and G.K.-M.; project administration, G.K.-M.;

funding acquisition, G.K.-M. All authors have read and agreed to the published version of the manuscript.

Funding: This research was funded by the National Research Foundation, grant number 116355, and the Department of Science and Innovation Africa Health Research and Innovation Programme in partnership with the South African Medical Research Council, grant number 96148.

Institutional Review Board Statement: The study was conducted in accordance with the Declaration of Helsinki and approved by the Health Science Research Ethics Committee of the University of the Free State (protocol code UFS-HSD2019/1574/2611-0003, 15 July 2023).

Informed Consent Statement: Informed consent was obtained from all subjects involved in the study.

Data Availability Statement: Data are not available as this would compromise respondents' anonymity.

Acknowledgments: Raymond Tweheyo is thanked for contributing to the data analysis.

Conflicts of Interest: The authors declare no conflicts of interest. The funders had no role in the design of the study; in the collection, analyses, or interpretation of data; in the writing of the manuscript; or in the decision to publish the results.

References

1. World Health Organization. *mhGAP Humanitarian Intervention Guide (mhGAP-HIG): Clinical Management of Mental, Neurological and Substance Use Conditions in Humanitarian Emergencies*; WHO: Geneva, Switzerland, 2015; ISBN 9789241548922.
2. Qin, X.; Hsieh, C.R. Understanding and addressing the treatment gap in mental healthcare: Economic perspectives and evidence From China. *Inquiry* **2020**, *57*, 46958020950566. [CrossRef] [PubMed]
3. World Health Organization. *Comprehensive Mental Health Action Plan 2013–2030*; WHO: Geneva, Switzerland, 2021.
4. Heunis, J.C.; Schneider, H. Integration of ART: Concepts, policy and practice. *Acta Acad.* **2006**, *2006* (Suppl. S1), 256–285.
5. World Health Organization. *The World Health Report: Make Every Mother and Child Count*; WHO: Geneva, Switzerland, 2005.
6. Kozlowska, O.; Lumb, A.; Tan, G.D.; Rea, R. Barriers and facilitators to integrating primary and specialist healthcare in the United Kingdom: A narrative literature review. *Future Healthc. J.* **2018**, *5*, 64–80. [CrossRef] [PubMed]
7. Nguyen, T.; Tran, T.; Tran, H.; Tran, T.; Fisher, J. Challenges in integrating mental health into primary care in Vietnam. In *Innovations in Global Mental Health*; Okpaku, S., Ed.; Springer: Cham, Switzerland, 2019.
8. Martinez, W.; Galván, J.; Saavedra, N.; Berenzon, S. Barriers to integrating mental health services in community-based primary care settings in Mexico City: A qualitative analysis. *Psychiatr. Serv.* **2017**, *68*, 497–502. [CrossRef]
9. Topp, S.M.; Abimbola, S.; Joshi, R.; Negin, J. How to assess and prepare health systems in low- and middle-income countries for integration of services—A systematic review. *Health Policy Plan.* **2018**, *33*, 298–312. [CrossRef]
10. Stein, D.J. A new mental health policy for South Africa. *S. Afr. Med. J.* **2014**, *104*, 115–116. [CrossRef]
11. Pillay, Y. State of mental health and illness in South Africa. *S. Afr. J. Psychol.* **2019**, *49*, 463–466. [CrossRef]
12. Republic of South Africa. *Mental Health Care Act No. 17 of 2002*; South Africa Government Gazette: Pretoria, South Africa, 2012; Volume 449, p. 24024.
13. World Health Organization. *Mental Health Care Law: Ten Basic Principles*; WHO: Geneva, Switzerland, 1996; WHO/MNH/MND/96.9.
14. Silva, G.A.D.; Cardoso, A.J.C.; Bessoni, E.; Peixoto, A.D.C.; Rudá, C.; Silva, D.V.D.; Branco, S.M.J. Deinstitutionalization and autonomy: Outcomes from a Brazilian mental health policy. *Cien Saude Colet* **2022**, *27*, 101–110. [CrossRef]
15. Szabo, C.P.; Kaliski, S.Z. Mental health and the law: A South African perspective. *BJPsych Int.* **2017**, *14*, 69–71. [CrossRef]
16. Funk, M.; Saraceno, B.; Drew, N.; Faydi, E. Integrating mental health into primary health care. *Ment. Health Fam. Med.* **2008**, *5*, 5–8.
17. World Health Organization. *World Mental Health Report. Transforming Mental Health for All*; WHO: Geneva, Switzerland, 2022; ISBN 9789240049338.
18. Statistics South Africa. *Non-Communicable Diseases in South Africa, 2008–2018*; Statistics South Africa: Pretoria, South Africa, 2023.
19. Kenge, A. The challenge of NCD prevention and control in South Africa and other developing countries. In *Proceedings and Recommendations of the 2022 National Research for Health Summit, 22–23 November 2022*; National Health Research Committee: Benoni, South Africa, 2022.
20. National Department of Health. *National Mental Health Policy Framework and Strategic Plan 2013–2020*; NDoH: Pretoria, South Africa, 2013.
21. Naledi, T.; Barron, P.; Schneider, H. Primary health care in SA since 1994 and implications of the new vision for PHC re-engineering. In *South African Health Review 2022*; Padarath, A., Moeti, T., Eds.; Health Systems Trust: Durban, South Africa, 2023; pp. 17–28.
22. National Department of Health. *National Mental Health Policy Framework and Strategic Plan 2023–2030*; NDoH: Pretoria, South Africa, 2023.
23. Sorsdahl, K.; Petersen, I.; Myers, B.; Zingela, Z.; Lund, C.; van der Westhuizen, C. A reflection of the current status of the mental healthcare system in South Africa. *SSM—Ment. Health* **2023**, *4*, 100247. [CrossRef]

24. Ahuja, S.; Hanlon, C.; Chisholm, D.; Semrau, M.; Gurung, D.; Abdulmalik, J.; Mugisha, J.; Mntambo, N.; Kigozi, F.; Petersen, I.; et al. Experience of implementing new mental health indicators within information systems in six low- and middle-income countries. *BJPsych Open* **2019**, *5*, e71. [CrossRef] [PubMed]
25. Lund, C.; Petersen, I.; Kleintjes, S.; Bhana, A. Mental health services in South Africa: Taking stock. *Afr. J. Psychiatry* **2012**, *15*, 402–405. [CrossRef] [PubMed]
26. Freeman, M.C. Global lessons for deinstitutionalisation from the ill-fated transfer of mental health-care users in Gauteng, South Africa. *Lancet Psychiatry* **2018**, *5*, 765–768. [CrossRef] [PubMed]
27. Scher, M. Inquest begins over South African mental health failings. *Lancet* **2021**, *398*, 288. [CrossRef]
28. Docrat, S.; Besada, D.; Cleary, S.; Daviaud, E.; Lund, C. Mental health system costs, resources and constraints in South Africa: A national survey. *Health Policy Plan.* **2019**, *34*, 706–719. [CrossRef]
29. Setona, K.R.; Sehularo, L.A.; Mokgaola, I.O. Challenges faced by mental health nurse specialists in North West, South Africa. *Afr. J. Nurs. Midwifery* **2020**, *22*, 17.
30. Tansella, M. Making mental health services work at the primary level. *Bull. World Health Organ.* **2000**, *78*, 501–502.
31. Foo, C.; Shrestha, P.; Wang, L.; Du, Q.; García-Basteiro, A.L.; Abdullah, A.S.; Legido-Quigley, H. Integrating tuberculosis and noncommunicable diseases care in low- and middle-income countries (LMICs): A systematic review. *PLoS Med.* **2022**, *19*, e1003899. [CrossRef]
32. Kigozi-Male, G.; Heunis, C.; Engelbrecht, M.; Tweheyo, R. Possible depression in new tuberculosis patients in the Free State province, South Africa. *S. Afr. J. Infect. Dis.* **2024**, *39*, 653. [CrossRef]
33. Collins, P.Y.; Kline, S. A historic moment for mental health integration in HIV and tuberculosis programmes. *Lancet Psychiatry* **2022**, *9*, 936–937. [CrossRef] [PubMed]
34. Granberg, A.; Matérne, M.; Lundqvist, L.O.; Duberg, A. Navigating change—managers' experience of implementation processes in disability health care: A qualitative study. *BMC Health Serv. Res.* **2021**, *21*, 571. [CrossRef] [PubMed]
35. Hosseini-Moghaddam, F.; Mohammadpour, A.; Bahri, N.; Mojalli, M. Nursing managers' perspectives on facilitators of and barriers to evidence-based practice: A cross-sectional study. *Nurs. Open* **2023**, *10*, 6237–6247. [CrossRef] [PubMed]
36. Malakoane, B.; Chikobvu, P.; Heunis, C.; Kigozi, G.; Kruger, W. Health managers and community representatives' views of a system-wide intervention to strengthen public healthcare in the Free State, South Africa. *Afr. Health Sci.* **2023**, *23*, 747–764. [CrossRef]
37. Malakoane, B.; Heunis, J.C.; Chikobvu, P.; Kigozi, G.; Kruger, W.H. Public health system challenges in the Free State, South Africa: A situational appraisal to inform health systems strengthening. *BMC Health Serv. Res.* **2020**, *20*, 58. [CrossRef]
38. World Health Organization. *Everybody Business: Strengthening Health Systems to Improve Health Outcomes. WHO's Framework*; WHO: Geneva, Switzerland, 2007; ISBN 9789241596077.
39. World Health Organization. *Monitoring the Building Blocks of Health Systems: A Handbook of Indicators and Their Measurement Strategies*; WHO: Geneva, Switzerland, 2010; ISBN 978921564052.
40. Mounier-Jack, S.; Griffiths, U.K.; Closser, S.; Burchett, H.; Marchal, B. Measuring the health systems impact of disease control programmes: A critical reflection on the WHO building blocks framework. *BMC Public Health* **2014**, *14*, 278. [CrossRef]
41. de Savigny, D.; Adam, T. *Systems Thinking for Health Systems Strengthening*; WHO: Geneva, Switzerland, 2009; ISBN 9789241563895.
42. Mutale, W.; Bond, V.; Mwanamwenge, M.T.; Mlewa, S.; Balabanova, D.; Spicer, N.; Ayles, H. Systems thinking in practice: The current status of the six WHO building blocks for health system strengthening in three BHOMA intervention districts of Zambia: A baseline qualitative study. *BMC Health Serv. Res.* **2013**, *13*, 291. [CrossRef]
43. Andersson, G.Z.; Reinius, M.; Eriksson, L.E.; Svedhem, V.; Esfahani, F.M.; Deuba, K.; Rao, D.; Lyatuu, G.W.; Giovenco, D.; Ekström, A.M. Stigma reduction interventions in people living with HIV to improve health-related quality of life. *Lancet HIV* **2020**, *7*, e129–e140. [CrossRef]
44. DeSanto, D.; Velen, K.; Lessells, R.; Makgopa, S.; Gumede, D.; Fielding, K.; Grant, A.D.; Charalambous, S.; Chetty-Makkan, C.M. A qualitative exploration into the presence of TB stigmatization across three districts in South Africa. *BMC Public Health* **2023**, *23*, 5. [CrossRef]
45. Hines, A.C.; Rose, A.L.; Regenauer, K.S.; Brown, I.; Johnson, K.; Bonumwezi, J.; Ndamase, S.; Ciya, N.; Magidson, J.F.; Myers, B. "Early in the morning, there's tolerance and later in the day it disappears"—The intersection of resource scarcity, stress and stigma in mental health and substance use care in South Africa. *Camb. Prism. Glob. Ment. Health* **2024**, *11*, e45. [CrossRef]
46. Statistics South Africa. *Census 2022*; Statistical Release P0.301.4; Statistics South Africa: Pretoria, South Africa, 2022.
47. Ndlovu, N.; Gray, A.; Mkhabela, B.; Myende, N.; Day, C. Health and related indicators. In *South African Health Review 2022*; Padarath, A., Moeti, T., Eds.; Health Systems Trust: Durban, South Africa, 2023; pp. 108–122.
48. Janse van Rensburg, A.; Petersen, I.; Wouters, E.; Engelbrecht, M.; Kigozi, G.; Fourie, P.; van Rensburg, D.; Bracke, P. State and non-state mental health service collaboration in a South African district: A mixed methods study. *Health Policy Plan* **2018**, *33*, 516–527. [CrossRef] [PubMed]
49. Hlatshwako, T.G.; Shah, S.J.; Kosana, P.; Adebayo, E.; Hendriks, J.; Larsson, E.C.; Hensel, D.J.; Erausquin, J.T.; Marks, M.; Michielsen, K.; et al. Online health survey research during COVID-19. *Lancet Digit. Health* **2021**, *3*, e76–e77. [CrossRef] [PubMed]
50. Rossouw, T.M.; Wassenaar, D.; Kruger, M.; Blockman, M.; Hunter, A.; Burgess, T. Research ethics support during the COVID-19 epidemic: A collaborative effort by South African Research Ethics Committees. In *South African Health Review 2021*; Govender, K., George, G., Padarath, A., Moeti, T., Eds.; Health Systems Trust: Durban, South Africa, 2021; pp. 163–172.

51. Braun, V.; Clarke, V. Using thematic analysis in psychology. *Qual. Res. Psychol.* **2006**, *3*, 77–101. [CrossRef]
52. World Medical Association. WMA Declaration of Helsinki. Ethical Principles for Medical Research Involving Human Subjects. Available online: https://www.wma.net/policies-post/wma-declaration-of-helsinki-ethical-principles-for-medical-research-involving-human-subjects/ (accessed on 19 August 2024).
53. Shisana, O.; Stein, D.J.; Zungu, N.P.; Wolvaardt, G. The rationale for South Africa to prioritise mental health care as a critical aspect of overall health care. *Compr. Psychiatry* **2024**, *130*, 152458. [CrossRef]
54. National Department of Health. *Referral Policy for South African Health Services and Referral Implementation Guidelines*; NDoH: Pretoria, South Africa, 2013.
55. Petersen, I.; Bhana, A.; Campbell-Hall, V.; Mjadu, S.; Lund, C.; Kleintjies, S.; Hosegood, V.; Flisher, A.J. Mental Health and Poverty Research Programme Consortium. Planning for district mental health services in South Africa: A situational analysis of a rural district site. *Health Policy Plan.* **2009**, *24*, 140–150. [CrossRef]
56. Bimerew, M.; Korpela, M.; Adejumo, O. District facility managers' perspectives of mental health information processing and utilisation at primary care level in the Western Cape. *Afr. J. Phys. Act. Health Sci.* **2014**, *20* (Suppl. S1), 445–459.
57. Than, M.W.; Zaw, N.T.; Minn, K.; Saw, Y.M.; Kiriya, J.; Jimba, M.; Win, H.H.; Shibanuma, A. Assessing depressive symptoms among people living with HIV in Yangon city, Myanmar: Does being a member of self-help group matter? *PLoS ONE* **2021**, *16*, e0248807. [CrossRef]
58. Chingono, R.; Kasese, C.; Miles, S.; Busza, J. 'I was in need of somewhere to release my hurt': Addressing the mental health of vulnerable adolescent mothers in Harare, Zimbabwe, through self-help groups. *Glob. Health Action* **2022**, *15*, 2040151. [CrossRef]
59. Vickery, A. 'It's made me feel less isolated because there are other people who are experiencing the same or very similar to you': Men's experiences of using mental health support groups. *Health Soc. Care Com.* **2022**, *30*, 2383–2391. [CrossRef]
60. Korhonen, J.; Axelin, A.; Stein, D.J.; Seedat, S.; Mwape, L.; Jansen, R.; Groen, G.; Grobler, G.; Jörns-Presentati, A.; Katajisto, J.; et al. MEGA Consortium/Research Team. Mental health literacy among primary healthcare workers in South Africa and Zambia. *Brain Behav.* **2022**, *12*, 2807. [CrossRef]
61. McInnes, S.; Halcomb, E.; Ashley, C.; Kean, A.; Moxham, L.; Patterson, C. An integrative review of primary health care nurses' mental health knowledge gaps and learning needs. *Collegian* **2022**, *29*, 540–548. [CrossRef] [PubMed]
62. Fukunaga, R.; Moonan, P.K. Mental health and tuberculosis—Holding our breath in isolation. *Emerg. Infect. Dis.* **2024**, *30*, 627–628. [CrossRef]
63. Department of Health. Adult Primary Care Clinical Tool 2023. Available online: https://knowledgehub.health.gov.za/elibrary/adult-primary-care-apc-clinical-tool-2023 (accessed on 9 September 2024).
64. Chayama, K.L.; Hufstedler, E.; Whittle, H.J.; Nápoles, T.M.; Seligman, H.; Madsen, K.; Frongillo, E.A.; Weiser, S.D.; Palar, K. How food support improves mental health among people living with HIV: A qualitative study. *PLoS ONE* **2023**, *18*, e0282857. [CrossRef] [PubMed]
65. Ojo, T.; Ruan, C.; Hameed, T.; Malburg, C.; Thunga, S.; Smith, J.; Vieira, D.; Snyder, A.; Tampubolon, S.J.; Gyamfi, J.; et al. HIV, tuberculosis, and food insecurity in Africa—A syndemics-based scoping review. *Int. J. Environ. Res. Public Health* **2022**, *19*, 1101. [CrossRef]
66. Mash, R.J.; Schouw, D.; Daviaud, E.; Besada, D.; Roman, D. Evaluating the implementation of home delivery of medication by community health workers during the COVID-19 pandemic in Cape Town, South Africa: A convergent mixed methods study. *BMC Health Serv. Res.* **2022**, *22*, 98. [CrossRef]
67. Mugisha, J.; Abdulmalik, J.; Hanlon, C.; Petersen, I.; Lund, C.; Upadhaya, N.; Ahuja, S.; Shidhaye, R.; Mntambo, N.; Alem, A.; et al. Health systems context(s) for integrating mental health into primary health care in six Emerald countries: A situation analysis. *Int. J. Ment. Health Syst.* **2017**, *11*, 7. [CrossRef]
68. Mathias, K.; Bunkley, N.; Pillai, P.; Ae-Ngibise, K.A.; Kpobi, L.; Taylor, D.; Joag, K.; Rawat, M.; Hammoudeh, W.; Mitwalli, S.; et al. Inverting the deficit model in global mental health: An examination of strengths and assets of community mental health care in Ghana, India, Occupied Palestinian territories, and South Africa. *PLoS Glob. Public Health* **2024**, *4*, e0002575. [CrossRef]
69. Wolvaardt, G.; Johnson, S.; Cameron, D.; Botha, B.; Kornik, S. Challenges and constraints at district management level. In *South African Health Review 2013/14*; Padarath, A., English, R., Eds.; Health Systems Trust: Durban, South Africa, 2014; pp. 81–92.
70. Marais, D.L.; Petersen, I. Health system governance to support integrated mental health care in South Africa: Challenges and opportunities. *Int. J. Ment. Health Syst.* **2015**, *9*, 14. [CrossRef]
71. Chen, X.; Du, L.; Wu, R.; Xu, J.; Ji, H.; Zhang, Y.; Zhu, X.; Zhou, L. The effects of family, society and national policy support on treatment adherence among newly diagnosed tuberculosis patients: A cross-sectional study. *BMC Infect. Dis.* **2020**, *20*, 623. [CrossRef]
72. Nabunya, P.; Bahar, O.S.; Chen, B.; Dvalishvili, D.; Damulira, C.; Ssewamala, F.M. The role of family factors in antiretroviral therapy (ART) adherence self-efficacy among HIV-infected adolescents in southern Uganda. *BMC Public Health* **2020**, *20*, 340. [CrossRef]
73. Dhaliwal, J.S.; Chan, L.G.; Goh, J.C.B.; Koh, K.H.E.; Wong, C.S. Mental health and implications for antiretroviral adherence in a multiethnic Asian cohort. *Sex. Transm. Infect.* **2022**, *98*, 497–502. [CrossRef] [PubMed]
74. Levy, N. Taking responsibility for responsibility. *Public Health Ethics* **2019**, *12*, 103–113. [CrossRef] [PubMed]
75. Madlala, D.; Joubert, P.M.; Masenge, A. Community mental health literacy in Tshwane region 1: A quantitative study. *S. Afr. J. Psychiatry* **2022**, *28*, a1661. [CrossRef]

76. World Health Organization. Health Literacy. Available online: https://www.who.int/news-room/fact-sheets/detail/health-literacy (accessed on 5 August 2024).
77. Wiedermann, C.J.; Barbieri, V.; Plagg, B.; Marino, P.; Piccoliori, G.; Engl, A. Fortifying the foundations: A comprehensive approach to enhancing mental health support in educational policies amidst crises. *Healthcare* **2023**, *11*, 1423. [CrossRef] [PubMed]
78. Deribew, A.; Tesfaye, M.; Hailmichael, Y.; Negussu, N.; Daba, S.; Wogi, A.; Belachew, T.; Apers, L.; Colebunders, R. Tuberculosis and HIV co-infection: Its impact on quality of life. *Health Qual. Life Outcomes* **2009**, *7*, 105. [CrossRef]
79. Audet, C.M.; Ngobeni, S.; Graves, E.; Wagner, R.G. Mixed methods inquiry into traditional healers' treatment of mental, neurological and substance abuse disorders in rural South Africa. *PLoS ONE* **2017**, *12*, e0188433. [CrossRef]
80. Van Rooyen, D.; Pretorius, B.; Tembani, N.M.; ten Ham, W. Allopathic and traditional health practitioners' collaboration. *Curationis* **2015**, *38*, 1495. [CrossRef]
81. Campbell-Hall, V.; Petersen, I.; Bhana, A.; Mjadu, S.; Hosegood, V.; Flisher, A.J.; MHaPP Research Programme Consortium. Collaboration between traditional practitioners and primary health care staff in South Africa: Developing a workable partnership for community mental health services. *Transcult. Psychiatry* **2010**, *47*, 610–662. [CrossRef]

International Journal of
*Environmental Research
and Public Health*

MDPI

Review

Digital Health Technologies for Diabetic Foot Ulcers: A Systematic Review of Clinical Evidence, Access Inequities, and Public Health Integration

Tatiana Cristina Dias de Oliveira [1], Alana Ferreira de Oliveira [1], Laila de Castro Araújo [1], Maria Pantoja Moreira de Sena [2], Valéria de Castro Fagundes [3], Phelipe Augusto Rabelo Paixão [1], Stefani Gisele Bastos Dornas [1], Clarisse Andrade Sales [4], Ana Paula Simões Castro [4], Patricia Alves de Mendonça Cavalcante [4] and Luann Wendel Pereira de Sena [1,4,*]

[1] Graduate Program in Family Health, Federal University of the South and Southeast of Pará, Maraba 68507-590, Brazil
[2] Postgraduate Program in Tropical Diseases, Federal University of Pará, Belem 66075-110, Brazil
[3] Faculty of Medical Sciences of Pará, Para 38405-320, Brazil
[4] Postgraduate Program in Biodiversity and Biotechnology, Federal University of the South and Southeast of Pará, Maraba 68507-590, Brazil
* Correspondence: luannsena@unifesspa.edu.br; Tel.: +55-91981177718

Abstract

Diabetic foot ulcers are among the most severe complications of diabetes mellitus, disproportionately affecting populations in low- and middle-income countries. Digital health technologies have emerged as promising tools for prevention, diagnosis, and management; however, their effectiveness, usability, and applicability within public health systems remain insufficiently defined. This systematic review aimed to critically synthesize the clinical effectiveness, perceived usability, and methodological quality of digital interventions for the care of individuals with diabetes-related foot ulcers. A comprehensive search was performed in PubMed, Scopus, Web of Science, Embase, and Google Scholar for studies published between 2012 and 2024. Eighteen studies met the inclusion criteria, encompassing mobile health applications, wearable sensor devices, artificial intelligence-based tools, and telehealth platforms. Methodological quality was assessed using the Mixed Methods Appraisal Tool. Artificial intelligence-driven approaches demonstrated high diagnostic accuracy, with sensitivity and specificity above 90% for ulcer detection and classification. Mobile applications showed positive effects on self-efficacy, glycemic control, and adherence to preventive foot care, while usability scores were consistently high. Wearable sensor devices demonstrated potential for reducing ulcer recurrence, though supporting evidence remains limited. Across studies, recurrent methodological limitations included small sample sizes, absence of control groups, lack of economic evaluations, and barriers related to digital literacy and interoperability between systems. Most investigations were conducted in high-income countries, with limited consideration of public health contexts such as the Brazilian Unified Health System. In conclusion, digital health technologies show promise in improving the care of individuals with diabetes-related foot complications but face significant challenges regarding scalability, equity of access, and integration into public healthcare systems. Future research should prioritize context-adapted designs, robust clinical trials, and economic evaluations to inform health policies and support the rational adoption of these tools within universal health coverage frameworks. PROSPERO registration number: CRD420251023152.

Keywords: diabetic foot; health technology; mobile health applications; digital health

1. Introduction

Diabetic foot ulcers (DFU) are among the most severe and recurrent complications of diabetes mellitus, affecting 15–25% of patients during their lifetime [1]. They account for up to 85% of non-traumatic lower-limb amputations and are closely linked to functional decline, increased mortality, and substantial economic burden, particularly in low- and middle-income countries (LMICs) [2,3].

Despite advances in management—including surgical debridement, advanced wound dressings, and intensive glycemic control—recurrence rates remain high, with nearly 40% of patients experiencing a new ulcer within one year of initial healing [4]. In health systems with limited infrastructure and workforce shortages, such as those in parts of Latin America, these challenges are compounded by barriers to early diagnosis, continuity of care, and patient education.

In response, digital health technologies have gained prominence in clinical practice. These include mobile applications for self-care, wearable sensors for early detection of plantar changes, artificial intelligence (AI)-driven systems for automated triage, and telehealth platforms for remote monitoring [5–7]. When effectively implemented, such tools can expand access to healthcare, reduce hospitalizations, and strengthen disease surveillance in both urban and rural populations.

However, the literature demonstrates marked heterogeneity in the technologies evaluated, the outcomes measured, and the methodological quality of studies [8,9]. Moreover, most innovations are developed in high-income countries (HICs) and often fail to address structural barriers typical of public health systems, including low digital literacy, poor internet connectivity, fragmented electronic health records, and limited regulatory frameworks for digital innovation.

Thus, beyond clinical efficacy, it is essential to examine how digital interventions interact with public health governance, resource allocation, and equity of access—particularly within universal health systems such as the Brazilian Unified Health System (SUS). As digital health strategies become central to chronic disease management, their implementation must be critically appraised in terms of system capacity, workforce readiness, and the ethical implications of technological exclusion.

Against this backdrop, the present systematic review critically synthesizes current evidence on digital health technologies for the prevention, monitoring, and treatment of DFU. The review emphasizes clinical effectiveness, usability, and methodological rigor, while also addressing broader implications for access, equity, and health system integration in resource-constrained contexts.

2. Methods

This systematic review was conducted in accordance with the Preferred Reporting Items for Systematic Reviews and Meta-Analyses (PRISMA 2020) guidelines. The protocol was prospectively registered in the PROSPERO database (CRD420251023152). All methodological steps were performed independently by two trained reviewers to ensure transparency, reproducibility, and methodological rigor. Discrepancies were resolved by consensus with a third reviewer [10].

2.1. Data Sources and Search Strategy

A comprehensive literature search was conducted in PubMed/MEDLINE, Scopus, and Web of Science. The search covered studies published between 1 January 2012, and

15 April 2025, reflecting a 13-year period of rapid expansion in digital health technologies applied to diabetic foot care.

The search strategy combined controlled vocabulary (Medical Subject Headings [MeSH] and Health Sciences Descriptors [DeCS]) with free-text terms, organized into three domains: (i) clinical condition ("diabetes mellitus," "diabetic foot," "foot ulcer"); (ii) digital technologies ("mobile applications," "electronic health," "mobile health," "artificial intelligence," "wearable sensors"); and (iii) intervention functionalities ("self-care," "health education," "remote monitoring," "psychometric validation"). Boolean operators ("AND," "OR") were used to combine terms, and the syntax was adapted to each database. The complete search strategy is provided in Supplementary Material File S1.

Gray literature was also screened through Google Scholar, restricted to the first 60 results ranked by relevance. Reference lists of included articles were manually examined to identify additional eligible studies, and the ClinicalTrials.gov registry was consulted. Non-peer-reviewed documents (e.g., preprints, patents, dissertations, and technical reports) were excluded.

2.2. Eligibility Criteria

This review included empirical studies with human participants diagnosed with type 1 or type 2 diabetes mellitus, evaluating digital health technologies for the prevention, detection, monitoring, education, or remote support of plantar foot ulcers. Eligible interventions comprised mobile health applications, wearable sensors, artificial intelligence (AI)-based systems, digital platforms, and clinical decision-support tools.

Studies were required to report at least one clinical outcome (e.g., ulcer incidence or recurrence, wound-healing time, glycemic control) or one psychometric outcome (e.g., usability, self-efficacy, adherence to foot care, technology acceptance). Only articles published between January 2012 and April 2025 were considered.

Exclusion criteria included publications not in English, Portuguese, or Spanish; literature reviews, editorials, letters, or conference abstracts; studies using animal models or computer simulations without clinical validation; and studies lacking measurable clinical or psychometric outcomes.

2.3. Study Selection

The study selection followed three sequential steps: (i) removal of duplicates, (ii) screening of titles and abstracts, and (iii) full-text assessment. The Rayyan QCRI platform was used to enable blinded screening and decision tracking [11]. Two independent reviewers (T.C.D.d.O. and A.F.d.O.) performed the selection, achieving a Cohen's kappa coefficient of 0.84, which indicates substantial agreement. Discrepancies were resolved by a third reviewer (L.W.P.d.S.). When full texts were unavailable, corresponding authors were contacted via institutional email or through the ResearchGate platform.

2.4. Data Extraction

Data extraction was conducted using a structured Microsoft Excel® spreadsheet, pilot-tested on five randomly selected studies. Two reviewers (T.C.D.d.O. and A.F.d.O.) independently extracted the data, and discrepancies were resolved through discussion with a third reviewer (L.W.P.d.S.).

Extracted variables included study identification (first author, year), country of origin, study design, sample characteristics, type of digital technology, clinical and operational outcomes, psychometric instruments, and main findings.

2.5. Methodological Quality Assessment

The methodological quality of included studies was assessed using tools appropriate to each study design. Randomized controlled trials were evaluated with the Cochrane Risk of Bias 2.0 (RoB 2.0), which covers randomization, deviations from intended interventions, missing data, outcome measurement, and reporting bias. Non-randomized studies were assessed with the Risk Of Bias In Non-randomized Studies of Interventions (ROBINS-I), which examines seven domains including confounding, participant selection, and selective reporting.

Observational studies were appraised using the Newcastle–Ottawa Scale (NOS), covering selection, comparability, and outcome assessment. For studies involving technological development, psychometric validation, or qualitative methods, checklists from the Joanna Briggs Institute (JBI) were applied. Psychometric studies were further evaluated for content validity, internal consistency (e.g., Cronbach's alpha ≥ 0.80), and statistical robustness.

Reporting guidelines—including the Consolidated Standards of Reporting Trials (CONSORT), Strengthening the Reporting of Observational Studies in Epidemiology (STROBE), and Quality Assessment of Diagnostic Accuracy Studies (QUADAS)—were also used to support methodological appraisal.

All assessments were independently conducted by two reviewers (A.F.d.O. and L.W.P.d.S.) following prior calibration on a pilot set of studies. Discrepancies were resolved by consensus. Risk of bias was classified as high when two or more domains showed "critical risk," moderate when one critical or multiple concerns were identified, and low otherwise.

2.6. Data Synthesis

Given the heterogeneity in study design, population characteristics, technologies evaluated, and outcomes measured, a meta-analysis was not feasible. Instead, a narrative and systematic synthesis was performed in accordance with the Synthesis Without Meta-analysis (SWiM) framework.

To enable structured comparison, studies were grouped by primary type of digital technology: (i) mobile health applications and platforms, (ii) artificial intelligence (AI)-based algorithms and computer vision systems, (iii) wearable sensors and embedded medical devices, and (iv) integrated platforms or clinical decision-support systems. Within each category, outcomes were classified into three domains: clinical outcomes (e.g., ulcer healing, recurrence, glycemic control [HbA1c]); operational outcomes (e.g., treatment adherence, frequency of use, user engagement); and psychometric outcomes (e.g., usability, self-efficacy, perceived usefulness, satisfaction).

Two reviewers independently analyzed and interpreted the findings, with discrepancies resolved through discussion. Summary tables were developed to facilitate cross-category comparisons. Although statistical pooling of effect sizes was not possible, consistent patterns were identified and critically examined, including limitations in external validity and implications for public health policy and digital equity.

3. Results

3.1. Search Results

The systematic search of PubMed, Scopus, and Web of Science initially identified 95 records. After duplicate removal, 49 unique studies remained. Title and abstract screening excluded 46 records that did not meet the predefined eligibility criteria. The full texts of the remaining 45 studies were then assessed for eligibility, of which 27 were excluded due to lack of clinical or psychometric outcomes, ineligible populations, use of non-digital technologies, or incompatible study designs.

In total, 18 studies met all inclusion criteria and were retained for this systematic review [2,12–28]. The selection process, conducted in accordance with the Preferred Reporting Items for Systematic Reviews and Meta-Analyses (PRISMA 2020) guidelines, is illustrated in Figure 1.

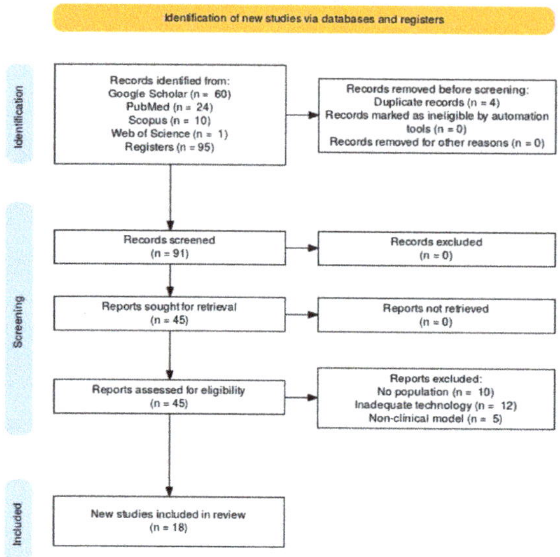

Figure 1. Study selection flowchart through literature search.

3.2. Characteristics of the Included Studies

The included populations varied considerably in sample size, age distribution, and clinical complexity. Samples ranged from healthy young adults, primarily recruited for device validation, to individuals with diabetes mellitus presenting with recurrent plantar ulcers, peripheral neuropathy, prior lower-limb amputations, and multiple cardiovascular or metabolic comorbidities. Most studies included middle-aged or elderly participants, reflecting the demographic profile most affected by DFU. Several also reported concomitant medication use, particularly antidiabetic agents (insulin, oral hypoglycemic drugs), cardiovascular therapies (antihypertensives, statins, antiplatelet agents), and treatments for neuropathic pain, all of which may influence ulcer healing, recurrence risk, and adherence to digital interventions.

Sample sizes ranged from single-patient case reports to large image datasets used for computational model training and validation. The digital technologies evaluated were categorized into four groups: (i) mobile health applications and platforms (e.g., INTELLIN®, MyFootCare, Minuteful, CARPeDia, Swift Medical Connect); (ii) artificial intelligence (AI) algorithms and computer vision systems (e.g., Faster Region-Based Convolutional Neural Network [R-CNN], Support Vector Machine [SVM], DenseNet, Mask R-CNN, Region-Based Fully Convolutional Network); (iii) wearable sensors and embedded devices, including smart insoles (Orpyx®), sensorized boots with inertial measurement units, and plantar thermometry systems (TempStat™); and (iv) clinical decision-support systems, often integrated with electronic medical records and used in outpatient care.

Each category presented distinct strengths and limitations. Mobile applications were widely accessible and user-friendly, improving self-management and adherence, but their effectiveness depended on sustained engagement and digital literacy. AI-based systems achieved the highest technical performance, often surpassing 90% accuracy for ulcer detection and classification, though their generalizability was constrained by small datasets and lack of external validation. Wearable sensors enabled continuous monitoring of plantar pressure and temperature, supporting early detection of recurrence risk, but faced challenges of cost, usability, and long-term adherence. Clinical decision-support systems enhanced professional decision-making when integrated with electronic records, although their direct impact on outcomes remained less validated and depended on interoperability and infrastructure. No single technology emerged as universally superior; instead, complementary or hybrid approaches may offer the most comprehensive solutions for DFU care.

Outcomes were classified into four domains: (i) clinical (ulcer recurrence, progression, new ulcer incidence); (ii) technical (accuracy, sensitivity, specificity, intersection over union [IoU], mean average precision [mAP]); (iii) operational (treatment adherence, user engagement, frequency of image transmission, interaction time); and (iv) psychometric (usability, satisfaction, perceived value).

Of the 18 studies included, 7 employed validated psychometric instruments, such as the System Usability Scale (SUS), EuroQol five-dimension instrument (EQ-5D), Technology Acceptance Model (TAM), self-efficacy scales (Cronbach's alpha ≥ 0.82), and adapted tools including the National Patient Survey and the OPUS scale [2,12,17,20,23,25,27]. The remaining 11 relied on non-standardized qualitative analyses, ad hoc questionnaires, or lacked structured psychometric assessment, limiting comparability and reproducibility [13–16,18,19,21,22,24,26,28].

AI-based approaches demonstrated high technical performance, with accuracy above 90% for ulcer detection and classification, comparable to experienced clinical evaluators [16,29]. Nonetheless, most studies used small datasets under controlled conditions, limiting external validity. Performance may vary in real-world clinical environments, where image quality, population heterogeneity, and workflow integration are critical. Large-scale, multicenter validation is therefore required before clinical adoption.

Mobile health applications targeting education and self-care were associated with improved self-efficacy, adherence, and glycemic control, including significant reductions in glycated hemoglobin (HbA1c) [23]. Plantar sensor technologies proved effective for early detection of pressure and temperature changes, enabling timely interventions such as offloading and footwear adjustments [14,25]. However, long-term adherence was inconsistent, influenced by comfort, device durability, and daily usability. Most studies also involved small samples and short follow-up, limiting evidence strength. Still, plantar sensors hold promise as cost-effective adjuncts to clinical monitoring in high-risk populations.

Key methodological limitations included socioeconomic barriers (restricted access to mobile devices, poor connectivity), low digital literacy, technical failures in system interoperability, and small sample sizes that undermined statistical power and generalizability [8,23,30–34].

Table 1 presents a summary of the key methodological characteristics and empirical findings of the studies included in this systematic review.

Table 1. Characteristics of the included studies.

Authors/Year	Study Location	Study Design	Population	Technology Used	Outcomes Assessed	Psychometric Instruments	Main Findings
Hazenberg et al./2012 [12]	Netherlands and Germany	Prospective feasibility study with four-month home follow-up	22 patients with DM1 or DM2, peripheral neuropathy and plantar deformities; mean age 60 years	The Portable Foot Imaging Device (PFID) provides high-resolution plantar imaging with automatic data transmission via modem.	Technical feasibility, clinical utility of images, quality of life and usability	EQ-5D, VAS (0–10) for usability	High lesion detection rate; usability VAS 7–9; slight improvement in EQ-5D; use <6 min
Wang et al./2015 [13]	USA	Methodological study with experimental evaluation of system	30 simulated and 34 real wounds in patients with DM2	Android app with optical box, automatic segmentation via Mean-Shift and K-means (GPU acceleration)	Segmentation accuracy, RYB classification, processing time	Validation by three experts, MCC index	Satisfactory segmentation (MCC = 0.736); average time of 15s per image; viable for near real-time use
Lazo-Porras et al./2016 [14]	Lima, Peru	Randomized, controlled clinical trial, with blinding of the evaluator (protocol)	Adults (18–80 years) with T2DM, risk 2 or 3 (IWGDF), pedal pulse present, with cell phone and consent	TempStat™ (plantar thermometry) + SMS/audio sending with self-care guidance	Primary: 12-month ulcer incidence; Secondary: TempStat™ adherence, engagement, and thermal response	Not applicable	Not applicable (study protocol)
Wang et al./2017 [15]	USA	Technological development and initial validation (computer system)	Real clinical images of ulcers captured via smartphone (number of patients not specified)	ML system: superpixels (SLIC), color descriptors, texture, DSIFT-BoW, and two-stage SVM	Accuracy in ulcer segmentation, feasibility on smartphones for remote monitoring	Not applicable	High accuracy in automated detection; feasibility on mobile devices; reduction in false positives/negatives

Table 1. *Cont.*

Authors/Year	Study Location	Study Design	Population	Technology Used	Outcomes Assessed	Psychometric Instruments	Main Findings
Goyal et al./2019 [16]	United Kingdom	Methodological study of development and validation of predictive models with deep learning	1775 images of feet with ulcers and 105 healthy ones	Faster R-CNN (InceptionV2), SSD (InceptionV2/MobileNet), R-FCN (ResNet101) with transfer learning	Accuracy, speed and IoU for real-time DFU detection	Not applicable	Faster R-CNN InceptionV2: mAP 91.8%, IoU 95.5%, 48 ms/img; SSD-MobileNet: 30 ms, mAP 83.6%; 80% accuracy via Jetson TX2/Android
Wijesinghe et al./2019 [17]	Sri Lanka	Development and evaluation of prototype with technical validation and usability	5 experts and 10 participants	Prototype consisting of a smartphone-based application (IDA app) integrated with a cloud telehealth platform, combined with deep learning algorithms (DenseNet-201, ResNet-18, VGG-16) and Mask R-CNN for image analysis; hardware included smartphone camera and data transmission modules	Accuracy in DR and DFU classification, segmentation, image retrieval, usability	System Usability Scale (SUS)	Accuracy >98% (DR), >97% (DFU); mAP >87% (segmentation), >99% (retrieval DR); SUS 88.5; better than 5 clinical
Zoppo et al./2020 [18]	Italy	Prospective, observational, comparative, non-randomized and monocentric clinical study	150 patients with chronic wounds (vascular, DFU and pressure)	Wound Viewer: AI with IR sensors, CMOS camera, LEDs, DT-CNN algorithm; AWS integration with GDPR/HIPAA	Area, depth, volume, WBP, tissue segmentation, diagnostic accuracy and comparison with other methods	Falanga WBP; confusion matrix; Kruskal–Wallis and Kolmogorov–Smirnov tests	97% bedside accuracy; measurements equivalent to conventional measurements ($p = 0.9$); error <14%; necrosis detected ≥7.3%; safe and non-invasive remote monitoring

Table 1. *Cont.*

Authors/Year	Study Location	Study Design	Population	Technology Used	Outcomes Assessed	Psychometric Instruments	Main Findings
Kong et al./2021 [19]	Canada	Clinical case study (case report)	Man, 57 years old, DM1, chronic ulcer, osteomyelitis, multiple comorbidities (CAD, CKD, PAD, previous amputation)	Swift Medical App—Patient Connect (Computer Vision, Calibrated Images, Encrypted Data, HIPAA/FDA Compliant)	Primary: wound evolution; Secondary: adherence, reduced consultations, cost/time, self-care, infection management	Not applicable	Images sent increased (2→39); effective control of 3 infections; reduction in time (~3 h) and cost (~US$50/visit); patient reported platform as educational and empowering
Bahaadinbeigy et al./2022 [20]	Iran	Methodological study in four phases (development and evaluation)	15 experts (Delphi) and 4 healthcare professionals (usability)	Telemedicine system in ASP with SQL database and SSL security protocol	Information needs, system usability, user satisfaction	Validated questionnaire (α = 0.952) + satisfaction questionnaire by experts	System with 75 essential items (registration, prescription, communication); 26 usability problems identified
Haycocks et al./2022 [21]	United Kingdom	Prospective feasibility study, mixed approach	15 patients with DM and healed diabetic foot ulcer	INTELLIN® (mHealth) app with monitoring, engagement and Markov model for cost–utility	Ulcer recurrence, SINBAD score, self-reference, usability, cost-effectiveness	Qualitative collection without validated instruments	53% with relapse (mean 273 days), mean SINBAD 2.1, no self-referral, high usability, ICER £20,000/QALY with ≥5% reduction in relapse, socioeconomic barriers limited adherence
Cassidy et al./2023 [22]	United Kingdom and New Zealand	Multicenter, prospective, observational, clinical proof-of-concept study	81 patients with diabetes; 203 images (162 with ulcer, 41 without)	Low-cost smartphone-embedded AI for automated ulcer detection	Sensitivity, specificity, reliability ($K\alpha$)	Krippendorff's Kappa ($K\alpha > 0.80$) for AI agreement vs. human raters	Sensitivity 91.6%, specificity 92.4%, high $K\alpha$; performance comparable to clinical; feasibility of automated remote monitoring

Table 1. *Cont.*

Authors/Year	Study Location	Study Design	Population	Technology Used	Outcomes Assessed	Psychometric Instruments	Main Findings
Chen et al./2023 [23]	Taiwan	single-blind clinical trial	100 elderly people with DM2 (average age 67.6 years); 50 control and 50 intervention	Digital self-care program based on Self-Efficacy Theory with videos, games, LINE messages and calls	Self-efficacy, foot self-care, HbA1c	Self-Efficacy Scale (α = 0.82) and Self-Care Scale (α = 0.92), Chinese version	Significant improvement in intervention: self-efficacy (24.96→76.56), self-care (8.08→32.36), HbA1c reduction by 0.41% ($p < 0.001$); control with less improvement
Ferreira et al./2023 [2]	Brazil	Methodological study with development and validation of neural network and application	250 for training/validation and 141 for testing; all with DM in the APS of Minas Gerais	MLP neural network integrated into the CARPeDia app (JavaScript); 10 × 10 × 2 architecture	Accuracy, sensitivity, specificity, PPV, NPV; usability (SUS)	Cross-validation (10-fold), Friedman test, Dunn–Bonferroni; SUS (93.3/100)	Accuracy 85%, sensitivity 84%, specificity 89%; high usability; parsimonious and applicable model with customized report generation
Keegan et al./2023 [24]	Baltimore, USA	Prospective, quantitative pilot study with technological intervention (8 weeks)	25 patients with DFU and history of revascularization/podiatry; mean age 65.5 years; 60% men; 52% black	Healthy.io Minuteful app, a smartphone-based wound imaging system using calibration markers for standardized images, automatic cloud upload, and AI-driven analysis providing wound size/healing progression reports; enabled remote monitoring and patient self-scanning	Engagement, satisfaction, therapeutic approach, wound reduction, healing, failures and technical support	Non-validated instrument (Likert + open questions developed by the team)	84% adhered to ≥1 scan, 20% completed all; 36% had adjusted conduct; mean wound reduction 41.6% (p = 0.005); 12% healed; 94.1% approved; technical and socioeconomic barriers

Table 1. *Cont.*

Authors/Year	Study Location	Study Design	Population	Technology Used	Outcomes Assessed	Psychometric Instruments	Main Findings
Park et al./2023 [25]	Texas, USA	Experimental study of technological validation (pilot)	14 healthy adults (mean age 31.6 ± 8.7 years; 64% women)	Orthopedic boot with IMU sensors, smartwatch, cloud-based clinical dashboard, wearable sensors for balance/gait	Adherence to use, postural stability (COM sway), step count, usability and acceptance	Adapted TAM questionnaire (5-point Likert, Q1–Q9)	Grip accuracy: 89.3%; improved stability ($p < 0.05$); step counting errors: 4.4% (slow), 36.2% (normal), 16% (fast); high acceptance, except aesthetics
Ploderer et al./2023 [26]	Australia	Prospective mixed methods study (predominantly qualitative), 3 months	12 patients with plantar ulcers (DM1/DM2), caregivers, access to Android smartphone	MyFootCare App (Android) with OpenCV and watershed algorithm for photo segmentation	Perception of value, engagement, barriers/facilitators to use and applicability	No validated psychometric scales applied; evaluation based on qualitative interviews and ad hoc Likert ratings (1–10) at weeks 0, 3, and 12	App perceived as useful; usage varied; facilitators: familiarity and support; barriers: usability, low digital literacy, limited image accuracy
Hellstrand et al./2024 [27]	Sweden	Randomized, patient-blinded, two-arm parallel clinical trial	100 patients with DM (47 intervention, 53 control; mean 66 ± 13 years), 2 evaluators (ort/prot)	CDSS for foot examination compared to traditional clinical examination	Patient satisfaction, professional experience, clinical interaction	National Patient Survey (modified) and OPUS	High satisfaction in both; OPUS without difference ($p = 0.78$); good usability; preserved professional-patient interaction
Matijevich et al./2024 [28]	USA	Prospective cohort study with illustrative case series	3 patients with T2DM, peripheral neuropathy, history of ulcers; ages 49–75; 2 with amputations	Orpyx®: sensory insoles with pressure, temperature and IMU sensors, with biofeedback via app	Plantar pressure, thermal variation, pre-ulcerative lesions, engagement and need for intervention	Adherence estimated by usage time, tracked steps, inactivity alerts, and interactions via RPM	No new ulcers in 8 months; pressure guided adjustments; temperature alone was insensitive; combined approach reinforced prevention and avoided recurrence

3.3. Quality Assessment

Among the randomized clinical trials (n = 3), Chen et al. [23] and Hellstrand Tang et al. [27] reported adequate randomization and partial blinding, minimizing potential performance bias. Only Chen et al. [23] explicitly described the use of intention-to-treat analysis. The protocol by Lazo-Porras et al. [14] was considered eligible; however, as no outcome data were available, a full methodological appraisal was not possible.

For studies focused on the development and validation of digital technologies (n = 9), quality appraisal considered detailed reporting of system architectures, use of cross-validation techniques (e.g., k-fold, external validation), and robust performance metrics such as accuracy, sensitivity, specificity, intersection over union (IoU), and mean average precision (mAP) [2,13,15–18,22,24,25]. Six studies applied either cross-validation or external testing, while three provided comprehensive descriptions of modeling strategies. Notably, Goyal et al. [16] and Ferreira et al. [2] explicitly acknowledged algorithmic limitations, enhancing transparency and reproducibility in computational analyses.

Studies evaluating wearable sensors or embedded medical devices (n = 4) [18,19,25,28] emphasized in-field clinical validation, use of objective indicators of user engagement (e.g., duration of use, number of alerts generated), and integration with mobile platforms or electronic health records. Park et al. [25] and Matijevich et al. [28] reported the most rigorous protocols in this category, although heterogeneity in engagement metrics limited direct comparability.

In usability and perception studies (n = 6) [2,12,17,23,25,27], validated psychometric instruments were frequently applied, including the System Usability Scale (SUS), Technology Acceptance Model (TAM), EuroQol five-dimension instrument (EQ-5D), and adapted tools such as the National Patient Survey and the OPUS scale. Mean scores consistently exceeded 80, indicating high acceptability. In contrast, two studies relied solely on non-standardized qualitative methods or ad hoc questionnaires and were thus classified as presenting a moderate risk of descriptive bias [19,26].

One study (n = 1), Haycocks et al. [21], employed a mixed-methods design that combined quantitative outcomes (e.g., SINBAD score, cost–utility analysis using Markov modeling) with qualitative usability evaluation. However, the absence of validated psychometric instruments and a formal methodological framework for qualitative analysis led to classification as moderate risk.

Overall, studies were stratified into three levels of bias risk: (i) low risk, assigned to 13 investigations with robust design, validated outcome measures, and well-defined populations (e.g., Chen et al. [23], Ferreira et al. [2], Zoppo et al. [18]); (ii) moderate risk, assigned to four studies with limitations such as small sample sizes, absence of control groups, or reliance on unvalidated instruments (e.g., Ploderer et al. [19], Kong et al. [24], Keegan et al. [26], Haycocks et al. [21]); and (iii) high or undefined risk, attributed to the protocol by Lazo-Porras et al. [14] and to studies that did not adequately report psychometric assessment strategies.

Table 2 provides a structured synthesis of methodological validation, use of psychometric instruments, and risk-of-bias assessment across all included studies, complementing the narrative description and facilitating rapid cross-study comparison.

Table 2. Sintese Quality assessment.

Study	Type of Study	Methodological Validation	Use of Psychometric Instruments	Bias Assessment
Hazenberg et al., 2012 [12]	Feasibility study with sensors	EQ-5D, time of use, practical evaluation	EQ-5D; VAS	Low

Table 2. *Cont.*

Study	Type of Study	Methodological Validation	Use of Psychometric Instruments	Bias Assessment
Wang et al., 2015 [13]	Algorithm with optical box	MCC; expert testing	Not applicable	Low
Lazo-Porras et al., 2016 [14]	Clinical trial protocol	Protocol without final data	Not applicable	High/Undefined
Wang et al., 2017 [15]	Automated segmentation system	High accuracy; technical validation	Not applicable	Low
Goyal et al., 2019 [16]	Deep learning with external validation	Detailed architecture and mAP/IoU	Not applicable	Low
Wijesinghe et al., 2019 [17]	AI-powered telehealth	mAP, classification superior to clinical	SUS	Low
Zoppo et al., 2020 [18]	Comparative clinical study	Comparison with gold standards	WBP, robust statistical analysis	Low
Kong et al., 2021 [19]	Clinical case report	Narrative drawing	Not applicable	Moderate
Bahaadinbeigy et al., 2022 [20]	Telemedicine system (Delphi)	4-phase assessment; validated questionnaire	Cronbach's alpha = 0.952	Low
Haycocks et al., 2022 [21]	Feasibility study with mixed approach	SINBAD score, absence of self-reference, economic analysis with Markov model	Non-standardized qualitative analysis	Moderate
Cassidy et al., 2023 [22]	Computer Vision and AI	Kappa, sensitivity, specificity	Kα (Krippendorff)	Low
Chen et al., 2023 [23]	Randomized clinical trial	Randomization and partial blinding; ITT mentioned	SUS and validated scales	Low
Ferreira et al., 2023 [2]	Technological validation with RNAs	Cross-validation and statistical testing	SUS	Low
Keegan et al., 2023 [24]	Pilot study of digital intervention	Clinical and operational results	Questionnaire not validated	Moderate
Park et al., 2023 [25]	Technological validation with sensors	Accuracy, engagement, technical validation	Adapted TAM	Low
Ploderer et al., 2023 [26]	Qualitative study with app	Thematic analysis without structured method	Likert 1–10; no validated scale	Moderate
Hellstrand et al., 2024 [27]	Randomized clinical trial	Randomization and partial blinding	OPUS; Modified national scale	Low
Matijevich et al., 2024 [28]	Prospective cohort with sensors	Continuous collection, engagement, adherence	Adherence via objective data	Low

4. Discussion

To our knowledge, this is the first systematic review to comprehensively synthesize evidence on digital health technologies applied to the prevention, detection, and management of diabetic foot ulcers (DFU). The findings indicate that mobile applications, wearable sensors, artificial intelligence (AI)-based algorithms, and integrated platforms hold considerable potential to enhance diagnostic accuracy, promote patient engagement, and enable remote lesion monitoring across diverse care settings.

AI-based interventions emerged as the most technically advanced. Studies employing convolutional neural networks (CNNs)—including Faster R-CNN, Mask R-CNN—and DenseNet architectures reported sensitivity and specificity above 90%, approaching or surpassing the diagnostic performance of clinical specialists. Despite these promising results, most studies were limited by small datasets, absence of external validation, and scarce evidence of real-world implementation. Variability in image quality, device resolution, and workflow integration further constrained generalizability. Standardization of datasets and adherence to frameworks such as CONSORT-AI and STARD-AI are essential to strengthen reproducibility and reliability.

Mobile applications demonstrated improvements in self-care, treatment adherence, and glycemic control, particularly when grounded in behavioral models such as Bandura's Theory of Self-Efficacy. For example, Chen et al. [23] reported significant increases in self-efficacy scores and reductions in glycated hemoglobin among users of an educational platform. These tools are low-cost and accessible, making them attractive in public health contexts. However, their effectiveness depends heavily on sustained engagement and digital literacy. Socioeconomic inequalities, lack of device compatibility, and poor internet connectivity remain critical barriers, especially in low-resource and older populations. Gaps in digital literacy, rural connectivity, and affordability further reinforce inequities in access.

Sensor-based technologies, including smart insoles and thermal or pressure monitoring systems, provided continuous and objective detection of plantar load and temperature variations—risk factors strongly associated with ulcer recurrence. Studies such as Matijevich et al. [28] reported recurrence prevention benefits during longitudinal follow-up. Nonetheless, limited sample sizes, lack of control groups, non-standardized adherence measures, and issues of cost, comfort, and durability reduced scalability. Long-term adherence was frequently undermined by integration challenges with daily routines.

Emerging imaging modalities, such as infrared thermography and automated wound measurement, remain exploratory but show potential for broader integration. For instance, Wijesinghe et al. [16] developed an AI-powered telehealth prototype that combined retinal and DFU imaging, achieving >97% classification accuracy. Despite strong technical performance, these approaches remain underrepresented in the literature, warranting further validation in diverse clinical contexts.

Assessments of usability and user perception revealed substantial methodological heterogeneity. While some studies employed validated instruments such as the System Usability Scale (SUS), others relied on non-standardized questionnaires or qualitative assessments, limiting comparability. Haycocks et al. [21], for example, relied exclusively on non-validated self-reported data, while Ploderer et al. [26] applied Likert scales without psychometric validation. These weaknesses underscore the importance of employing culturally adapted and validated tools, particularly for low-literacy and digitally vulnerable populations.

Geographical disparities were also evident. Most studies originated from high-income countries (e.g., United States, United Kingdom, Canada), where research focused primarily on technical validation and usability under controlled conditions. In contrast, studies from low- and middle-income countries (LMICs), such as Brazil and Peru, emphasized barriers related to infrastructure, health equity, and system integration, particularly within universal health systems such as the Brazilian Unified Health System (SUS). These systems face persistent challenges, including the absence of standardized national digital health protocols, fragmented electronic infrastructures, and insufficient policy frameworks for innovation.

Another critical gap is the paucity of robust economic evaluations. Only a minority of studies assessed cost-effectiveness, cost–utility, or organizational impact in real-world settings. Such analyses are crucial for decision-makers in resource-constrained contexts, where evidence of economic value is essential to justify technology adoption and guide rational allocation of scarce resources. Without this, innovations risk remaining confined to pilot projects.

Comparative synthesis across technology categories suggests complementary strengths and limitations. Mobile applications are accessible but dependent on literacy and engagement. AI systems achieved the highest diagnostic accuracy (>90%) but require larger, more diverse datasets and multicenter validation. Wearable sensors provide continuous monitoring but face adherence, usability, and cost barriers. Imaging-based modalities remain exploratory but present opportunities for integration into hybrid digital ecosystems. No single technology emerged as universally superior; instead, hybrid or integrated strategies appear most promising for comprehensive, equitable, and sustainable DFU management.

Despite the enthusiasm surrounding digital health, this review identified significant methodological limitations. Few studies employed randomized controlled designs or intention-to-treat analyses, and statistical modeling was often limited. The wide variation in outcomes—spanning computational metrics (e.g., accuracy, sensitivity), clinical endpoints (e.g., recurrence, healing time), and psychometric measures (e.g., usability, self-efficacy)—precluded meta-analysis and hampered comparability. Furthermore, while age and medication use were frequently reported, few studies explored their influence on technology adoption, adherence, or clinical outcomes, representing critical gaps for future research.

Methodological quality appraisal indicated that most studies presented low or moderate risk of bias. Investigations with robust designs, validated outcomes, and well-defined populations (e.g., Chen et al. [23], Ferreira et al. [2], Zoppo et al. [18]) were classified as low risk. Conversely, studies with small samples, lack of control groups, or reliance on unvalidated instruments (e.g., Kong et al. [19], Ploderer et al. [26], Haycocks et al. [21]) were deemed moderate risk. The protocol by Lazo-Porras et al. [14] was considered high or undefined risk due to the absence of outcome data.

Among the strengths of this review are the comprehensiveness of the search strategy, critical appraisal stratified by technology type, outcome domain, and study design, and the use of validated tools for bias assessment across diverse methodological frameworks. Limitations include the exclusion of studies in non-Latin languages and heterogeneity in reporting standards, which limited comparability. Future reviews should adopt mixed-methods approaches and advanced synthesis frameworks such as SWiM (Synthesis Without Meta-analysis), supplemented by sensitivity analyses.

In summary, digital health technologies represent a transformative frontier in DFU management. Yet their integration into clinical practice requires more than technical validation: it demands investment in digital infrastructure, development of standardized protocols, establishment of regulatory frameworks, and robust economic and implementation studies. Only through such measures can these innovations be scaled equitably and sustainably within real-world health systems.

5. Conclusions

Digital health technologies for diabetic foot ulcer (DFU) care have shown promising results in both prevention and remote monitoring. Artificial intelligence (AI)–based tools achieved high diagnostic accuracy in detecting and segmenting foot ulcers, while mobile health applications—particularly those grounded in behavioral models—improved self-efficacy, self-care behaviors, and glycemic control. Wearable sensors integrated into digital platforms demonstrated potential for reducing ulcer recurrence among high-risk patients.

Nevertheless, significant gaps remain. Most studies were limited by small sample sizes, lack of control groups, absence of external validation for computational models, and reliance on non-standardized psychometric instruments. These methodological weaknesses reduce robustness and reproducibility, restricting safe translation into real-world clinical practice.

Future research should prioritize randomized controlled trials, long-term follow-up, and comprehensive economic evaluations. Importantly, digital interventions must be adapted to the structural and operational realities of public health systems, particularly in low- and middle-income countries (LMICs), where inequities and resource constraints are most pronounced. In this context, health authorities operating under universal health coverage models—such as the Brazilian Unified Health System (SUS)—should advance a strategic agenda for digital health integration. This includes investments in interoperable and scalable platforms integrated with health information systems, capacity-building initiatives to strengthen digital literacy and care coordination in primary care, and the development of regulatory frameworks and public policies that promote equitable access to digital tools for vulnerable populations.

Such measures are essential not only to foster technological innovation but also to ensure that digital health functions as a mechanism for inclusion, access, and quality care—rather than as an additional driver of exclusion—within health systems committed to universality, equity, and comprehensiveness.

Supplementary Materials: The following supporting information can be downloaded at: https://www.mdpi.com/article/10.3390/ijerph22091430/s1, File S1: Search criteria for articles in the databases.

Author Contributions: Conceptualization, T.C.D.d.O. and A.F.d.O.; methodology, L.d.C.A. and L.W.P.d.S.; validation, M.P.M.d.S. and L.W.P.d.S.; formal analysis, V.d.C.F. and C.A.S.; investigation, P.A.R.P. and A.P.S.C.; resources, L.W.P.d.S.; data curation, S.G.B.D.; writing—original draft preparation, L.W.P.d.S.; writing—review and editing, T.C.D.d.O.; visualization, M.P.M.d.S. and P.A.d.M.C.; supervision, L.W.P.d.S. All authors have read and agreed to the published version of the manuscript.

Funding: This research received no external funding.

Conflicts of Interest: The authors declare no conflicts of interest.

References

1. Lee, S.H.; Kim, S.H.; Kim, K.B.; Kim, H.S.; Lee, Y.K. Factors Influencing Wound Healing in Diabetic Foot Patients. *Medicina* **2024**, *60*, 723. [CrossRef] [PubMed]
2. Ferreira, A.C.B.H.; Ferreira, D.D.; Barbosa, B.H.G.; de Oliveira, U.A.; Padua, E.A.; Chiarini, F.O.; Lopes, M.H.B.d.M.; Premaor, M.O. Neural network-based method to stratify people at risk for developing diabetic foot: A support system for health professionals. *PLoS ONE* **2023**, *18*, e0288466. [CrossRef]
3. Armstrong, D.G.; Tan, T.W.; Boulton, A.J.M.; Bus, S.A. Diabetic Foot Ulcers: A Review. *JAMA* **2023**, *330*, 62–75. [CrossRef] [PubMed]
4. Armstrong, D.G.; Boulton, A.J.M.; Bus, S.A. Diabetic Foot Ulcers and Their Recurrence. *N. Engl. J. Med.* **2017**, *376*, 2367–2375. [CrossRef]
5. Lung, C.W.; Wu, F.L.; Liao, F.; Pu, F.; Fan, Y.; Jan, Y.K. Emerging technologies for the prevention and management of diabetic foot ulcers. *J. Tissue Viability* **2020**, *29*, 61–68. [CrossRef]
6. Rosa, C.; Marsch, L.A.; Winstanley, E.L.; Brunner, M.; Campbell, A.N.C. Using digital technologies in clinical trials: Current and future applications. *Contemp. Clin. Trials* **2021**, *100*, 106219. [CrossRef] [PubMed]

7. Kumar Pendyala, S. Real-Time Analytics and Clinical Decision Support Systems: Transforming Emergency Care [Internet]. Available online: www.ijfmr.com (accessed on 10 July 2025).
8. Deniz-Garcia, A.; Fabelo, H.; Rodriguez-Almeida, A.J.; Zamora-Zamorano, G.; Castro-Fernandez, M.; del Pino Alberiche Ruano, M.; Solvoll, T.; Granja, C.; Schopf, T.R.; Callico, G.M.; et al. Quality, Usability, and Effectiveness of mHealth Apps and the Role of Artificial Intelligence: Current Scenario and Challenges. *J. Med. Internet Res.* **2023**, *25*, e44030. [CrossRef]
9. Bastardo, R.; Pavão, J.; Rocha, N.P. Methodological Quality of User-Centered Usability Evaluation of Digital Applications to Promote Citizens' Engagement and Participation in Public Governance: A Systematic Literature Review. *Digital* **2024**, *4*, 740–761. [CrossRef]
10. Page, M.J.; McKenzie, J.E.; Bossuyt, P.M.; Boutron, I.; Hoffmann, T.C.; Mulrow, C.D.; Shamseer, L.; Tetzlaff, J.M.; Akl, E.A.; Brennan, S.E.; et al. The PRISMA 2020 statement: An updated guideline for reporting systematic reviews. *BMJ* **2021**, *372*, 71. [CrossRef]
11. Ouzzani, M.; Hammady, H.; Fedorowicz, Z.; Elmagarmid, A. Rayyan-a web and mobile app for systematic reviews. *Syst. Rev.* **2016**, *5*, 210. [CrossRef]
12. Hazenberg, C.E.V.B.; Bus, S.A.; Kottink, A.I.R.; Bouwmans, C.A.M.; Schönbach-Spraul, A.M.; van Baal, S.G. Telemedical home-monitoring of diabetic foot disease using photographic foot imaging—A feasibility study. *J. Telemed. Telecare* **2012**, *18*, 32–36. [CrossRef]
13. Wang, L.; Pedersen, P.C.; Strong, D.M.; Tulu, B.; Agu, E.; Ignotz, R. Smartphone-based wound assessment system for patients with diabetes. *IEEE Trans. Biomed. Eng.* **2015**, *62*, 477–488. [CrossRef]
14. Lazo-Porras, M.; Bernabe-Ortiz, A.; Sacksteder, K.A.; Gilman, R.H.; Malaga, G.; Armstrong, D.G.; Miranda, J.J. Implementation of foot thermometry plus mHealth to prevent diabetic foot ulcers: Study protocol for a randomized controlled trial. *Trials* **2016**, *17*, 206. [CrossRef] [PubMed]
15. Wang, L.; Pedersen, P.C.; Agu, E.; Strong, D.i.M.; Tulu, B. Area Determination of Diabetic Foot Ulcer Images Using a Cascaded Two-Stage SVM-Based Classification. *IEEE Trans. Biomed. Eng.* **2017**, *64*, 2098–2109. [CrossRef]
16. Goyal, M.; Reeves, N.D.; Rajbhandari, S.; Yap, M.H. Robust Methods for Real-Time Diabetic Foot Ulcer Detection and Localization on Mobile Devices. *IEEE J. Biomed. Health Inform.* **2019**, *23*, 1730–1741. [CrossRef]
17. Wijesinghe, I.; Gamage, C.; Perera, I.; Chitraranjan, C. A Smart Telemedicine System with Deep Learning to Manage Diabetic Retinopathy and Foot Ulcers. In *MERCon 2019—Proceedings, 5th International Multidisciplinary Moratuwa Engineering Research Conference*; Institute of Electrical and Electronics Engineers Inc.: New York, NY, USA, 2019; pp. 686–691.
18. Zoppo, G.; Marrone, F.; Pittarello, M.; Farina, M.; Uberti, A.; Demarchi, D.; Secco, J.; Corinto, F.; Ricci, E. AI technology for remote clinical assessment and monitoring. *J. Wound Care* **2020**, *29*, 692–706. [CrossRef]
19. Kong, L.Y.; Ramirez-Garcialuna, J.L.; Fraser, R.D.J.; Wang, S.C. A 57-year-old man with type 1 diabetes mellitus and a chronic foot ulcer successfully managed with a remote patient-facing wound care smartphone application. *Am. J. Case Rep.* **2021**, *22*, e933879-1–e933879-7. [CrossRef]
20. Bahaadinbeigy, K.; Sheikhtaheri, A.; Fatehi, F.; Moulaei, K. Development and Usability Evaluation of a Telemedicine System for Management and Monitoring of Patients with Diabetic Foot. *Health Inf. Res.* **2022**, *28*, 77–88. [CrossRef] [PubMed]
21. Haycocks, S.; Cameron, R.; Edge, M.; Budd, J.; Chadwick, P. Implementation of a novel mHealth application for the management of people with diabetes and recently healed foot ulceration: A feasibility study. *Digit. Health* **2022**, *8*, 20552076221142103. [CrossRef]
22. Cassidy, B.; Hoon Yap, M.; Pappachan, J.M.; Ahmad, N.; Haycocks, S.; O'Shea, C.; Fernandez, C.J.; Chacko, E.; Jacob, K.; Reeves, N.D. Artificial intelligence for automated detection of diabetic foot ulcers: A real-world proof-of-concept clinical evaluation. *Diabetes Res. Clin. Pract.* **2023**, *205*, 110951. [CrossRef] [PubMed]
23. Chen, S.M.; Wu, C.J. Investigating the effects of digital foot self-management program on enhancing self-efficacy and self-care behavior among community-dwelling older adults with type 2 diabetes: A randomized controlled trial. *Digit Health* **2023**, *9*, 20552076231220791. [CrossRef] [PubMed]
24. Keegan, A.C.; Bose, S.; McDermott, K.M.; Starks White, M.P.; Stonko, D.P.; Jeddah, D.; Lev-Ari, E.; Rutkowski, J.; Sherman, R.; Abularrage, C.J.; et al. Implementation of a patient-centered remote wound monitoring system for management of diabetic foot ulcers. *Front. Endocrinol.* **2023**, *14*, 1157518.
25. Park, C.; Mishra, R.; Vigano, D.; Macagno, M.; Rossotti, S.; D'Huyvetter, K.; Garcia, J.; Armstrong, D.G.; Najafi, B. Smart Offloading Boot System for Remote Patient Monitoring: Toward Adherence Reinforcement and Proper Physical Activity Prescription for Diabetic Foot Ulcer Patients. *J. Diabetes Sci. Technol.* **2023**, *17*, 42–51. [CrossRef]
26. Ploderer, B.; Clark, D.; Brown, R.; Harman, J.; Lazzarini, P.A.; Van Netten, J.J. Self-Monitoring Diabetes-Related Foot Ulcers with the MyFootCare App: A Mixed Methods Study. *Sensors* **2023**, *23*, 2547. [CrossRef]
27. Hellstrand Tang, U.; Tranberg, R.; Sundberg, L.; Scandurra, I. How do patients and healthcare professionals experience foot examinations in diabetes care?—A randomised controlled study of digital foot examinations versus traditional foot examinations. *BMC Health Serv. Res.* **2024**, *24*, 1387. [CrossRef]

28. Matijevich, E.; Minty, E.; Bray, E.; Bachus, C.; Hajizadeh, M.; Liden, B. A Multi-Faceted Digital Health Solution for Monitoring and Managing Diabetic Foot Ulcer Risk: A Case Series. *Sensors* **2024**, *24*, 2675. [CrossRef] [PubMed]
29. Zhou, G.X.; Tao, Y.K.; Hou, J.Z.; Zhu, H.J.; Xiao, L.; Zhao, N.; Wang, X.-W.; Du, B.-L.; Zhang, D. Construction and validation of a deep learning-based diagnostic model for segmentation and classification of diabetic foot. *Front. Endocrinol.* **2025**, *16*, 1543192. [CrossRef] [PubMed]
30. de Morais, G.H.D.; de Araújo, J.F.; Mendes, A.D.C.M.; da Silva, C.B. Letramento digital em saúde: Capacidades, desafios e impactos na autonomia do indivíduo. *Cad. Pedagógico* **2025**, *22*, e13122. Available online: https://ojs.studiespublicacoes.com.br/ojs/index.php/cadped/article/view/13122 (accessed on 15 July 2025). [CrossRef]
31. Shiferaw, K.B.; Roloff, M.; Waltemath, D.; Zeleke, A.A. Guidelines and Standard Frameworks for AI in Medicine: Protocol for a Systematic Literature Review. *JMIR Res. Protoc.* **2023**, *12*, e47105. [CrossRef]
32. Lu, T.; Lin, Q.; Yu, B.; Hu, J. A systematic review of strategies in digital technologies for motivating adherence to chronic illness self-care. *npj Health Syst.* **2025**, *2*, 13. Available online: https://www.nature.com/articles/s44401-025-00017-4 (accessed on 15 July 2025). [CrossRef]
33. Cruchinho, P.; López-Franco, M.D.; Capelas, M.L.; Almeida, S.; Bennett, P.M.; da Silva, M.M.; Teixeira, G.; Nunes, E.; Lucas, P.; Gaspar, F. Translation, Cross-Cultural Adaptation, and Validation of Measurement Instruments: A Practical Guideline for Novice Researchers. *J. Multidiscip. Healthc.* **2024**, *17*, 2701–2728. [CrossRef] [PubMed]
34. Montgomery, R.M. Evaluating Health Technologies in the Brazilian Public and Supplementary Health Systems: Policy, Economic, and Public Health Implications [Internet]. 2025. Available online: https://www.preprints.org/manuscript/202502.0657/v1 (accessed on 15 July 2025).

MDPI AG
Grosspeteranlage 5
4052 Basel
Switzerland
Tel.: +41 61 683 77 34

International Journal of Environmental Research and Public Health Editorial Office
E-mail: ijerph@mdpi.com
www.mdpi.com/journal/ijerph